Comprehensive Manuals of Surgical Specialties

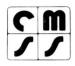

Richard H. Egdahl, editor

Byron J. Masterson

Manual of Gynecologic Surgery

With contributions by Kermit E. Krantz, William J. Cameron,
James W. Daly, Jamil A. Fayez, and Ernest W. Franklin III

Includes 192 color illustrations

Springer-Verlag
New York   Heidelberg   Berlin

Comprehensive Manuals of Surgical Specialties, Volume 4

SERIES EDITOR

Richard H. Egdahl, M.D., Ph.D., Professor of Surgery, Boston University Medical Center, Boston, Massachusetts 02118

AUTHOR

Byron J. Masterson, M.D., Professor, Department of Obstetrics and Gynecology, University of Kansas Medical Center, College of Health Sciences and Hospital, Kansas City, Kansas 66103

CONTRIBUTORS

William J. Cameron, M.D., Professor and Vice-Chairman, Department of Obstetrics and Gynecology, University of Kansas Medical Center, College of Health Sciences and Hospital, Kansas City, Kansas 66103

James W. Daly, M.D., Professor, Department of Obstetrics and Gynecology, University of Florida College of Medicine, Gainesville, Florida 32610

Jamil A. Fayez, M.D., Professor, Department of Obstetrics and Gynecology, University of Missouri–Kansas City School of Medicine, Kansas City, Missouri 64108

Ernest W. Franklin III, M.D., Director, Foundation for Gynecologic Oncology, Atlanta, Georgia 30342

Kermit E. Krantz, M.D., Professor and Chairman, Department of Obstetrics and Gynecology, University of Kansas Medical Center, College of Health Sciences and Hospital, Kansas City, Kansas 66103

MEDICAL ILLUSTRATOR

Deanne McKeown, Design and Illustration Section, Learning Resources Division, University of Kansas Medical Center, College of Health Sciences and Hospital, Kansas City, Kansas 66103

Library of Congress Cataloging in Publication Data

Main entry under title:
Manual of gynecologic surgery.

  (Comprehensive manuals of surgical specialties ; v. 4)
  Includes bibliographies and index.
  1. Gynecology, Operative. I. Masterson, Byron J.
[DNLM: 1. Genital diseases, Female—Surgery—Handbooks.
WP660 M421m]
RG104.M34   618   78-32118

ISBN 0-387-90372-0   Springer-Verlag   New York   Heidelberg   Berlin
ISBN 3-540-90372-0   Springer-Verlag   Berlin   Heidelberg   New York

This book is dedicated to my family.

Editor's Note

Comprehensive Manuals of Surgical Specialties is a series of surgical manuals designed to present current operative techniques and to explore various aspects of diagnosis and treatment. The series features a unique format with emphasis on large, detailed, full-color illustrations, schematic charts and photographs to demonstrate integral steps in surgical procedures.

Each manual focuses on a specific region or topic and describes surgical anatomy, physiology, pathology, diagnosis and operative treatment. Operative techniques and stratagems for dealing with surgically correctable disorders are described in detail. Illustrations are primarily depicted from the surgeon's viewpoint to enhance clarity and comprehension.

Other volumes in preparation:

Manual of Lower Gastrointestinal Surgery
Manual of Urologic Surgery
Manual of Vascular Surgery
Manual of Cardiac Surgery
Manual of Liver Surgery
Manual of Soft Tissue Tumor Surgery
Manual of Orthopaedic Surgery
Manual of Upper Gastrointestinal Surgery
Manual of Plastic Surgery
Manual of Ambulatory Surgery

Richard H. Egdahl

Preface

The *Manual of Gynecologic Surgery* is a comprehensive guide for operative decision-making and technique in female pelvic surgery. For a wide array of problems requiring surgical intervention, this volume examines the anatomy, preoperative evaluation, surgical strategy, details of technique, postoperative management, and anticipated results. The management of operative complications and injuries to bowel, urinary system, and pelvic vessels is discussed.

This volume is divided into three sections: ambulatory, vaginal, and abdominal surgery. The ambulatory section will be particularly useful to the family physician. The abdominal section explains complication management for the gynecologist whose surgical background may not include gastrointestinal or urinary tract surgery. The section on ovarian surgery contains additional data for the general surgeon who may encounter unexpected ovarian lesions. Although the book should be most useful to gynecologic residents-in-training and practicing gynecologists, it will also be of use to general surgeons who perform gynecologic operations and to all physicians who perform ambulatory gynecologic procedures.

The operative techniques depicted are currently used procedures based on the newer concepts of wound healing and suturing, utilizing modern surgical instrumentation. When several techniques are available, the author's personal preference is described.

This book, which was produced by the project manager system, represents the efforts of 21 persons in three cities. Christine G. Williamson managed the project with drive, understanding, and skill. She was responsible also for coordinating information retrieval, organizing the chapters, and editing the text.

To maintain artistic uniformity, Deanne McKeown illustrated the entire book. The preliminary sketches were prepared from notes and sketches made in the operating room during actual performance of the techniques described. After thorough graphic and anatomic research, they were reviewed by the author, then skillfully rendered in color. The final transparent watercolor plates present visual communication of the essence of the surgical procedures included here.

A full-time research staff comprised of Dr. William Hamilton, Scott Smith, and David Wright, reference librarian, abstracted references from the medical literature for the last 10 years on each topic. This large amount of data was narrowed to as few references as possible, consistent with the intent of each chapter. These efforts contributed to the constant reviewing and updating of the text during its 15 months of preparation.

My three fellows, Drs. Tom Snyder, Tom Sullivan, and Javier Magrina, were helpful in correlating, reviewing, and retrieving valuable information. In addition, their contribution to the improved level of surgical care on the gynecologic surgical service is appreciated.

My Section Manager, Felicia Weiner, successfully coordinated my various clinic and operating room schedules, speaking engagements, and university and other obligations to provide me the time necessary for the writing of this book. The advice and encouragement of A. J. Yarmat, Ph.D., Director of Communications for the University of Kansas, also contributed to the development of this book.

Byron J. Masterson

Acknowledgments

My medical career has been encouraged at every turn by my two principal surgical teachers, Dr. Kermit E. Krantz and Dr. Felix Rutledge. They have supported me at each step of my career and in every endeavor. I trust this book merits that confidence.

I am indebted to Dr. Hugh Stephenson, who interested me as a medical student in experimental vascular surgery and showed me how crucial the finer points of technique were in the success of a surgical procedure; to Drs. Carl Moore and Herbert Goldberg, who showed me the pleasure in an academic pursuit; and to Drs. Glover Copher, Eugene Bricker, John Spratt, Ernesto Ego-Aguirre, Bill Spanos, Harold Gainey, Vernon Colpitts, Joe Lucci, Bill Peterson, Sam Montello, Tom McGuire, Bill Jewell, John Weigel, and all the other surgeons with whom I have scrubbed and learned during my surgical experience.

I wish to thank Dr. Richard Egdahl, who first suggested that the publisher and I get together for this volume, and Dr. Hugh Barber, who encouraged me to use a straightforward writing format. Thanks also to Dr. Dick Mattingly, who suggested that the manual concept was worthwhile, and to John Lewis for guidance in the initial stage of this work. I also wish to thank Ron Pfost and Bernard Brown who consistently encouraged me when the task seemed impossible. Finally, my thanks to Springer-Verlag for their superb staff and wise counsel during the production of this book.

Contents

Ambulatory Surgery

The ambulatory surgical procedure is no different than the inpatient procedure and is accompanied by the same preoperative visit, explanation of the procedure, appropriate operative permission forms, a brief note concerning the procedure, and postoperative instructions.

It is important to establish standard protocols for each procedure performed on an ambulatory surgical service. For example, prepare preoperative setup instructions accompanied by instrument lists and glossy photographs of properly arranged instruments. Keep these instructions in the surgical area so that the instruments will be available to the surgeon in a complete and consistent fashion. As most of the procedures described herein are performed on the patient who is awake and alert, it is important there be no confusion or inappropriate delays. The surgical area should be relatively quiet and talking among surgical staff limited to professional matters.

The patient must be handled in a sympathetic and understanding manner with repeated reassurance. The patient often has no standard for comparison and must be assured that the procedure is progressing satisfactorily.

During the office visit preceding the surgical procedure, advise the patient to have someone accompany her home if the procedure involves sedation or possible significant blood loss. The patient is given a printed instruction sheet which contains the "do's and don'ts" following such surgical procedure and a description of anticipated side effects, such as the amount of bleeding to be noted. Phone numbers where the physician may be reached after office hours, a prescription for pain medication, and a return appointment is provided when the patient is sent home following the procedure.

Investigation of the most common gynecologic symptoms of pelvic pain or abnormal vaginal bleeding and the performance of various surgical procedures, including sterilizations, are well managed in the ambulatory patient. Specific techniques are considered in the sections to follow.

Vulvar Ambulatory Surgery

The biopsy is the hallmark of the successful management of vulvar lesions and is satisfactorily accomplished in the ambulatory patient. Although cancer of the vulva is rare and represents approximately 4% of carcinoma found in the gynecologic patient, early detection by biopsy of the vulvar lesion is mandatory.[8]. Vulvar cancer cure rates closely approximate the stage of disease when first seen, and early diagnosis is only possible with biopsy of a suspicious vulvar lesion. Biopsies vary from a small punch biopsy obtained with a disposable 3-mm punch to elliptical biopsies as performed with small sharp scissors and thumb forceps. Large lesions such as psoriasis or areas of hypertrophic disease are studied with a punch biopsy; the smaller lesions such as solid nodules, nevi, and small discrete neoplastic processes are best totally excised and submitted for pathologic examination.

Punch Biopsy of Vulvar Lesions

Dermatologic punch biopsies are quite satisfactorily performed in the ambulatory patient (Figures 1.1 and 1.2). Instruct the patient to cut the hair with scissors in the area of the lesion before the surgery; no shaving is required. Colored preparation solutions are not recommended as they prevent a clear definition of the area for biopsy purposes. Toluidine blue staining of the vulva is occasionally useful to outline such areas of abnormal cellular activity and may be used when definite lesions are difficult to outline. Remember that toluidine blue does not stain Paget's disease effectively.

On dismissal the patient is given separately packaged 4 × 4 inch

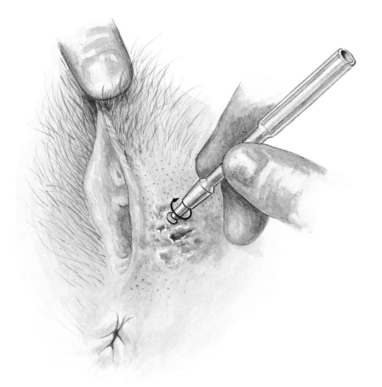

FIGURE 1.1. Dermatologic punch biopsy. With the patient in the lithotomy position, the skin is prepared with a Betadine (povidone–iodine) scrub of 1 min. Use a small wheal to initiate anesthesia as the vulva has a significant number of nerve fibers, particularly around the area of the hymen and urethra. The skin is fixed with the hand so that the punch will clearly go through into the subcutaneous tissues without difficulty. A 3-mm dermal punch is directed into an area of the lesion that seems well vascularized. The punch is circled in a clockwise fashion until there is a release of resistance, indicating that the punch blade is in the subcutaneous tissues. Remove the punch.

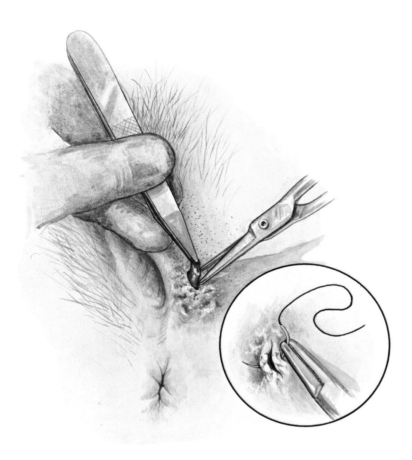

FIGURE 1.2. Pull the disk of tissue upward with the thumb forceps. The deeper portion is cut sharply with disposable scissors. Inset: Close the defect produced with 4-0 absorbable suture. No dressing is required.

gauze pads. Ice cubes in a disposable plastic bag will reduce the swelling which accompanies most vulvar procedures and reduces pain. Most late bleeding can be managed at home with pressure. The patient is dismissed to return in 1 week after the pathological examination of tissues has been completed. Any additional therapy needed for the vulvar lesion diagnosed by biopsy may be planned during the return visit.

Excisional Biopsy of Vulvar Lesions
Excisional biopsy is accomplished in a similar fashion (Figure 1.3). In performing the excisional biopsy remember that local anesthesia does not prevent the patient from perceiving traction as adjoining areas of skin are mobilized. Instruct the patient that she will have no pain but may have some sensation of the area being pulled upward.

Marsupialization of Bartholin's Gland
Infection of Bartholin's gland, which destroys the duct, is a common clinical occurrence. Such glandular epithelium continues to secrete until back pressure prevents a further secretion, producing an encapsulated cyst. This cyst of Bartholin's gland lies just beneath the skin and is easily accessible for drainage. Simple drainage procedures have been employed for a number of years; however, the contracture of the stab wound obstructs the drainage site and the patient develops the cystic structure again, often with secondary infection leading to abscess formation. Marsupialization avoids resealing of the surgical defect by careful suturing of the epithelium of the skin to the margin of the cyst wall, producing a sinus tract. Such incisions should be as large as the cyst wall will allow; they will greatly decrease the chance of recurrence. The normal process of wound healing with contrac-

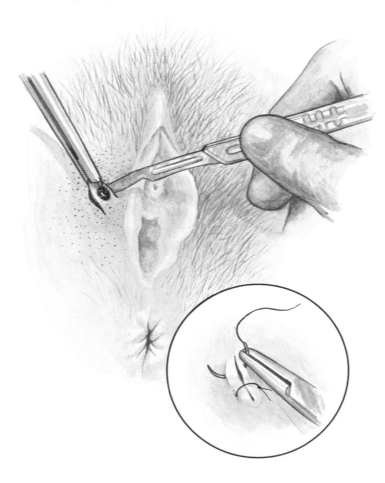

FIGURE 1.3. Excisional biopsy. Cut sufficient hair from the vulva to allow exposure of the wound area. With the patient in the lithotomy position, prepare the skin with a Betadine solution (povidone–iodine) and infiltrate 1% Xylocaine into the base of the area to be exercised with a disposable syringe and a 23-gauge needle. Allow 2 min for the anesthesia to take effect, then excise the area around the lesion. Two millimeters of normal appearing skin should surround the lesion and its base should be completely covered by underlying tissues. Bleeders in the base of the incised lesion will usually stop with pressure. Close the elliptical defect with a 4-0 chromic suture if mucosal or a monofilament nylon suture if on the cutaneous surface. Several small mosquito clamps should be available as the vulva is a very vascular area.

ture will diminish the size of the sinus tract and, if small, will obstruct its outflow (Figures 1.4 and 1.5).

It is the intent of the procedure to produce a smooth epithelial surface. Crushing of the gland margin or the use of excessive suture material will incur scar formation with subsequent contracture and closing of the opening into the gland. A small sampling of the cyst wall may be obtained for pathological examination and any solid nodules in the area should, of course, be biopsied. Ice cubes in a disposable plastic bag are useful to avoid additional pain from swelling. It is of interest that in a series of 700 lesions of Bartholin's gland treated surgically at the Mayo Clinic between 1910 and 1947, only 7 primary carcinomas were found, an incidence of 1%.[2]

Bartholin's Gland Abscess

In addition to Bartholin's gland cyst, patients may present with an acute abscess involving Bartholin's gland. Whether preceded by an infected cyst or an acute inflammatory process, the drainage procedure is, most often, all that can be done for these patients. Patients do have acute pain and the purulent material in the abscess is often under some pressure.

The patient is placed in the lithotomy position and the skin over the cyst is prepared with a Betadine scrub. After the area has been infiltrated with 1% Xylocaine, the gland is incised and a defect of 1 to 2 cm is produced. While a No. 11 Bard-Parker knife is often supplied in the usual set for drainage of abscesses, the author prefers a blade with a rounded margin so that an actual incision of larger size may be made rather than a single small stab wound. Often margins of such a stab wound bleed due to the acute inflammatory nature of the process; however, suture material is best

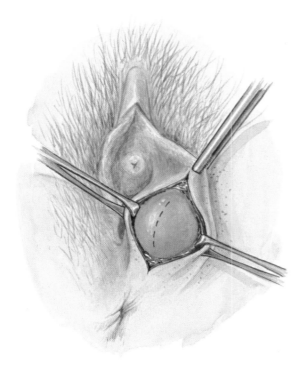

FIGURE 1.4. Marsupialization of Bartholin's gland. The patient is placed in the lithotomy position, the hair over the area to be incised is cut with scissors, and the skin over the cyst is carefully prepared with a Betadine solution (povidone–iodine). The area over the incision site is infiltrated with 1% Xylocaine and 2 min is allowed for the anesthesia to become effective. Advise the patient that she will feel some pressure. Using a sharp knife, incise the skin and the cyst to produce a 2- or preferably 3-cm defect.

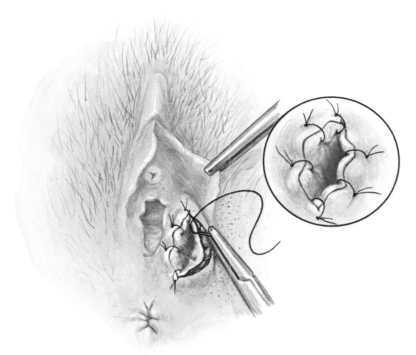

FIGURE 1.5. Grasp the margins of the cyst wall with a small mosquito clamp and suture the margin with 4-0 absorbable suture. The incision in the gland should be as large as practical to avoid stricture with subsequent reformation of the gland abscess. Should a large abscess be present initially, perform a simple incision as outlined without suturing the margins of the gland. No packs or drains are used in this wound. The patient is to return in 1 week.

avoided if possible. The patient will experience immediate relief of her discomfort.

Cultures of purulent material should be taken; however, they usually do not produce a discrete pathogen. The purulent material may have a most disagreeable odor, particularly if anaerobic bacteria have been prominent in the infection producing the abscess, and a large plastic bag should be immediately available in which to place soiled dressings and sponges to minimize office odor. If significant cellulitis surrounds the abscess, an antibiotic should be administered for 5 days. Metronidazole is useful if the odor suggests anaerobic bacteria; however, drainage will produce prompt

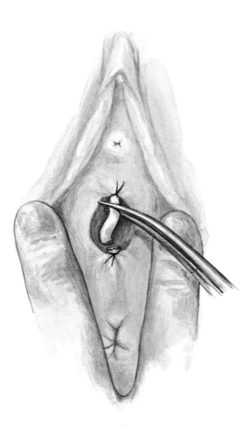

FIGURE 1.6. A common hymeneal abnormality is a simple strand connecting the anterior and posterior hymen. The area is scrubbed with a Betadine solution (povidone–iodine). Xylocaine jelly is applied over the mucosa and the proximal segments are infiltrated with 1% Xylocaine. After a 2-min wait, 3-0 Vicryl suture is tied snugly about each end and the intervening mucosal strip is excised.

resolution without any additional medication in most patients. The patient may be instructed to apply hot soaks to the area to promote resolution of cellulitis.

Hymenal Lesions

Lesions of the lower vagina that require surgical intervention include abnormalities of the hymen. The hymen is richly endowed with a nerve supply but can be operated on under local anesthesia without difficulty (Figure 1.6). Local anesthesia is also used in patients who have strictures after vaginal surgery or other hymenal abnormalities that are to be dilated. The patient is given a vaginal dilator—either a plastic syringe container or a manufactured dilator—for home use after the first dilation.

Imperforate hymen, while rare, does occur and should be treated; however, these patients need further diagnostic studies if a large pelvic mass has been produced by trapped menstrual fluid. A great amount of time and effort should be expended to minimize the psychological impact of this procedure in the adolescent female. She needs to be repeatedly told "she is normal" and steps need to be taken to ensure that this concept is reinforced at home.

Vaginal Ambulatory Surgery

With the increasing emphasis on preventive medicine, early vaginal lesions are being observed that formerly were often thought to be extensions of cervical or vulvar lesions. In Rutledge's series of 101 patients with primary vaginal cancer, 70 of the patients had invasive lesions with no previous history of cancer in the cervix or elsewhere and 31 of the patients had in situ vaginal cancer.[16] It is important, therefore, to biopsy vaginal lesions and submit tissues for pathological examination.

Nodular lesions or lesions suspected of being malignant in the upper vagina may be biopsied without any anesthesia as the upper vagina contains few nerve fibers. The patient is placed in the lithotomy position and prepped with aqueous Zephiran. Tischler biopsy forceps with a very sharp margin are used to good advantage in these vaginal lesions. If the lesion is mobile, it may be stabilized with a skin hook.

Duct cysts in the anterior vagina are also seen but should not be approached in the ambulatory patient because of the need for careful study to exclude upper urinary tract abnormalities. The cyst, unless symptomatic or associated with progressive upper urinary tract abnormalities, is best left alone.

Cervical Ambulatory Surgery

The number of available procedures for the management of cervical abnormalities has increased in recent years due to technological advancement. Thermal cautery is rarely used today and the crude biopsy forceps with tearing-type jaws are unsuitable for use in the patient who is awake and feels the traction of such pulling. As there are few nerve fibers in the cervix, procedures that do not disturb the endocervix may be accomplished without any supplementary anesthesia. The endocervix, however, contains numerous nerve fibers that transmit pain at the level of the internal os. Procedures that involve dilating the cervix require additional anesthesia.

Patients undergoing ambulatory procedures must have a diagnostic Papanicolaou smear performed during a prior office visit. It must be emphasized, however, that patients with a negative Papanicolaou smear may have a cervical malignancy. In the study by Maisel et al. on the reliability of the Papanicolaou smear in the diagnosis of cervical cancer, it was demonstrated that 4.3% of the patients with a tissue diagnosis of cancer or atypical hyperplasia of the cervix had a negative Papanicolaou smear. This is particularly true in patients with advanced cancer of the cervix.[13] These data confirm the need for definitive cervical biopsies prior to cryosurgery or other cervical procedures when gross cervical abnormalities are noted.

Cervical Biopsy

The need for cervical biopsies has decreased with the increasing use of colposcopic examination; however, patients who present with complaints of bleeding following intercourse, spotting, grossly visible lesions, or a diagnosis of endometrial cancer require a cervical biopsy, as do those patients requiring pathological confirmation of the colposcopic diagnosis.

To perform the cervical biopsy, very sharp, easily directed cervical biopsy forceps are essential (Figure 1.7). The author recommends Tischler-type forceps with a pistol-grip handle. The Kevorkian biopsy punch forceps are often suggested; however, the bite is small, the jaw is delicate, and they are, in the author's opinion, inadequate for general use. A stronger and more sturdy instrument such as the Younge or Tischler biopsy forceps is recommended. A long needle holder, long thumb forceps, a supply of 00 chromic gut suture with a sharp needle, and long scissors are packaged in the surgical area. Schiller's stain is useful in the office to direct the operator toward areas that do not stain and often consist of abnormal epithelium.

Cervical Polypectomy

Patients with a cervical polyp may present with abnormal vaginal bleeding or excessive watery vaginal discharge. According to Aaro and Jacobson, endocervical polyps are rarely malignant, as demonstrated in their series of 1009 patients in which only 2 patients had malignant polyps. Nonetheless,

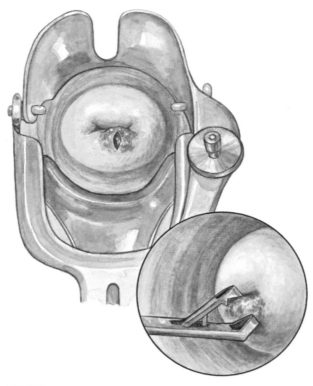

FIGURE 1.7. Cervical biopsy. The patient is instructed that she may feel some pressure but pain will be minimal. A vaginal speculum with an adequate light source is placed in the vagina, exposing the area to be biopsied. If Tischler biopsy forceps are used, which have sharp pointed jaws, no tenaculum need be placed on the cervix. If other biopsy forceps are used, a tenaculum is needed to stabilize the cervix. The lesion is biopsied with a large sharp bite of the forceps and the specimen is placed directly into formalin. Multiple lesions may be biopsied simultaneously and these must be individually identified. Unless a specific lesion is present, the areas at 3 o'clock and 9 o'clock are not used for routine biopsy sites as the descending branch of the cervical artery is present and bleeding will occur. If bleeding does occur a suture may be placed in the ambulatory patient without difficulty. The patient is asked to return in 1 week for review of her biopsy findings.

the polyp should be excised and submitted for pathological examination.[1] In addition, the endocervix and endometrium should be studied by aspiration biopsy at the time of polyp excision.

With the patient in the lithotomy position, the cervix is prepared with aqueous Zephiran and the polyp is removed with sharp biopsy forceps as described in the section on cervical biopsy. Frequently, however, the polyp may be of such size that the base cannot be grasped with the biopsy forceps. In this instance, a tonsil snare is quite useful; the wire is slipped into the cervix and passed about the base of the polyp, and the polyp amputated. It is again emphasized that the polyp may have produced no symptoms whatsoever and the bleeding the patient experienced may be due to a lesion elsewhere in the uterus.

Cervical Strictures

Cervical strictures may be handled on an outpatient basis. If adequate egress is present for menstrual fluid it is rarely necessary to dilate the cervix. The usefulness of dilation in dysmenorrhea is open to some doubt. If the cervix needs to be dilated in order to accept a small endometrial curette or other surgical instrumentation, anesthesia is provided as previously discussed.

Cryosurgery

Cryosurgery is the technique of causing cell death by freezing the tissues. The basic purpose of cryosurgery of the cervix is to destroy the cystic cervical glands; the epithelium then lies on the cervical stroma in the absence of the cystic structures, which tend to get infected and promote a persistent discharge.

Cryosurgery is effectively performed in the ambulatory patient and does not require local anesthesia. The patient is placed in the lithotomy position and a speculum is inserted into the vagina. The vagina and cervix are cleansed with cotton pledgets soaked in aqueous Zephiran. The cryoprobe is placed in the area to be treated and the machine is turned on (Figure 1.8). The duration of the freezing differs according to the cryoprobe used and the lesion being treated; however, the purpose of the treatment is to destroy the lesion and to allow the freezing process to extend into the area of normal tissue. Average freezing time is 2 to 3 min. Once this is accomplished, the probe is defrosted and removed from the cervix.[17]

Patients having cryosurgery are advised to avoid intercourse for 2 weeks and are instructed that a profuse watery discharge may follow. Such discharge may occur for approximately 6 weeks. Healing is aided by the application of intravaginal antibiotic cream, either triple sulfa or Furacin cream.

Take great care to avoid performing cryosurgery in patients with acute cervicitis and perimetritis. Administer antibiotics for 1 week prior to

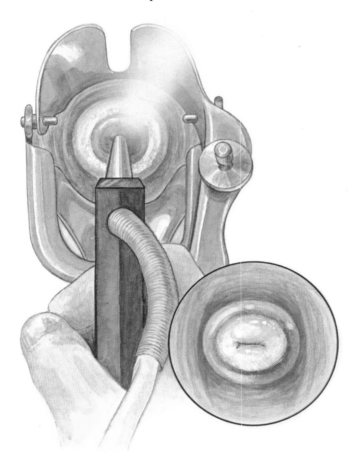

FIGURE 1.8. Cryosurgery. As large a speculum as possible is placed in the vagina to keep the vaginal epithelium from rolling in toward the cervix, which may become adherent to the probe. The probe is coated with K-Y jelly or some similar substance and is placed firmly against the cervix and turned on.

cryosurgery to avoid the development of acute pelvic inflammatory disease, which occasionally progresses to abscess formation.

Cryosurgery in the management of carcinoma in situ has been proposed by Creasman et al. [4,5] and Townsend and Ostergard.[18] Such methods of management should be limited to those patients who are most reliable in their follow-up, as there is a significant incidence of recurrent cervical intraepithelial neoplasia in these patients.

Colposcopy

The colposcope, as described in Europe in the late 1920s by Hinselman, is a useful diagnostic instrument. The author prefers to use the colposcope to suggest areas where biopsy would be most informative. While there have been innumerable symposia and seminars on the use of colposcopy held about the country, the key is still to confirm each diagnosis that involves a neoplastic process with tissue biopsy. Such biopsies should be large enough for the pathologist to orient and should be representative of the lesion observed. The large, sharp biopsy forceps that have been described previously are appropriate for this purpose.

While there are several colposcopes available in the author's clinic for research, laser, and diagnostic purposes, a small stand-mounted colposcope is most useful in office practice. It requires no special wiring, occupies little space in the office, and may be easily moved from one examining room to another.

Colposcopic examination requires no special preparation. The patient should have had a cytological examination prior to colposcopy, with the results available to the physician. There are several techniques described by Dexeus et al. for the visualization of the cervical epithelium,[7] but the author prefers the following as a simple and rapid means of obtaining the maximum information.

The patient is placed in the lithotomy position for usual examination; the speculum is placed in the vagina after the examiner has carefully observed that no lesions are being hidden by the blades of the speculum; and the upper vagina is inspected for changes associated with diethystilbestrol administration and other abnormalities.

The cervix is irrigated with 3% acetic acid by means of a small spray bottle, thus avoiding the trauma of constant swabbing with cotton pledgets. Following application of the acetic acid (approximately 30 to 45 sec should be allowed for the full changes to occur in the cervix), the epithelium, where intraepithelial neoplasia is active, will become opaque. Repeatedly moisten the cervix as the examination is performed. The entire examination usually requires less than 10 min.

The normal components of the cervix to be noted in a colposcopic examination are the epithelium, the cervical stroma, the underlying vessels, and the transformation zone. The epithelium, in its normal state, is transparent until intraepithelial neoplastic disease occurs; it then opacifies, producing the changes illustrated in Figure 1.9. It is important that the entire squamocolumnar junction be visualized. Aids to visualization include the endocervical speculum and the use of cottom swabs to hold up the anterior cervix. If the squamocolumnar junction is totally visualized, no further diagnostic studies are necessary, as documented in a recent study by Urcuyo et al.[19] In the absence of such visualization, it is mandatory to perform an endocervical curettage, and conization should also be considered. The reader is referred to the text by Dexeus et al. for an exhaustive presentation of the numerous colposcopic abnormalities from a histologic point of view.[7]

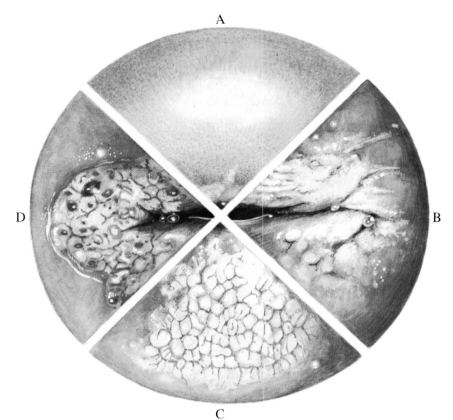

FIGURE 1.9. Changes seen on colposcopy. **A.** Normal cervical epithelium is transparent and glistening and overlies the small uniformly shaped capillaries. **B.** Cervicitis is recognized by the irregularity of the squamocolumnar junction with the nodularity produced by underlying cysts caused by an obstruction of the outflow of the mucus of the cervical clefts. The absence of any abnormal vessels and epithelial thickening is apparent. **C.** Mosaicism appears as tile-like plaques covering an area of the cervix. The abnormal vessels lying between these plaques are apparent and contrast sharply with the regular appearance of the cervical vessels. **D.** Grossly abnormal cervical vessels and epithelium should be biopsied. Colposcopic abnormalities suggesting malignancy are markedly tortuous and irregular vessels, thickened white epithelium of irregular consistency, and destruction of underlying stroma.

After the cervix has been carefully studied and the abnormalities noted, a drawing is made of sufficient size such that these areas may be carefully identified in the future. Representative biopsies are taken and labeled from the different sites of the cervix. A description of the epithelium, transformation zone, epithelial abnormalities, and character of the vessels should be noted.

The patient is instructed to return in 1 week for the results of the colposcopic biopsies. If no abnormalities are present, no additional biopsies need be taken, but if the patient has varying degrees of intraepithelial neoplasia or any other abnormalities, then obtain several biopsies. Small lesions are completely excised with the biopsy forceps, thus requiring no additional therapy. Bleeding from the biopsy sites may be treated with silver nitrate stick, a suture if necessary, vaginal pack, or a solution of ferrous subsulfate. (This is a caustic solution and should not be allowed to come in contact with the vaginal epithelium but simply the area in the cervix. It is most effective if the blood can be minimized and the solution applied directly to the small bleeding sites.)

It is again emphasized that liberal use of the colposcopically directed biopsy will greatly improve the management of cervical intraepithelial neoplasia in the ambulatory gynecologic patient. The neglect of biopsies in favor of colposcopic examination alone will produce clinical disasters because some crucial lesions will be missed in their earliest states.

Laser Therapy

Laser therapy is an increasingly popular technique in gynecologic ambulatory surgery. Intraepithelial neoplastic lesions on the surface of the cervix that can be well visualized and the small recurrence of intraepithelial neoplasia in the apex of the vault are handled in a painless fashion in the clinic without the need for general anesthesia or hospitalization. This procedure is cost effective and appears to produce a low recurrence rate after therapy.

The carbon dioxide laser is able to destroy cervical intraepithelial neoplasia on the cervix and vagina due to its ability to direct high-intensity energy at a precisely controlled depth. It is extremely important that the exact nature of the process being treated be known, and this information can only be obtained through careful colposcopic examination combined with multiple, well-placed biopsies and study by competent pathologists. The laser requires a direct and complete view of the lesion. In the absence of these requirements, the laser is indeed a dangerous instrument. If, however, these lesions are carefully studied and visualized, the carbon dioxide laser appears effective.

The author's clinic uses the carbon dioxide laser. Its activity is directed by a small green dot which is moved about the cervix with a small director that focuses the split beam on the vaginal lesion (Figure 1.10). Lesions are reduced to carbon dioxide and oxygen with no residual; therefore, should a virus genome or other abnormality be in the nucleic acids, no residual remains to produce neoplastic change. Areas so treated are very dry. Specific techniques and treatment times depend on the specific instrument used, and such data must be completely studied before the laser is used.

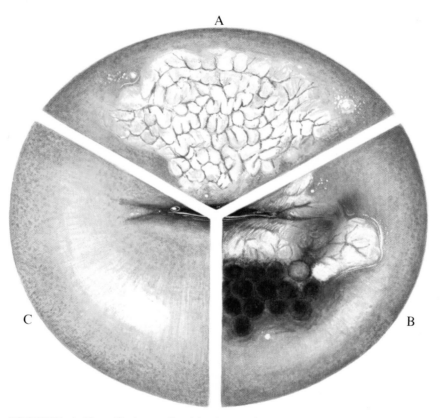

FIGURE 1.10. Carbon dioxide laser therapy. **A.** This cervix has abnormal epithelium at the squamocolumnar junction. These lesions will histologically appear as severe dysplasia. **B.** The small green dot is the laser beam director. The small blackened areas are the char remaining after the laser treatment. Each of these is a single laser firing. The char will extend to the stroma destroying the epithelium. Remember that the laser is of no benefit in lesions that extend inside the squamocolumnar junction or in instances where direct visualization of the entire lesion is not possible. **C.** View taken 6 weeks after laser therapy shows the destruction of the abnormal epithelium. Such areas must be carefully followed with colposcopic and confirming cytological examinations.

A comment must be made regarding diethylstilbestrol patients. It is the author's belief that these patients are overtreated. With the infrequent development of clear cell cancers in these patients, an estimated 0.1 to 1 in 1000,[9] there is little reason to treat the upper vaginal tract, and observation is sufficient. There is no current evidence to suggest that the laser should be used to remove areas of adenosis in the upper vagina and the author does not recommend it for this purpose.

Long-term follow-up data on the use of the laser in cervical intraepithelial neoplasia are just being accumulated and the literature should be watched carefully by anyone using the laser.

Uterine Ambulatory Surgery

In view of the increasing interest in the early diagnosis of endometrial cancer, it is fortunate that access to the uterine cavity is readily available. The diagnostic procedures outlined below are quite amenable to the ambulatory patient, which facilitates frequent investigation of the endometrium.

Uterine Sound

A common procedure performed in the ambulatory gynecologic patient in the uterus is the placement of a uterine sound. The procedure is preceded by careful palpation of the pelvis to determine the direction of the uterus and its cavity. No preparation or anesthesia is needed, but the patient is advised that she may have a sensation of cramping. The sound should be one that bends and can be directed to conform to the uterine cavity. The sound should have centimeter marks on it so that the distance in the uterus may be carefully measured. The presence of small submucous fibroids or uterine cavity abnormalities and the presence or absence of the uterus in a pelvic mass can be determined by this simple technique.

Endometrial Aspiration Biopsy

The endometrial aspiration biopsy is a simple, relatively painless, inexpensive, and accurate technique for histologic diagnosis of endometrial abnormalities. It has essentially replaced dilatation and curettage as a diagnostic measure. Successful biopsy is anticipated in 89% of patients, with a 95.5% accuracy rate reported.[20] The Papanicolaou smear cannot be relied upon for screening of endometrial cancer, as documented by Burk et al.,[3] making this additional study mandatory in the patient over the age of 30 with abnormal bleeding, in the patient receiving estrogen, and in other groups at risk for endometrial cancer. Contraindications are cervical stenosis, pregnancy, and acute or subacute pelvic inflammatory disease.

The author prefers an endometrial diagnostic device of his own design* to obtain tissue from the endometrial cavity (see Figure 1.15, p. 18). This device consists of a lightweight hand-held suction unit incorporating a disposable collection chamber with an attached narrow-gauge malleable curette. The curette has a sharp cutting edge on three sides protected by a rounded tip for safe insertion. The shaft of the curette is marked in centimeters so that it may be used simultaneously as a sound.

There is no need for a cervical tenaculum if the direction of the cavity is easily determined, but if marked retroversion or anteversion is present, a tenaculum may facilitate curette introduction (Figure 1.11).

* Masterson endometrial diagnostic device, Codman and Shurtleff, Inc., Randolph, Mass.

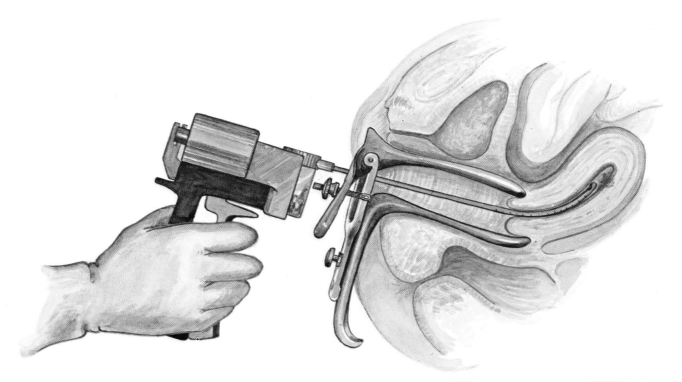

FIGURE 1.11. Endometrial aspiration biopsy. Gently insert the curette after determining the direction of the uterus by palpation and cleaning the cervix with Betadine or aqueous Zephiran. Note the uterine depth in centimeters, and remove and bend the cannula as needed to conform to the uterine position. Move the curette downward systematically through all four quadrants of the uterine cavity while repeatedly compressing the handle. Observe the tissue collecting in the container. When a thorough investigation is complete, remove the device and aspirate fixative to recover any tissue in the curette. Remove the collection vial, place the vial cap, and discard the curette unit.

Endometrial tissue analysis is preferable to cytological study as it provides greater diagnostic accuracy particularly in precursor lesions and has a much lower false negative rate. Two millimeter cannulas make biopsy available for the older patient with a small atrophic cervix.

If no tissue is obtained with aspiration biopsy, one will rarely find any tissue with a dilatation and curettage. Jonas has shown excellent correlation between outpatient endometrial aspiration biopsy without anesthesia and inpatient dilatation and curettage under general anesthesia.[10] McGuire, in an earlier study, documented a 94% accuracy rate of endometrial biopsy.[14]

When endometrial cells are required for cytological study, the Isaacs aspiration syringe is useful and well designed.

Although the author's clinic has a hysteroscope available, little practical application has been found for it nor does it significantly add to the information needed in clinical practice.

Dilatation and Curettage

The safety of dilatation and curettage on an outpatient basis is well established. Kennedy noted no serious complications in 1,000 office curettages[12] and its use was emphasized as early as 1925 by Kelly.[11] Mengert and Slate[15] and Daichman and Mackles[6] have also reported sizable series of dilatations and curettages performed on an outpatient basis without significant injury. Curettage is used mostly for complications of pregnancy such as incomplete abortion or in those patients who need associated cervical dilatation.

No shaving is necessary and if the no-touch technique is used, extensive draping is not required. Premedication consisting of meperidine hydrochloride (Demerol), 75 mg given as the patient arrives in the operating area, is useful. A Betadine preparation of the perineum and vagina is done prior to insertion of the weighted speculum. When indicated, cervical biopsies are done after the tenaculum is placed on the cervix.

The paracervical area may be infiltrated with 5 ml of 1% Xylocaine without epinephrine to block pain sensation from the endocervix. A brief period of discussion with the patient after its injection will serve to reassure the patient and allow time for the local anesthesia to become effective. Sound the uterus and record its depth. Gently curette the endocervix, remembering that this is the area with the most nerve fibers. A small Heaney curette is useful in this instance. Dilate the cervix to accept a medium size dilator and in turn a medium size curette, and curette the cavity. Bend the curette to conform to the uterine sound, which has previously been made to conform to the direction of the uterine cavity (Figures 1.12 through 1.14).

If the curettage is done for an incomplete abortion, it is not usually necessary to dilate the cervix, but check the cavity with polyp forceps for retained tissue. Remember that patients who have had incomplete abortions should be typed and administered RhoGAM to prevent isoimmunization.

If uterine perforation is discovered, check it with a sound. Pass the sound through the margins of the suspected perforation. If the perforation is in the midline and manipulations of the uterus have been gently performed, further problems are uncommon.

If the uterine perforation is lateral the possibilities of concealed hemorrhage exist. Introduction of the laparoscope will document the injury to adjacent viscera. If injury of the bladder, colon, small bowel, or other structures exists immediate laparotomy is necessary.

Following uncomplicated dilatation and curettage the patient is dismissed to return to the office in 1 week for follow-up visit and review of the pathological findings. Histologic diagnoses found on outpatient curettage are listed in Table 1.1.

Note that most patients who have curettages performed for menorrhagia have benign endometrial abnormalities. Seventy percent of the patients

TABLE 1.1. Histologic Diagnoses

Diagnosis	No. of Patients
Progestational	165
Proliferative	109
Hyperplasia	37
Atrophic or inactive	35
Carcinoma	10
Endometrial polyp	10
Endocervical polyp	7
Incomplete abortion (unrecognized)	7
Tuberculosis	1
Insufficient tissue	44

From Mengert, W. F., and Slate, W. G.: *Am. J. Obstet. Gynecol.* **79**:727–735, 1960.

15

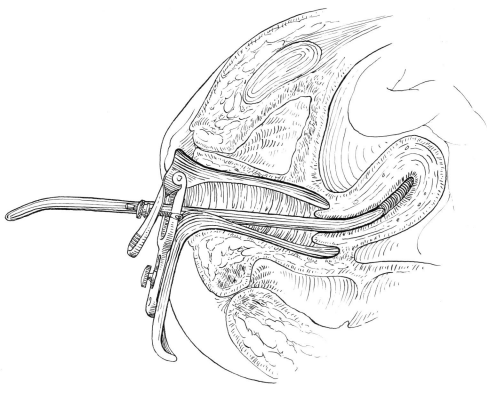

FIGURE 1.12.

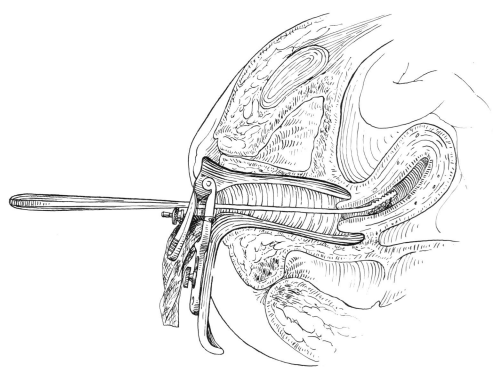

FIGURE 1.13.

with menorrhagia or metromenorrhagia have a normal bleeding pattern following dilatation and curettage alone. Patients who have a progestational endometrium will not need additional endocrine therapy. Treat patients who have hyperplastic endometrium of benign type or proliferative endometrium with 100 mg progesterone in oil.

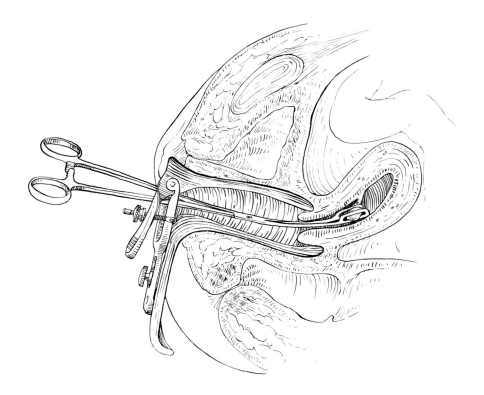

FIGURE 1.14.

APPENDIX   Standard Surgical Instruments

Ambulatory Surgery
  Gloves
  Drapes
  Light source
  1% Xylocaine with epinephrine
  1% Xylocaine jelly
  Aqueous Zephiran
  3% acetic acid
  Betadine scrub
  Cotton pledgets
  Gauze squares
  Specimen containers
  Sutures, assorted sizes
  Schiller's solution
  Toluidine blue
  Ferrous subsulfate
  Silver nitrate

Vulvar Biopsy, Bartholin's Gland
Marsupialization, and Hymenal Surgery
  3-mm disposable punch
  Adson-Brown thumb forceps
  Needle holder
  Suture scissors
  2 Allis clamps
  Knife
  3 Mosquito hemostats
  Vaginal dilator

Vaginal and Cervical Surgery
  Biopsy forceps
  Thumb forceps, long
  Needle holder, long

Colposcopy
  Spray bottle of 3% acetic acid
  Long Procto-type applicators
  Sponges
  Small Q-tips
  Skin hooks
  Biopsy forceps
  Endocervical curette
  Speculum

Endometrial Biopsy
  Endometrial aspiration biopsy kit,
    2 mm and 3 mm (see Figures 1.11
    and 1.15)
  Uterine sound

Dilatation and Curettage
  Tenaculum
  Graduated uterine sounds
  Graduated uterine dilators
  Heaney curette
  Medium sharp curette
  Randal stone forceps
  Weighted speculum

17

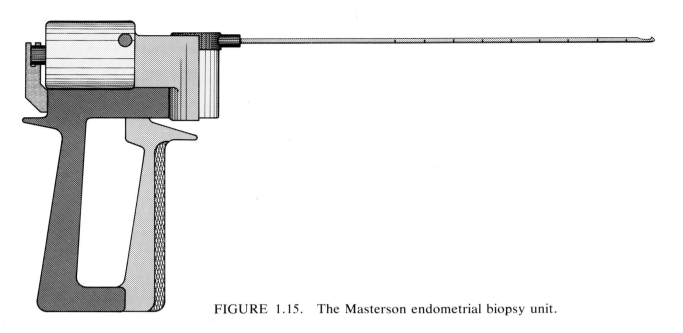

FIGURE 1.15.   The Masterson endometrial biopsy unit.

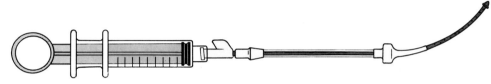

FIGURE 1.16.   Isaacs aspiration syringe.

References

1. Aaro, L.A., Jacobson, L.J., and Soule, E.H.: Endocervical polyps. *Obstet. Gynecol.* **21:**659–665, 1963.
2. Bowing, H.H., Fricke, R.E., and Kennedy, T.J.: Radium therapy for carcinoma of Bartholin's glands. *Am. J. Roentgenol.* **61:**517–529, 1949.
3. Burk, J.R., Lehman, H.F., and Wolf, F.S.: Inadequacy of Papanicolaou smears in the detection of endometrial cancer. *N. Engl. J. Med.* **291:**191–192, 1974.
4. Creasman, W.T., and Parker, R.T.: Management of early cervical neoplasia. *Clin. Obstet. Gynecol.* **18:**233–245, 1975.
5. Creasman, W.T., Weed, J.C., Curry, S.L., et al.: Efficacy of cryosurgical treatment of severe cervical intraepithelial neoplasia. *Obstet. Gynecol.* **41:**501–505, 1973.
6. Daichman, I., and Mackles, D.: Diagnostic curettage—A 13-year study of 585 patients. *Am. J. Obstet. Gynecol.* **95:**212–218, 1966.
7. Dexeus, S.J., Carrera, J.M., Coupez, F.: *Colposcopy* (Austin, K.L., transl.). Philadelphia, Saunders, 1977.
8. DiSaia, P.H., Morrow, C.P., and Townsend, D.E.: Cancer of the corpus. In: *Synopsis of Gynecologic Oncology.* New York, Wiley, 1975.
9. Herbst, A.L., Cole, P., Colton, T., et al.: Age-incidence and risk of diethylstilbestrol-related clear cell adenocarcinoma of the vagina and cervix. *Am. J. Obstet. Gynecol.* **128:**43–50, 1977.
10. Jonas, H.S.: Early diagnosis of endometrial cancer. In Masterson, B.J. (ed.): *Proceedings of Symposium on New Developments in Gynecologic Cancer.* Lawrence, Kansas, University of Kansas Printing Service, 1978.
11. Kelly, J.A.: Curettage without anesthesia on the office table. *Am. J. Obstet. Gynecol.* **9:**78–80, 1925.
12. Kennedy, C.R.: After office hours. *Obstet. Gynecol.* **17:**128–134, 1961.

13. Maisel, F.J., Nelson, H.B., Ott, R.E., et al.: Papanicolaou smear, biopsy, and conization of cervix. *Am. J. Obstet. Gynecol.* **86:**931–936, 1963.
14. McGuire, T.H.: Efficacy of endometrial biopsy in the diagnosis of endometrial carcinoma. *Obstet. Gynecol.* **19:**105–107, 1962.
15. Mengert, W.F., and Slate, W.G.: Diagnostic dilatation and curettage as an outpatient procedure. *Am. J. Obstet. Gynecol.* **79:**727–731, 1960.
16. Rutledge, F.: Cancer of the vagina. *Am. J. Obstet. Gynecol.* **97:**635–649, 1967.
17. Townsend, D.E.: Cryosurgery. *Obstet. Gynecol. Annu.* **4:**331–345, 1975.
18. Townsend, D.E., and Ostergard, D.R.: Cryocauterization for preinvasive cervical neoplasia. *J. Reprod. Med.* **6:**55–60, 1971.
19. Urcuyo, R., Rome, R.M., and Nelson, J.H.: Some observations on the value of endocervical curettage performed as an integral part of colposcopic examination of patients with abnormal cervical cytology. *Am. J. Obstet. Gynecol.* **128:**787–792, 1977.
20. Walters, D., Robinson, D., Park, R.C., et al.: Diagnostic outpatient aspiration curettage. *Obstet. Gynecol.* **46:**160–164, 1975.

Selected Bibliography

Blaustein, A. (ed.): *Pathology of the Female Genital Tract.* New York, Springer-Verlag, 1977.

2 Laparoscopy

William J. Cameron

Laparoscopy, although not a new procedure, did not gain momentum, especially in the United States, until the development of optics and fiberoptic light bundles in 1952 made it both practical and popular. Laparoscopy now accounts for the majority of all gynecologic operations and is second only to abortion in the United States in its frequency as a surgical procedure.

The following indications for laparoscopy are accepted by most gynecologists:

Suspected pelvic mass
Suspected ectopic pregnancy
Chronic pelvic pain
Symptomatic retroversion of the uterus
Evaluation of tubal disease
Infertility
Unexplained fever
Unexplained anemia
Second-look procedure for carcinoma of the ovary
Intersex problems
Evaluation of uterine anomalies prior to definitive surgery
Confirmation of uterine perforation
Search for ectopic intrauterine device
Female sterilization
Research purposes

The following operations are performed via laparoscopy:

Evaluation of the pelvis in infertility with tubal insufflation
Adhesiolysis
Ovarian biopsy
Biopsy of lesions on peritoneal or uterine surface
Uterine suspension
Fimbriolysis
Aspiration of ovarian cysts
Division of uterosacral ligaments
Removal or fulguration of tubal pregnancies
Sterilization by clips, bands, rings, or fulguration

Guidance of a needle for upper abdominal biopsies, chiefly liver
Removal of ectopic intrauterine devices, splints, or tubal hoods
Fulguration of uterine perforation

Complications that have been reported include superficial abdominal wall infections, hematoma formation, bowel burns, laceration of mesenteric vessels, pneumo-omentum, mesosalpingeal vessel hemorrhage, inadvertent round ligament fulguration, gas emboli, thermal injury to blood vessels, introduction of the trocar or cannula into the gut, blood vessel, or sacrum, puncture of the urinary bladder, skin burns (especially abdominal wall burns, which can necrose and slough), and cardiac arrest, with and without fatality. Most of these complications occur during the process of creating a pneumoperitoneum, introducing the trocar, or using electrocoagulation. Meticulous attention to training, equipment, position, anesthesia, and methodology will decrease the complication rate to an extremely low level (2 to 6 per 1000 cases).[2]

There has been such a proliferation of laparoscopic equipment that enumeration is impossible. The basic pieces of equipment necessary are a light source with a fiberoptic cable, an insufflation chamber with a dial recording the pressure at the end of the insufflating needle, a cannula for creation of the pneumoperitoneum, a trocar with sleeve, the laparoscope itself, a smaller diameter cannula and sleeve for a second puncture, and various instruments that may be used through the second cannula or through the second channel of the operating laparoscope. The latter would include specialized instruments for manipulation, fulguration, division of adhesions, biopsy, aspiration, grasping, and the like.

Preoperative Preparation

General anesthesia is favored by most laparoscopists. A "balanced" anesthetic that employs induction with sodium thiopental (Pentothal) followed by nitrous oxide–oxygen mixture, a succinylcholine drip, and endotracheal intubation is probably the best all-around method. However, the procedure has been performed with local anesthetic or regional blocks, including epidural and spinal. All methods are quite satisfactory. The choice of anesthetic depends on the patient, the procedure, the physician, and the availability of the anesthetic. Although the vast majority of laparoscopists employ carbon dioxide as the insufflating gas, nitrous oxide is also perfectly dependable and may be slightly less irritating to the peritoneum.

Some think it advantageous to prepare their patients with a bowel preparation as if for intravenous pyelogram.[3] Others feel that simethicone given the morning of the procedure reduces intrabowel gas, increasing visibility.[1]

Operative Technique

The position of the patient is important since the vagina and cervix should be available for manipulation, especially for infertility studies. Various instruments have been designed to affix the cervix, to manipulate the uterine fundus, and to insufflate transcervically. Although the procedure can be done with the patient in the supine position, the author favors a low dorsilithotomy position for ease of bladder drainage and cervical manipulation. The patient is fully draped except for the lower abdomen and perineum and placed at 15 degrees of Trendelenburg.

The abdomen, perinuem, vagina, and cervix are scrubbed with an antiseptic preparation. Shaving the pubic hair is unnecessary. The urinary bladder is drained with a straight catheter; we have not found a need for an indwelling catheter since most procedures are not that time consuming. The patient is draped as mentioned above. With a No. 11 or No. 15 knife blade a transverse or vertical incision approximately 10 mm long is made in the umbilicus (Figure 2.1). The incision should be through skin only. In the intraumbilical area, the fascia is extremely close to the surface because of the paucity of subcutaneous fat here. This makes an ideal place to enter the abdominal cavity, but at the same time the blood vessels of the omentum and mesentery are also close to skin, so care must be taken to keep the incision superficial.

The creation of the pneumoperitoneum is probably the most critical step in the entire procedure. The abdomen is grasped in the midline just below the incision and elevated as high as possible. This tenting of the anterior abdominal wall develops a *potential* space between the peritoneum and the underlying structures. It is not necessary to use towel hooks or other clamps for this elevation, even in the obese. The cannula, which has a retractable blunt stylet and a pointed sleeve, is directed slightly caudad, at approximately 30 degrees from the vertical. The cannula must be held by the barrel so that the spring-retractable stylet is not impeded. The needle is then thrust firmly through the abdominal wall. Some laparoscopists irrigate with saline at this point, or by opening the insufflating valve the gas pressure at the needle point can be read on the dial of the insufflating cham-

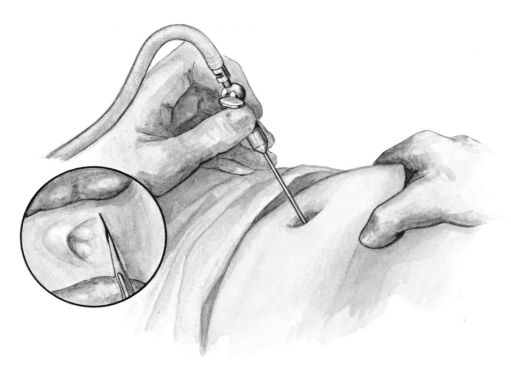

FIGURE 2.1.   Elevation of the lower abdominal wall creates a potential space for the placement of the insufflating needle. Note that the valve is in the off position and that the operator's fingers are holding the hub of the needle, allowing the spring-loaded stylet to be retracted when going through dense tissue. The angle of the needle is approximately 30 degrees from the vertical aimed toward the cul-de-sac. Inset: The operator's fingers spread the lower umbilical fold so that the knife blade slides cleanly through the skin only. The incision may be made vertically if preferred.

ber. In most machines, this pressure should be approximately 8 to 14 mm Hg. If it is even slightly higher than that, it probably represents a faulty puncture. The needle should be moved, withdrawn somewhat, and otherwise manipulated to obtain the desired pressure.

It is always preferable to perform another puncture than to insufflate gas when there is doubt as to the needle's location. When the correct placement is achieved, instead of immediately releasing the abdominal wall, the operator should wait until a bubble of the insufflating gas has formed around the cannula. Then the abdomen is slowly returned to its normal state and insufflation is continued. The amount of gas needed to develop the pneumoperitoneum varies greatly depending on the operator, the weight and parity of the patient, and the muscle tone of her abdominal wall. A high-parity patient with a lax abdominal wall requires more gas than a low-parity young person with a strong abdominal wall. Approximately 2,500 ml is an average but many operators will use more than that depending on the intraabdominal pressure, which should not exceed 24 mm Hg.

When the pneumoperitoneum is optimal, a sharp pyramid-ended trocar and trocar sleeve are placed in the same incision (Figure 2.2). The trocar is removed, leaving the sleeve in place. The trumpet valve can be depressed momentarily, allowing gas to escape, confirming its intraperitoneal position. The laparoscope is attached to the light source and introduced through the trocar sleeve with the laparoscopist looking through the laparoscope as it enters the abdominal cavity. It is unwise to place the laparoscope into the sleeve without observing through it as one is unaware what lies opposite the end of the sleeve.

Both the single-puncture and double-puncture techniques can be used. In the single-puncture method, a channel in the operating laparo-

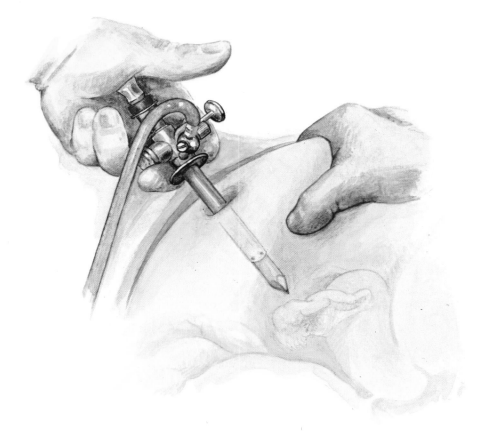

FIGURE 2.2. The abdominal wall is stabilized and elevated by the operator's hand and the trocar and its sleeve are aimed at the cul-de-sac in the pocket of gas formed by insufflation. The blunt end of the trocar nestles in the operator's palm and the thrusting motion is nontwisting and firm, not spastic.

23

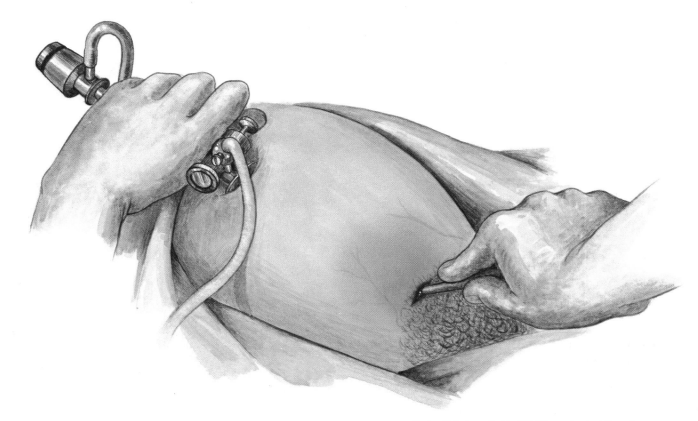

FIGURE 2.3. Holding the laparoscopy light against the anterior abdominal wall allows transillumination and visualization of the superficial inferior epigastric vessels. The laparoscope also serves as a splint under the abdominal wall so that the operating trocar may be pushed in against its resistance. Note the finger along the shaft of the operating trocar preventing inadvertent deep puncture.

scope allows the introduction of instruments to accomplish the intent of the operator. In the two-puncture technique, the operating room lights are dimmed and the laparoscope is brought up and held against the abdominal wall for transillumination (Figure 2.3). A 6 mm incision is made in an avascular area at or below the pubic hairline. The operating trocar and sleeve are placed in this incision.

Specialized instruments can be placed in the sleeve remaining after withdrawal of the trocar. Peritubal adhesions can be lysed with small scissors (Figure 2.4), an ovarian biopsy can be taken with other forceps (Fig-

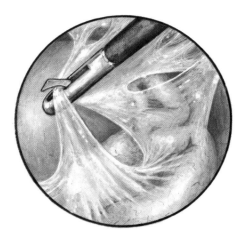

FIGURE 2.4. The small cobweb-like adhesions may be dissected and rarely cause bleeding requiring coagulation, but the patient should be on a groundplate in case a vascular adhesion is cut. Note the kinking of the oviduct and the adhesions overlying the ovary immediately below.

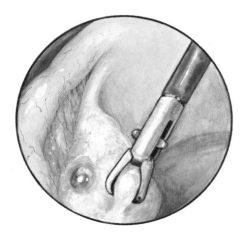

FIGURE 2.5. Note the suspensory ligament of the ovary anteriorly and the oviduct running superiorly. A corpus luteum cyst is seen on the surface of the ovary. The biopsy should include material from fairly deep within the cortex to be informative. The biopsy site need not be coagulated for hemostasis.

ure 2.5), an ovarian cyst aspiration can be performed with a needle, or sterilization can be accomplished by fulguration or with bands or clips.

Fulguration of oviducts for sterilization is probably most safely done with bipolar forceps so that the current does not course through the body of the patient but goes from one jaw of the forceps to the other, causing electrocoagulation between them. The oviduct is fulgurated in the isthmus with a "three-burn" technique (Figures 2.6 and 2.7). Even with bipolar forceps, and *especially* with unipolar forceps, care must be taken to see that the oviduct is elevated away from bowel. Prevention of one type of bowel burn hinges upon preventing condensation of current at a point where it might affect the bowel: When current is applied to the oviduct with a unipolar

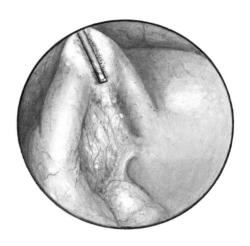

FIGURE 2.6. Tubal cauterization for sterilization: the three-burn procedure. The oviduct is grasped in its isthmic portion and thoroughly cauterized.

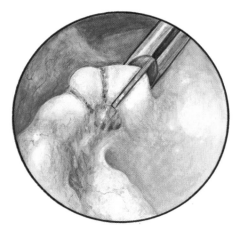

FIGURE 2.7. The isthmus of the tube is thoroughly cauterized in three areas immediately adjacent to each other. The tube does not need to be divided as the results are not improved by the additional surgery. Note the suspensory ligament of the ovary and the ovary immediately inferior to the oviduct.

25

system, it courses through the oviduct in all directions. If the end of the oviduct is touching adjacent bowel, the current becomes condensed at that point and this increase in density can cause a burn of the bowel wall in the area where fimbria touches it. This phenomenon has actually been observed. The danger is minimized by the use of the bipolar forceps system and they are highly recommended. **Caution:** When using bipolar forceps, the patient should be on a ground plate so that one may switch to a unipolar system if necessary. If electrocoagulation of bleeding vessels is necessary, the bipolar forceps is an unsatisfactory instrument. One should remove the forceps, put in a coagulation instrument, and switch to a unipolar circuit.

If, during fulguration of oviducts or other structures, one fails to see the blanching that normally occurs, resist the impulse to simply increase the current. Instead, withdraw the instrument and check all wiring connections, ground cords, plugs, plates, and so forth. Some small defect will usually be found in the circuitry which has escaped the attention of the operating room staff. When the defect is rectified, fulguration can then be accomplished with relative safety. Those wishing to pursue the matter of the various types of circuitry and their effects are referred to Chapter 4 by Loffer and Pent in the text *Laparoscopy*.[2]

Uterine suspension in cases of markedly symptomatic retroversion can be easily performed via laparoscopy. The only deviation from the procedure described above is that two operating cannulas are placed approximately 3 cm lateral of the midline. Grasping forceps are put through the sleeve, seizing each round ligament at its midpoint. The forceps, round ligament, and trocar sleeve are all withdrawn from the abdominal wall, exposing the round ligament, which is then sutured to the rectus sheath (Figure 2.8).

At the conclusion of the laparoscopic procedure, the small cannula sheath is removed, the laparoscope is removed, and the trumpet valve is depressed, allowing the gas to escape. As the pneumoperitoneum deflates, pressure is placed on the lower abdomen with the trocar sleeve in a nearly horizontal position, allowing egress of most of the insufflated gas. The trocar sleeve is then removed and the skin incision is closed with sutures of fine absorbable material. The patient is told that there are no restrictions on her activities but that she can anticipate tenderness in the paraumbilical area and might well experience pain in the shoulders due to subdiaphragmatic irritation from the remaining gas. She is dismissed ambulatory and told to resume full activity as she feels fit.

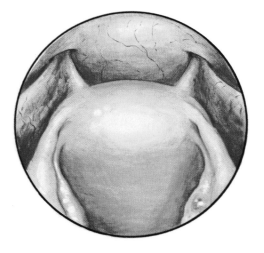

FIGURE 2.8. At the conclusion of the procedure, the midportion of round ligaments have been pulled through the abdominal wall and sutured with nonabsorbable material to the anterior rectus sheath anteverting the uterus. Note the vessels on the bladder in the midline.

In summary, a trained laparoscopist paying meticulous attention to detail involving the positioning of the patient, anesthesia, equipment, and performance of the procedure itself will have a successful outcome and a satisfied patient.

References

1. Buck, W.H.: Personal communication 1977.
2. Loffer, F.D., and Pent, D.: Statistics. In Phillips, J. (ed.): *Laparoscopy*. Baltimore, Williams & Wilkins, 1977, ch. 23.
3. Soderstrom, R., and Butler, J.: A critical evaluation of complications in laparoscopy. *J. Reprod. Med.* **10:** 245–246, 1973.

Selected Bibliography

Rioux, J., and Cloutier, D.: Basic principles of electrosurgery. In Phillips, J. (ed.): *Laparoscopy*. Baltimore, Williams & Wilkins, 1977, ch. 4.

Vaginal Surgery

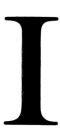

Wound Healing in Gynecologic Surgery

3

Gynecologists, like all surgeons, perform essentially three functions in surgical procedures: they incise tissue, perform some observation or task, and repair the wound created. The alterations in tissue incised, the changes produced by the implantation of foreign bodies such as prosthesis or suture material, and the response as the wound heals have been given little attention in the gynecologic literature. Our colleagues in the fields of plastic and general surgery have made monumental contributions to our understanding of these processes. Gynecologic surgeons should be conversant with the more recent literature, particularly the work of Drs. J. Engelbert Dunphy, Erle E. Peacock, and Walton Van Winkle. The following section draws heavily from these authors and their contributions to the art and science of surgery are appreciated.

Response to Injury

Inflammatory Phase

Whether one enters the patient with a single stroke of the sharp knife, with a scissor wound in the performance of an episiotomy, or through the insertion of the trocar in laparoscopy, the initial basic response to injury is the same and is called the *inflammatory* or *substrate phase* of wound healing. The magnitude of this inflammatory response varies in proportion to the trauma inflicted, being least with a knife, intermediate in a scissor wound, and greatest with blunt dissection. The addition of cautery, constant rubbing of the wound, traumatic clamping of tissue, and excess suture material all greatly accentuate the injury.

The initial response to incision is the release of blood from small vessels in the area. The vessels immediately respond with vasoconstriction; this vasoconstrictive period lasts for approximately 10 min. It is followed by general vasodilation of the area vessels. The cellular response begins immediately and leukocytes adhere to the endothelium of vessels in the area of injury. Within 1 hr the entire endothelium is covered with adherent polymorphonuclear leukocytes, erythocytes, and platelets. Active rouleaux formation plugs the small capillaries and further obstructs blood flow. Leakage of fluid also occurs directly between endothelial cells of the vessels, and the surgeon notices this as a clear serum bathing the wound edges. White blood cells actively migrate to the wound in approximately the same concentration as in the plasma. It would appear that the predominance of mononuclear cells found later in the wound is due to the shorter life of polymorphonuclear leukocytes. A hemostatic response occurs simultaneously with the vascular response and the plasma kinin system produces a local cycle of increased permeability. More platelets and fibrin are laid down, with the formation of blood clots.

Numerous substances are active in the vascular and inflammatory responses to the initial incision. Histamine, serotonin, kinins, and various chemotactic agents all play an active role. An additional group of substances quite active in the response to injury are prostaglandins E_1 and E_2. They have strong vasodilative and lymph flow–increasing properties and have a very prominent role as mediators of the acute inflammatory process. Note that certain drugs, among them aspirin, are potent inhibitors of prostaglandin synthesis.[10]

Secondary Phase

The initial phase of wound healing lasts from the time of the incision to the fourth day. During the later portion of this substrate phase, the cellular infiltrates into the area of the wound include polymorphonuclear leukocytes, lymphocytes, macrophages, and monocytes. Mast cells are present and are a source of heparin and a variety of enzymes. Remember that no wound strength is present during the early repair process, but a weak gel-like substrate of enzymes, fibrin, and white cells fills the space produced by the wound. Re-exploration in the immediate postoperative period therefore has little retardant effect on wound healing as no collagen strands linking the wound edges are present. Epithelium grows from both the wound edges and the bases of hair follicles if any adnexal structures remain in the wound.

Fibroplastic or Proliferative Phase

This phase of wound healing occurs during days 5 to 20. The key element during this phase is the fibroblast. While debated for many years, it appears from the work of Grillo and Potsaid that most fibroblasts arise locally.[4] This evidence was obtained by the use of the inhibitory effects of irradiation on fibroblasts. Design and repair of an incision in irradiated fields must accommodate the changes in the healing process caused by irradiation or serious wound complications arise.[4]

Fibroblasts actively synthesize collagen, which provides for the strength of the repair. Mucopolysaccharides are secreted as well, which may contribute to fibril orientation and proliferation.

The observation that the fibroblasts arise locally places great emphasis on the need for gentle wound construction and repair. These fibroblasts use the fibrin strands as scaffolding and begin to elaborate fibrous collagen precursor into the wound. Capillaries follow with fibroblasts, and new capillary formation is prominent. Capillaries are formed by endothelial budding and contain a plasminogon activator that produces fibrinolysis, and the fibrin net is removed. The wound is actively invaded with capillaries and fibroblasts. Collagen fibrils are laid down and cross-linkages occur which produce the rapidly increasing tensile strength of the wound. By the end of the 21st day, the wound has regained approximately 30% of its original tensile strength, a figure equal to the percentage provided by nonabsorbable sutures (Figure 3.1).

32

It is important to note that the wide scar is weaker than the narrow one. The ideal wound is a wound with normal tissues approximated by minimal new connective tissue formation.

Remodeling Phase

The final phase of wound healing is particularly active in the buttock, abdominal wall, and back. Wound healing then, is a process of protein synthesis subject to numerous modifying factors. Vitamin C deficiency, protein starvation, cortisone and nitrogen mustard administration, and irradiation have been shown to have retarding effects on wound healing. Edema and anoxia also have deleterious effects. Local infection severely disrupts the healing process and occurs when the number of bacteria exceeds the injured tissue's ability to deal with the bacterial population in the wound. The usual gynecologic patient does not suffer from malnutrition or protein deficiencies severe enough to retard healing. Cortisone usage is much less common in gynecologic patients than in, for example, patients with inflammatory diseases of the bowel. Anemia severe enough to produce anoxia is rare in clinical practice today, and congestive failure is usually detected and treated prior to surgery.

The most common retardant of repair in gynecologic surgery is injury from poor tissue handling, antiquated instruments, excessively sized, chemically reactive strangulating sutures, and poorly designed surgical procedures that fail to adhere to sound surgical practices based on modern wound repair data. The resultant trauma increases the infection rate, delays wound healing, and promotes formation of a weaker scar.

The procedures, instruments, suture selection, and pre- and postoperative recommendations presented in this manual are chosen and designed to interfere least with wound healing. As the surgeon can do little to accelerate wound healing, he can ill afford to retard its normal progression.

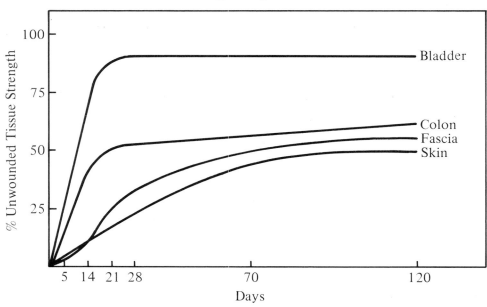

FIGURE 3.1. Adapted from: Van Winkle W., Salthouse T.N.: Biological response to sutures and principles of suture selection. Sommerville, N.J., Ethicon, 1976.

33

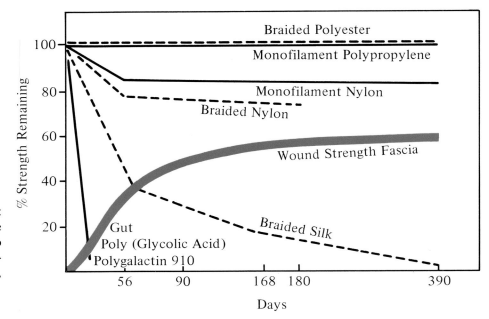

FIGURE 3.2. Adapted from: Van Winkle W., Salthouse T.N.: Biological response to sutures and principles of suture selection. Somerville, N.J., Ethicon, 1976.

Suture

Suture Materials

As surgical skills and techniques advance, suture selections become more important. Suture technology has not produced a perfect suture material but progress is being made. The ideal characteristics of nonreactivity, properly timed complete absorption, high tensile strength, and proper handling characteristics are not now available in any single suture material; therefore, the surgeon must be familiar with several suture types.

New suture materials are derived from poly(glycolic acid) (Dexon, Vicryl), polyamides (nylon), polyesters (Dacron), and polyolifins (Prolene). As textile technology advances, handling characteristics of these synthetic materials will improve; gut, cotton, and silk, which have served surgeons and their patients so well for so many years, will become less attractive.

Suture material is generally classified as absorbable and nonabsorbable in type. The term *nonabsorbable* suggests permanence and continued strength, but this is not necessarily the case. The filaments of 2-0 braided black silk, a nonabsorbable suture, are widely separated by fibroblasts 21 days after surgical implantation, and only 50% of the original strength of the suture remains at 50 days. Braided polyester, however, has little loss of tensile strength or fibril absorption after 1 year in tissue[12] (Figure 3.2).

Clinical practice requires not only proper material selection but correct choice of suture size as well. Tensile strength and knot-breaking strengths for various suture sizes are listed in Table 3.1.

It makes little sense to use sutures markedly stronger than the tissues in which they are placed (Table 3.2); hence, the large gut sutures (Nos. 0, 1, and 2) historically used in gynecologic surgery have little justification when tissue strength, knot-pulled breaking strength, and modern wound data are reviewed. The increasing quality, consistency, and strength of synthetic sutures makes possible the use of smaller diameter suture material: 3-0 absorbable suture has 40% less volume than 2-0, and 2-0 suture 36% less than 0[6]; 2-0 polygalactin 910 is approximately as strong as 0 chromic, permitting its substitution and a reduction in the volume of suture material left in the wound. Cutting the suture close to the knot also reduces the amount of suture material placed into the wound.

TABLE 3.1. Observed Average Knot-Pulled Breaking Strength

Suture	Strength (lb)	USP Requirements (lb)
Vicryl		
4-0	3.2	
3-0	5.0	
2-0	7.9	
0	10.8	
1	14.8	
Chromic catgut		
3-0	3.9	4.4
00	5.7	6.1
0	8.4	8.4
1	11.1	
Nurolon		
3.0	3.5	2.1
00	4.8	3.2
0	7.0	4.8
1	10	6.0

Courtesy of Russell W. Davis, Product Director, Ethicon, Somerville, N.J., 1978.

TABLE 3.2. Pull-out Strengths in Tissues

Tissue	Strength (lb)
Fat	0.44
Peritoneum	1.9
Muscle	2.8
Fascia	8.3

Adapted from Van Winkle, W., and Hastings, J. C.: *Surg. Gynecol. Obstet.* **135**:113–126, 1972.

Suture Selection

Specific suture selection for each procedure is noted in each chapter, but some generalizations are possible.

Retention sutures should be of large monofilament nylon or polyester for patient comfort and nonreactivity. To convince oneself of the variation in wound response to suture, the surgeon need only place a retention suture of large-diameter silk alongside one of monofilament nylon or polyester. Before the sutures are removed, a wide area of inflammatory response will be present around the silk suture, but little response will be noted with the monofilament suture. Monofilament polypropylene sutures require numerous knots, which does produce some mass of suture material, but this is negligible as the knot is outside the tissues. The ends of such large sutures can be irritating to the patient; however, the suture ends may be pulled into a cut portion of catheter. Place through-and-through retention sutures carefully so as to avoid the anastomosis between the superior and inferior epigastric arteries. Retention sutures placed through and through give great wound security. Kobak observed that Kennedy reported over 30,000 wounds without a dehiscence using retention sutures.[6]

Zero or 2-0 braided nylon is the author's choice for midline incision closure. Postelthwait reported that nylon causes the least tissue reaction[11] and Van Winkle and Salthouse noted no increase in experimental infections when braided nylon was compared to monofilament nylon.[12]

The use of absorbable sutures in midline abdominal wound closure would seem unwise after review of Figure 3.2, although good results have been reported.[1]

A wound closure is only as strong as the tissues in which the suture is placed, hence wide bites of tissue should be included in the outer arm of the Smead-Jones closure. A good rule of thumb is to place the sutures as far apart as they are from the wound edge.

Sutures placed in the Smead-Jones fashion are stronger than any other common closure technique. Larsen and Ulin measured the mean tensile strength of artificial wounds closed with 3-0 polyester in kilograms.[7] With the sutures placed in strong material, Smead-Jones closure failed at 39 kg and was 2 to 3 times as strong as the other types of closure. Continuous sutures failed at 18 kg and the single interrupted stitch at 22 kg.

For a suture to be effective in approximating tissue, the knot must be secure. Magilligan and DeWeese reported four square knots as the most stable configuration of those they tested.[8] In most clinical situations, three well placed square knots will suffice in braided nylon, Vicryl, or chromic suture.

Stainless steel wire of 2-0 (No. 28) gauge is a strong nonreactive suture. It cannot be used in thin patients and is being replaced by the new synthetic sutures for fascial closure.

Transverse wounds of the abdomen of the Pfannenstiel type have significant inherent strength and may be closed with a smaller suture. Continuous absorbable suture of 2-0 diameter is adequate for this fascial closure. If the patient has a transverse incision through all layers, use nonabsorbable sutures of 2-0 braided nylon. If a fine cosmetic scar is desired, close the transverse incision with 3-0 subcuticular monofilament polypropylene or nylon; 4-0 gut may be used, and while tissue reaction is greater, patients appreciate that no suture need be removed. The choice of transverse incision with a subcuticular closure and a few 5-0 or 6-0 monofilament nylon sutures to even any ridges produced by the subcuticular suture is most useful to provide a good cosmetic result. Bracing the wound margins with Steri-strips or collodian dressing will diminish stress on the wound edge, which will decrease scar width.

Use 3-0 braided nylon suture for ovarian arteries and uterine arteries and 2-0 or 3-0 absorbable suture for the vaginal cuff and cardinal ligaments. The use of very fine absorbable suture to close the vaginal cuff in vaginal and abdominal hysterectomy will greatly diminish the reaction noticed in the paravaginal tissues postoperatively. The hesitance to use nonabsorbable suture for vascular ligatures in the pelvis because of its tendency to form granulomas and extrude through the vaginal cuff does not pertain to braided nylon. Oral surgeons now use braided nylon in the mouth with great frequency and notice very little extrusion.[5] Nylon has some inherent antibacterial properties in the suture itself and will produce much less suture reaction in the pelvis than silk.[2] It does little good, however, to use a very fine suture if large traumatic needles are used. Carefully chosen fine-diameter intestinal needles produce much less trauma to tissues and are useful in performing gynecologic surgical procedures.

It is important to observe that while some suture materials and configurations of sutures are much less prone to be associated with infection than others, all suture material increases wound infection rate experimentally. The author does not close the subcutaneous tissues for this reason.

Bacteria can be recovered from the majority of surgical wounds, but the number of bacteria must exceed 10^6/g of tissue for clinical evidence of infection with most bacteria. If silk material is added to the experimental wound, 10^3 organisms/g will regularly produce clinical infection.[3] Close wounds with the minimum amount of the least reactive suture consistent with hemostasis, operative interest, and anatomic closure.

Surgical Instruments

The modern surgical hemostat dates from the work of Dr. Ambroise Pare in the mid 1500s. Surgical instruments became more traumatic in gyneco-

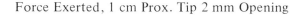

Force Exerted, 1 cm Prox. Tip 2 mm Opening

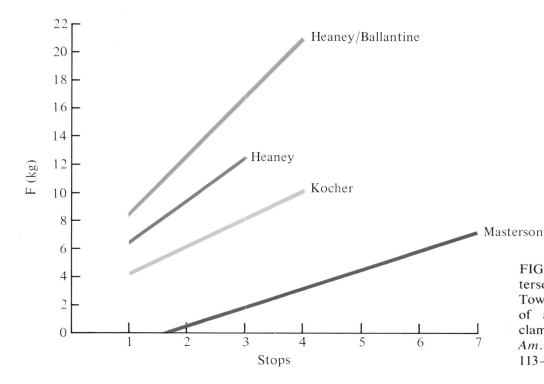

FIGURE 3.3. From: Masterson B.J., Sullivan T., Townsend P.R.: Development of a noncrushing vascular clamp for pelvic surgery. *Am. J. Obstet. Gynecol.* **132:** 113–115, 1978.

logic surgery and reached their acme with the angiothryptor of Kossman. The maximum compressive force available was sought and great tissue destruction was produced. The lack of blood, the absence of antibiotics, and the lethal nature of any infection acquired in surgery seemed to justify these forces. Modern wound healing data make it abundantly clear that the wound with the least trauma, dead tissue, and suture material has the most resistance to infection. This wound heals with greater strength than the wound that contains tissues compressed by surgical instruments of excessive force. The purpose of gynecologic surgical forceps is not the compression of tissues, but rather traction to increase exposure and to mobilize tissues into the field.

Select artery forceps of very fine construction with sharp points and a gentle pelvic curve. Adson or Gemini artery forceps 8 inches in length serve admirably for this purpose, and eight pairs should be available for pelvic surgical procedures. The jaws produce little trauma, the instrument is large enough such that it is not easily misplaced at the time of laparotomy, and its curved end is useful in suture passage.

The author has designed clamps for the parametria, vagina, pericolpos, pelvic arteries, and veins. The Masterson clamp* has nontraumatic teeth that sit in a jaw with minimal lateral motion, a strong box lock, and multiple wide-travel ratchets. This instrument produces minimal jaw pressure with effective tissue fixation and is available in $8\frac{1}{2}$- and 10-inch lengths with straight, curved, and right-angle jaw configurations. Heaney and Kocher clamps all produce excessive pressure in the tissues clamped with no greater purchase for traction. The trauma produced is remarkable when studied in the surgical laboratory.[9] Figure 3.3 illustrates relative pressures measured in the jaws of some of the clamps described.

* Codman and Shurtleff, Inc., Randolph, Mass.

Thumb forceps with serrated jaws should be available in short, medium, and long lengths (see Figure 3.4). Adson-Brown forceps provide excellent traction with minimal tissue trauma. Never grasp needles with thumb forceps as this destroys the teeth. When suturing, grasp tissues to be sutured with thumb forceps and curve the needle gently through the tissue; do not release the tissues by the thumb forceps. A common mistake of the fledgling surgeon is to release the tissues as soon as the needle has passed and grasp for the needle with the thumb forceps. This both destroys the thumb forceps and unnecessarily traumatizes tissues which are to be joined. The original purchase should remain in the thumb forceps and the needle holder should be returned to the position of function with the palm down, grasping the needle in the opposite tissues and completing the arc. If the thumb forceps are not removed, the needle will remain quite stationary in the tissue sutured and can be easily grabbed.

When reconstructive procedures are performed deep in the pelvis, very narrow long thumb forceps, such as the Debakey thumb forceps, are useful.

Dissection should be sharp wherever possible and knife handles of varying lengths are needed. The use of the knife handle as a dissector instead of the blade is a misuse of the instrument.

Fine dissecting scissors are a vital tool in pelvic surgery (Figure 3.4). The author prefers the short, fine-bladed, slightly rounded Metzenbaum scissors or Nelson chest scissors of delicate construction. Purchase excellent scissors and guard them from the less skilled surgeon. Use these scissors for dissection, not cutting vaginal or thick portions of tissue; have strongly constructed scissors for these purposes in both long and very long (12-inch) lengths.

Have needle holders available in short, medium, and long lengths (Figure 3.5). Very long delicate needle holders are needed for ureteral anastomosis. Jaw strength should be sufficient for holding both very fine and medium length needles. Avoid the use of very large needles in the pelvis, but occasionally a general closure needle is needed deep in the pelvis, and the jaws should be sufficient to handle this without springing. The surgeon may palm the needle holder without closing for more rapid suturing.

Hemostatic clip pliers of medium and long lengths are employed in pelvic surgery, and at least three pairs are necessary with sufficient clips to complete the procedures anticipated.

The key to pelvic surgery is exposure. The pelvis restricts mobility because of the rigid, bony formation and the proper retractors are most important in pelvic surgery (Figure 3.7).

Equally as important is a complete set of instruments for the very obese patient with a very deep pelvis. The Balfour retractors with very large deep blades are invaluable, as are at least two very long needle holders, thumb forceps, scissors, and artery forceps.

Glassman bowel forceps are useful, as are lightly constructed rubber-shod clamps. A complete list of these and other instruments is provided in the Appendix.

Finally, an auxiliary light source is a necessity for surgery in the deep recesses of the pelvis. A flexible fiberoptic cable light with a sterile transparent sleeve that slips over it is very functional in abdominal procedures, and a weighted speculum that transmits both light and suction is most useful in vaginal procedures.

APPENDIX   Instrument List

Vaginal Surgery
  Scissors
    2 — 7″ Metzenbaum (delicate) curved
    1 — 9″ Metzenbaum (delicate) curved
    1 — 6¾″ Mayo curved
    1 — Suture

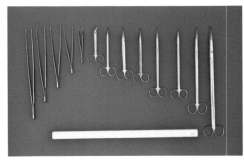

FIGURE 3.4.   Thumb forceps and scissors.

Thumb forceps
    2 — 4¾″, 6¼″, 8″ Adson-Brown
    2 — 8″, 1 × 2 teeth

Needle holders
    2—6″, 7″ Crile Wood (delicate)
    2 — 7″ Mayo Hegar
    1 — 9″ Julian

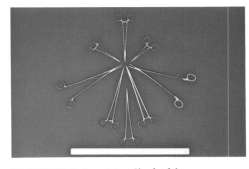

FIGURE 3.5.   Needle holders.

Clamps
    3 — 6¼″ Lahey thyroid tenaculum
    6 — 6¼″ Allis adair
    4 — 8″ Masterson curved
    4 — 8″ Masterson straight
    8 — 6¼″ Crile curved
    4 — 5½″ Crile straight
    2 — 8″ Allis
    4 — 8″ Gemini

Other
    Schubert uterine biopsy forceps
    Pratt uterine dilatator and curette
    Sponge forceps
    Uterine sounds
    Knife handle
    Basin
    Towel clips
    Neuro, pool, and tonsil suction tips
    Marking pen
    Fiberoptic light source
    Bipolar coagulator

  Retractors
    1 — Weighted vaginal speculum 1¾″ × 3″, 1¾ × 4″
    3 — Deaver 1″ × 9″
    1 — Sims vaginal retractor

Abdominal Surgery
  Scissors
    1 — 5½″ flat
    2 — 7″ Metzenbaum (delicate) curved
    2 — 9″, 11″ Nelson (delicate) curved
    1 — 10″, 11″ Metzenbaum (delicate) curved
    1 — 9″, 14″ heavy curved dissection
    1 — 4¾″ wire cutter
    1 — Potts cardiovascular right angle
    1 — Suture

  Thumb forceps
    2 — 4¾″, 6¼″, 8″ Adson-Brown
    2 — 9½″ Debakey
    2 — 8″, 1 × 2 teeth

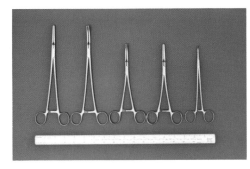

FIGURE 3.6.   Clamps.

Needle Holders
2 — 6″, 7″ Crile Wood (narrow jaw)
1 — 8¼″, 9″ Julian
2 — 9″, 10″ Wagenstein
1 — 10½″ Masson (delicate)

Clamps
4 — 5¼″ Crile straight
16 — 6¼″ curved delicate
16 — 5″ mosquito
8 — 8″ Gemini or Adson
4 — 8½″ Masterson straight
2 — 8½″ Masterson curved
4 — 10½″ Masterson straight
2 — 10½″ Masterson curved
4 — Sarot intrathoracic
2 — Glassman intestinal
2 — 8″ Allis and Babcock
2 — Hemostatic clip appliers medium and large

Retractors
3 — Double-hook skin tenaculum
1 — Balfour regular with shallow and deep blades, extra large
2 — Richardson small, medium, large
3 — Deaver 1″ × 12″
3 — Deaver 1½″ × 12″
3 — Deaver 3″ × 12″
1 — Deaver 3″ × 12″ × 7½″
1 — Deaver 5″ × 13″ × 7½″
2 — Deaver 1″ × 16″
2 — Harrington 2″ × 12″
1 — Harrington 2½″ × 12″
1 — Harrington 3¼″ × 10″
2 — Crushing vein retractor

Other
Sponge forceps
Knife holders
Basins
Towel clips
Neuro, pool, and tonsil suction tips
Marking pen
Fiberoptic abdominal light source
Bipolar coagulator

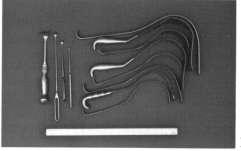

FIGURE 3.7.   Retractors.

References

1. Baggish, M.S., and Lee, W.K.: Abdominal wound disruption. *Obstet. Gynecol.* **46:**530–534, 1975.
2. Edlich, R.F., Panek, P.H., Rodeheaver, G.T. et al.: Physical and chemical configuration of sutures in the development of surgical infection. *Ann. Surg.* **177:**769–688, 1973.
3. Elek, S.D., and Conen, P.E.: The virulence of *Staphylococcus pyogenes* for man. A study of the problems of wound infection. *Br. J. Exp. Pathol.* **38:** 573–586, 1957.
4. Grillo, H.C., and Potsaid, M.S.: Studies in wound healing. IV. Retardation of contraction by local x-irradiation, and observations relating to the origin of fibroblasts in repair. *Ann. Surg.* **154:**741–750, 1961.
5. Hiatt, W.R.: Personal communication, 1978.
6. Kobak, M.W.: *Studies on the Abdominal Incision.* Springfield, Ill., Thomas, 1965.
7. Larsen, J.S., and Ulin, A.W.: Tensile strength advantage of the far-and-near suture technique. *Surg. Gynecol. Obstet.,* **131:**123–124, 1970.
8. Magilligan, D.J., and DeWeese, J.A.: Knot security and synthetic suture materials. *Am. J. Surg.* **127:**355–358, 1974.

9. Masterson, B.J., Sullivan, T.G., and Townsend, P.: Development of a non-crushing clamp for gynecology surgery. *Am. J. Obstet. Gynecol.* **132:**113–117, 1978.
10. Peacock, E.E., and Van Winkle, W.: Healing and repair of viscera. In: *Wound Repair*. Philadelphia, Saunders, 1976, ch. 12.
11. Postlethwait, R.W.: Long-term comparative study of nonabsorbable sutures. *Ann. Surg.* **171:**892–898, 1970.
12. Van Winkle, W., and Salthouse, T.N.: Biological response to sutures and principles of suture selection. Somerville, N.J., Ethicon, 1976.

Selected Bibliography

Dunphy, J.E., and Van Winkle, W.: Repair and regeneration. In: *The Scientific Basis for Surgical Practice*. New York, McGraw-Hill, 1960.
Peacock, E.E., and Van Winkle. W.: *Wound Repair*. Philadelphia, Saunders, 1976.

4 Cervical Conization

Conization of the uterine cervix was first described by Lisfranc in 1815 and the techniques, indications, and adjunctive procedures have been modified significantly since that time. Simms, in 1861, sutured the cervix, and Sturmdorf, in 1916, described his inverting suture.[8] The use of the cryostat for rapid diagnosis in conization specimens was popularized by Rutledge and Ibanez[6] and conization was most frequently used for diagnosis of abnormal cervical cytological specimens during the late 1960s. However, many of the previous indications for conization have been supplemented by new procedures made available by technological advancement. Conization is rarely indicated for the repair of cervical lacerations, and cryosurgery has replaced it in the management of symptomatic chronic cervicitis. Likewise, colposcopy with directed biopsy has reduced the number of conizations performed in the investigation of abnormal cervical cytologies by 90% in most gynecology–oncology services today.

Preoperative Evaluation

Modern indications for conization are adjuncts to the more central diagnostic procedure of colposcopy. The author feels that no one should investigate an abnormal vaginal cytology without colposcopy available. If colposcopy is unavailable, the patient is referred, not operated upon. If a gross cervical lesion is present, biopsy, not conization, is indicated. There is no rationale for performing conization in a patient with a large cervical cancer when an office biopsy is quite sufficient. The additional inflammatory response occasioned with conization renders radical surgery more hazardous and complicates radiation therapy.

Modern indications for cervical conization include abnormal cytological findings with normal colposcopic examination, colposcopic lesion which extends into the endocervix in the absence of a gross cancer, suspicious histologic findings on endocervical curettage not diagnostic of cancer, and colposcopic biopsy of microinvasion where more extensive disease is suspected; conization may also be employed as a method of primary therapy in a patient who does not wish hysterectomy and whose lesion is not amenable to laser. Due to the physiologic eversion of the cervix, conization is rarely indicated in pregnancy and colposcopy will prove to be quite accurate in most instances.[3]

42

Operative Technique

Place the patient in the lithotomy position and prepare and drape in the usual manner for vaginal surgery. The bladder is not emptied. Perform an examination under anesthesia. If colposcopic mapping of the known lesion is not available, colposcope the patient at the time of conization. Rubio and Thomassen evaluated the Schiller test in patients before conization and found false-positive Schiller test results in 32% of patients and false-negative results in 60%.[4] The Schiller test is therefore unreliable in planning the surgical margin of conization specimens.

The surgical technique is illustrated in Figures 4.1 through 4.3.

If bleeding occurs in the conization margins, reinject the margins with vasoconstrictive solution and pack Avitene into the conization defect. An

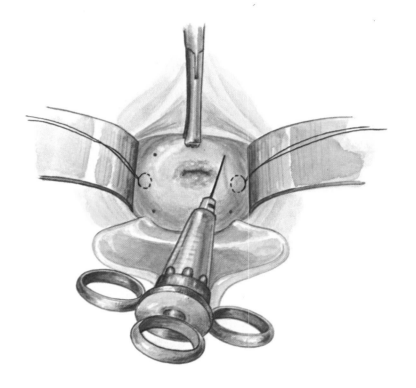

FIGURE 4.1. Bring the cervix down with a tenaculum and inject it with a solution of 1:100,000 epinephrine or 1:200,000 Neo-Synephrine (6 drops in 30 ml of saline). Place 2-0 Vicryl sutures deep enough in the lateral margins of the cervix at 3 and 9 o'clock to surround the descending cervical branch of the uterine artery as it courses downward into the cervix. Tie these sutures with a square knot and leave the ends long.

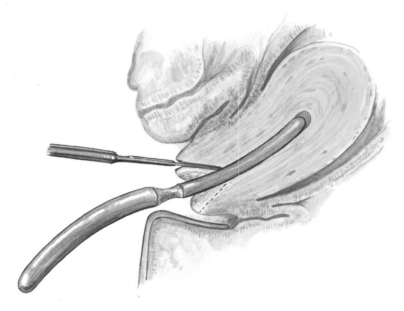

FIGURE 4.2. Insert a sound or No. 5 Hegar dilator into the cervix and with a No. 15 Bard-Parker blade sharply incise the specimen, using the dilator as a central focus for the end of the knife. It is important that a dilator or sound be used because many postconization bleeders have resulted from cutting across the central axis of the uterus with the tip of the blade and incising above the conization site deeply into the opposite uterine wall. Using an Allis clamp, grasp the cone as it is cut, pull it downward, and following excision place a suture at the 12 o'clock position in the conization specimen.

43

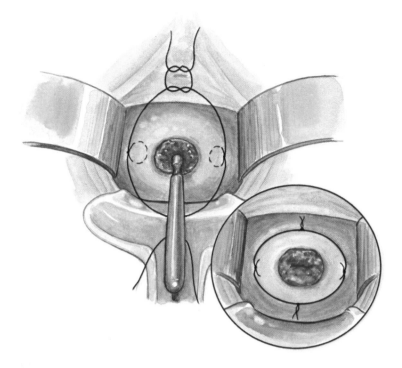

FIGURE 4.3. The endocervix and the endometrial cavity are curetted with a sharp curette as discussed in the section on Dilatation and Curettage in Chapter 1. The sound is replaced in the uterus and the ties are tied snuggly over a No. 5 sound to avoid stenosis and stricture. The sound is removed. Inset: The sutures are tied and the ends of the absorbable suture are cut.

alternative method with excellent reported results has been described by VillaSanta.[9] With the No. 5 dilator in place, tie sutures over the cervix and remove the dilator; having the dilator in place prevents occlusion of the endocervix. In using this method, VillaSanta reduced postcone bleeding by 90% and reported no cervical stenosis in 500 patients.

Following the conization, no pack is placed in the vagina. Avoid Sturmdorf sutures and mass ligature-type sutures as they produce necrosis and sloughing with intense reaction in the cervix, promoting delayed vaginal bleeding. Claman and Lee noted that any patient who bled in the hospital had a much greater liklihood of recurrence of more serious bleeding after discharge. In their series of 1,008 cases, the patients who were operated on by a less experienced surgeon, who were less than 30 years of age, and who had mass ligature or Sturmdorf and side stitches and vaginal packing had the highest incidence of complications, approaching 40%.[2] Furthermore, Claman and Lee documented an average complication rate of 25% and 10% postoperative bleeding, 3% morbidity, and 5% readmission rates.[2]

Rubio et al. noted no relationship between postcone hemorrhage and the size of the conization.[5] The purposes of the cone should be foremost in the surgeon's mind when performing a cone. If the procedure is therapeutic, then the conization follows, if possible, the margins of the lesion to be excised. If the lesion extends well up the endocervical canal, then the cone must extend well up into that area as well.

Postoperative Management

The patient is dismissed 48 hr after conization. If a catheter was necessary postoperatively, remove the catheter prior to discharge and place the patient on a urinary antiseptic such as nitrofurantoin macrocrystals (Macrodantin), 50 mg q.i.d. for 10 days. Instruct the patient to abstain from intercourse for 2 weeks and prescribe a vaginal cream such as triple sulfa cream, one-half an applicator every morning, for the first 10 days following conization.

The patient returns for a follow-up examination when the inflammatory changes have subsided, approximately 6 weeks after conization. If the patient has any abnormal cytology after conization, reconization may be performed, although the author recommends simple hysterectomy. If the conization was performed in a young woman for treatment of carcinoma in situ, careful cytological examinations are imperative. In the absence of abnormal cytology, routine follow-up and evaluation is in order, with a Papanicolaou smear every 3 months for the first year, at 6-month intervals in the second year, and yearly thereafter. If cytological studies are negative for the first year, the chance of recurrence is 0.4%.[1]

Results

Conization is quite accurate when compared to colposcopic biopsy or random punch biopsy. Cervical conization approaches 99% in accuracy in patients having abnormal epithelial lesions of the cervix; the 1% failure group consists of patients with unsuspected invasive cancer. Punch biopsy is less accurate because the smaller tissue sample, endocervical epithelial abnormalities, an atrophic cervix, and a small vagina make the biopsy difficult. When punch biopsies are obtained in a ring fashion with six to eight biopsies and subsequent curettage, biopsy may approach 94% accuracy; however, this is a significant number of biopsies and careful histologic examination is better achieved with conization.[7]

Conization is successfully used for therapy. Bjerre et al. performed cold-knife conization in 2,099 patients with abnormal Papanicolaou smears: 1,500 were found to have carcinoma in situ and conization alone was curative in 87% of these patients.[1] The cure rate did not depend on whether or not a resection margin was free of pathological epithelium. Of the 1,500 patients, 156 had an additional cytological abnormality; 8 of these patients were found to have invasive cancer. Others have followed conization with hysterectomy and found 22% to 27% of patients had residual carcinoma in situ in the hysterectomy specimen. While one might suspect that conization would greatly increase the risk of spontaneous abortion and premature delivery, Bjerre et al. reported an abortion increase from 12% to only 17% after conization; they also observed no increase in frequency of premature delivery due to conization.[1]

References

1. Bjerre, B., Gosta, E., Folke, L., et al.: Conization as only treatment of carcinoma in situ of the uterine cervix. *Am. J. Obstet. Gynecol.* **125:**143–152, 1976.
2. Claman, A.D., and Lee, N.: Factors that relate to complications of cone biopsy. *Am. J. Obstet. Gynecol.* **120:**124–128, 1974.
3. Ortiz, R., and Newton, M.: Colposcopy in the management of abnormal cervical smears in pregnancy. *Am. J. Obstet. Gynecol.* **109:**46–49, 1971.
4. Rubio, C.A., and Thomassen, P.: A critical evaluation of the Schiller test in patients before conization. *Am. J. Obstet. Gynecol.* **125:**96–99, 1976.
5. Rubio, C.A., Thomassen, P., and Kock, Y.: Influence of the size of cone specimens on postoperative hemorrhage. *Am. J. Obstet. Gynecol.* **122:**939–944, 1975.
6. Rutledge, F., and Ibanez, M.L.: Use of the cryostat in gynecologic surgery. *Am. J. Obstet. Gynecol.* **83:**1208–1213, 1962.

7. Selim, M.A., So-Bosita, J.L., Blair, O.M., et al.: Cervical biopsy versus conization. *Obstet. Gynecol.* **41:**177–182, 1973.
8. van Nagell, J.R., Parker, J.C., Hicks, L.P., et al.: Diagnostic and therapeutic efficacy of cervical conization. *Am. J. Obstet. Gynecol.* **124:**134–139, 1976.
9. VillaSanta, U.: Hemostatic "Cerclage" after knife conization of the cervix. *Obstet. Gynecol.* **42:**299–301, 1973.

Vaginal Hysterectomy

Vaginal hysterectomy was a common procedure before the turn of the century, at which time abdominal surgery became safer due to improved anesthetic techniques, blood transfusions, and antibiotics. Dr. N. Sproat Heaney of Chicago repopularized the use of vaginal hysterectomy as well as instruments for vaginal surgery.[15] The use of the vaginal hysterectomy procedure gradually increased and it is a common gynecologic procedure today. The proportion of hysterectomies performed vaginally varies with the personal choice and training of the surgeon; however, in general, 48% to 70% of hysterectomies are performed vaginally.[4,16]

Preoperative Evaluation

The indications for vaginal hysterectomy are pelvic relaxation, metromenorrhagia, leiomyoma uteri, carcinoma in situ, sterilization, dysmenorrhea, atypical adenomatous hyperplasia, and, though rare, adenomyosis, chronic cervicitis with discharge not responding to cryosurgery, and cervical stricture requiring dilatation. Occasionally adenocarcinoma of the endometrium is given as an indication for vaginal hysterectomy; however, the author prefers to explore the patient and remove the ovaries, which may not always be done through the vaginal route.

Pelvic Relaxation

Pelvic relaxation accounts for 40% of vaginal hysterectomies.[14] Vaginal hysterectomy combined with pelvic floor repair is the procedure of choice for uterine prolapse, enterocele, and cystocele. The surgeon must be aware that the addition of pelvic floor repair to vaginal hysterectomy in the young woman produces significant morbidity.

Metromenorrhagia

Metromenorrhagia accounts for 27% of vaginal hysterectomies.[14] Place these patients on oral iron therapy when seen preoperatively as the patient often has diminished body iron stores as well as anemia, and transfusions may be avoided by increasing the patient's hemoglobin preoperatively. Examine the uterine cavity and cervix for malignant disease preoperatively in patients with abnormal uterine bleeding. A negative cytological examination with a normal appearing cervix and a sampling of the endometrial and endocervical cavities by suction device or endometrial biopsy are adequate measures preoperatively. If instruments cannot be passed into the uterine cavity preoperatively, curettage at the time of surgery is indicated and any suspicious tissues are sent for frozen section. Any patient who has an abnormal appearing cervix requires a cervical biopsy.

Leiomyoma Uteri

The use of vaginal hysterectomy in the treatment of uterine leiomyoma varies greatly in the literature depending upon the choice of the individual gynecologic surgeon. Pratt and Gunnlaugsson have shown that morcellation may be accomplished with essentially the same blood loss but with a 9% increase in morbidity and minor complications.[15] The author feels that it is unnecessary to extend indications for vaginal procedures to include the removal of large pelvic masses. The route and incision which provides the best exposure will ultimately provide the best result. An abdominal incision gives superior exposure for uteri larger than 10 weeks in size. It is axiomatic that a morcellation procedure cannot be performed in any patient in whom the uterine cavity has not been carefully sampled and no possibility of intrauterine malignancy exists.

Carcinoma in Situ

Carcinoma in situ is treated by vaginal hysterectomy if the patient has completed her family. The lack of correlation of margins of in situ carcinoma and Schiller's stain is discussed in Chapter 4. The inaccuracy of Schiller's stain makes careful colposcopic mapping of the lesion and study of the upper vaginal mucosa essential prior to surgical removal. Any carcinoma in situ extending from the cervix onto the vagina is carefully marked with a marking pencil or outlined with a knife and excised at the time of vaginal hysterectomy by turning the cuff in. Fair sized margins of carcinoma in situ extending off the cervix may be excised in this fashion, producing very little defect in the upper vagina. No special resection or radical procedure is necessary in the treatment of carcinoma in situ and simple vaginal hysterectomy will suffice.

Sterilization

Vaginal hysterectomy is a recommended procedure in the young woman who has completed her family. Atkinson and Chappell reported good results in a series of patients who had vaginal hysterectomy for that purpose.[1] The patient may have an intrauterine device in place. Although Atkinson and Chappell observed no significant increase in morbidity in patients with an intrauterine device in place at the time of surgery,[1] the author recommends removal of the intrauterine device 2 weeks prior to surgery, as discussed in Preoperative Preparation.

Dysmenorrhea

Dysmenorrhea without desired potential childbearing capacity is a justifiable indication for vaginal hysterectomy. The absence of uterine descensus sometimes seen in patients who have a long history of dysmenorrhea is not a contraindication. Careful preoperative psychological evaluation is important. Patients with emotional problems and psychogenic dysmenorrhea do not benefit from surgery and will center their complaints in another gynecologic area or in a postoperative problem with resultant unhappy patient and surgeon.

Atypical Adenomatous Hyperplasia

This condition is easily treated with vaginal hysterectomy. There should be no confusion as to the possibility of adenocarcinoma being present. If there is any doubt, abdominal hysterectomy is the procedure of choice to allow for abdominal exploration.

Obesity

Obesity as an indication for vaginal rather than abdominal removal of the uterus has been carefully studied by Pitkin.[13] He reported a series of obese patients who did not have any additional risks in vaginal hysterectomy as compared to an associated nonobese series. The limiting factor in vaginal hysterectomy is of course not the soft tissues but rather the bony structure. Patients who have a wide pubic arch will have excellent exposure in vaginal surgery; however, if the patient has a very narrow subpubic arch, exposure may be limited and often the abdominal route is a better choice in these patients.

Contraindications

Coulam and Pratt have studied the effect of previous pelvic surgery in 621 patients who underwent vaginal hysterectomy.[5] There was no significant difference in morbidity, complications, time of hospitalization, frequency of morcellation, transfusion rate, or postoperative hemoglobin drop in this group of patients when compared with a group of 942 patients who had no prior pelvic surgical procedures. They concluded that choice of vaginal route depends on the characteristics of the pelvis and not on the prior surgical procedure. They found that if the uterus was mobile and vaginal supporting structures relaxed, vaginal hysterectomy was quite satisfactory.

If the patient has had radiation therapy for some unrelated disease process, vaginal surgery and pelvic floor repair are approached with great caution and in general are not performed.

If there is any confusion as to uterine mobility then the abdominal route is preferred, allowing the surgeon careful direct visualization in uterine removal.

Preoperative Preparation

If the patient has an intrauterine device in place, the surgeon should remove it 2 weeks prior to surgery and place the patient on aerobic and anaerobic spectrum antibiotics. Recent studies indicate that intrauterine device users have a three- to fivefold increased risk of pelvic inflammatory disease over nonusers.[11] This evidence confirms the need for prophylactic treatment of the patient for pelvic inflammatory disease prior to vaginal hysterectomy.

Preparation of the vagina prior to vaginal hysterectomy has been shown to be quite effective in reducing bacterial flora in the vagina.[12] The endocervix, however, frequently remains culture positive, and short-term prophylactic antibiotics such as the cephalosporins given prior to and at the time of surgery markedly decrease postoperative morbidity. There has been no increase in infections caused by resistant organisms nor does a prophylactic course of antibiotics predispose the patient to more severe or delayed infections.[10] Mayer and Gordon reported a decrease in febrile morbidity in vaginal hysterectomy patients from 43% to 8% with the prophylactic use of antibiotics.[9] Ledger et al. have shown that there is little difference in short-term and long-term antibiotic therapy,[8] but an essential finding in all studies is that the maximum benefit is obtained if the patient has an adequate level of antibiotics in her blood stream at the time the incision is made.

Operative Technique

The position of the patient is critical for additional exposure. The patient must be well down on the operating table with the buttocks protruding from the edge of the table. The surgeon must personally assure himself of this position prior to preparation of the patient. The patient's legs must be well up from the field. There are numerous types of stirrups, both with the leg directly extended and with the leg in an obstetric-type stirrup or suspended with straps. Regardless of the stirrup used, it is essential to have adequate padding and no pressure points to avoid injury to the peroneal nerve and other neurological injuries.

Occasionally one will have a patient in whom vaginal exposure is difficult. In this instance the patient may be placed in a Tredelenburg position or a lateral tilt position. A midline episiotomy may be used to increase exposure. Where additional manipulation is needed in the upper vagina, a large Schuchardt incision is performed in benign disease as well as for Schauta hysterectomy. Although significant exposure will be gained with this technique, the surgeon should be aware of the discomfort of a large Schuchardt incision and weigh this against the option of performing an abdominal hysterectomy and thus having the exposure needed.

The first assistant stands to the right of the surgeon if the surgeon is right-handed and the second assistant stands to the left. The scrub nurse will most conveniently pass instruments between the surgeon and the first assistant. Some surgeons prefer a small table affixed to the operating table for placement of instruments; the author finds this cumbersome. The second assistant can palm the suture scissors and the remainder of the instruments may be passed. The use of a large one-piece drape improves the draping and prevents large gaps. The author uses a half-sheet clipped to his lap and allows it to fall over his knees as well as a skin towel clipped to his back.

The room is equipped with a dual light source with a switch for varying intensities and a weighted speculum with suction and light source is useful.

Surgical instruments necessary for the vaginal hysterectomy include the following: narrow Deaver retractors, the longer length being particularly useful when removing tubes and ovaries; Adson-Brown forceps in medium and long lengths; and fine, long Metzenbaum scissors. Sharp strong scissors may be available, but most of the lower ligamentous structures can be cut with a knife. The author uses vaginal hysterectomy clamps of his own design (Masterson clamp) to minimize the tissue trauma while maintaining traction on the vascular structures to tie ligatures.

Many techniques for vaginal hysterectomy have been described varying from using no clamp to a triple-clamp technique. It is emphasized that the surgeon should strive for minimal trauma, maximal exposure, and the least amount of devitalized tissue remaining with the smallest possible amount of suture material left in the wound.

The operation is illustrated in Figures 5.1 through 5.11.

The use of T-tube drains and suction in vaginal hysterectomy has recently been proposed. Careful attention to minimizing dead tissue and the

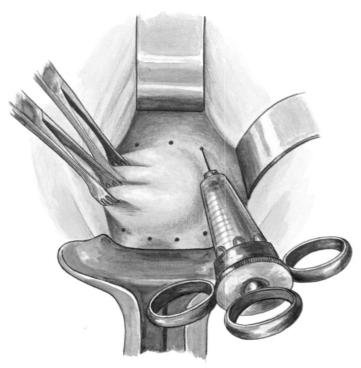

FIGURE 5.1. Empty the patient's bladder with a catheter. Insert a weighted speculum into the vagina with as long a blade as will stay fully in the vault. Place two Deaver retractors laterally in the vagina and two thyroid clamps well into the anterior and posterior lips of the cervix. The surgeon holds both of these in his left hand and injects a dilute solution of Neo-Synephrine in the approximate line of incision about the cervix. Liberally infiltrate the vaginal epithelium posteriorly to minimize vaginal bleeding.

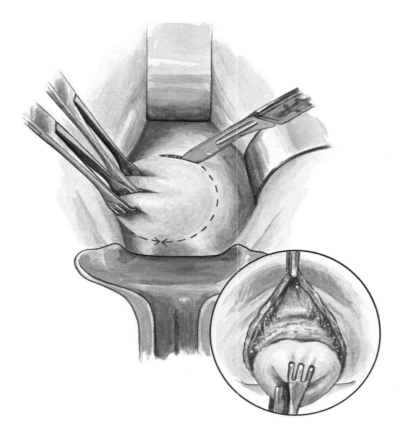

FIGURE 5.2. Using lateral traction, make a circumferential incision in the vaginal epithelium about the cervix. This incision is the crux of vaginal hysterectomy. It is made just as the vaginal epithelium sweeps upward from the cervix and deeply into the tissues beneath the vaginal epithelium but does not include the uterine muscle. A slight increase in resistance is felt as the knife blade enters the muscularis. To determine the lower limits of the bladder, pass a malleable sound, palpating it through the bladder wall. Mobilizing the uterus upward will indicate the posterior cul-de-sac margins and lateral traction will often show a bulge in the vagina where the cardinal ligaments sweep downward. Place strong upward traction on the bladder with Adson-Brown thumb forceps either singly or in tandem to allow introduction into the plane between the bladder and uterus. If the vaginal incision is too deep, one will dissect into myometrium with significant bleeding. If the incision is too shallow, one can dissect into the bladder muscle. The space is marked with some strands of connective and areolar tissue as one approaches the most inferior portion of the anterior cul-de-sac.

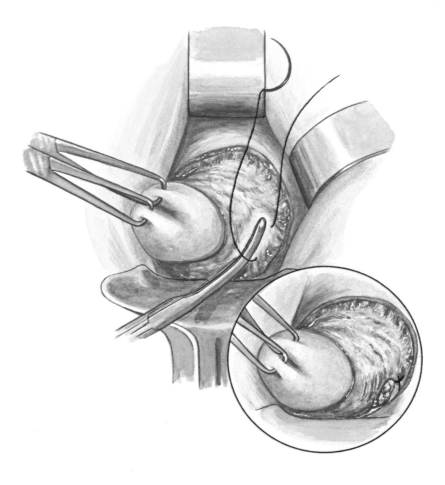

FIGURE 5.3. Strong traction is applied on the uterus and a Masterson clamp is placed on the lowermost portions of the supports of the uterus, namely the utero-sacral ligaments. The clamp is cut free with a knife and an absorbable suture of 2-0 Vicryl or chromic catgut is placed. Inset: Place a simple tie with three knots and cut the stitch near the knot. There is no reason to leave the ends of these sutures long, as each bit of suture left promotes infection in this area. The uterosacral ligament on the other side is handled in a similar fashion.

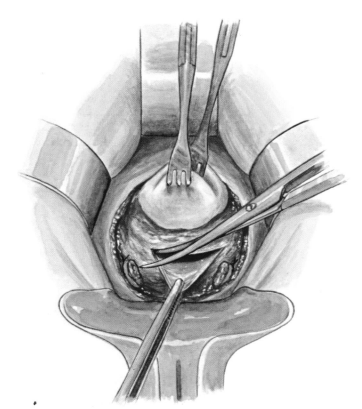

FIGURE 5.4. While the cul-de-sac may be entered in some patients before any ligamentous structures are ligated, frequently it is more easily visualized after the uterosacral ligaments are tied. The uterus is pulled upward and the posterior cul-de-sac is visualized and entered. If there is any question as to whether or not this is truely the cul-de-sac, palpation will confirm that it is peritoneum. It is entered more safely in the midline and is cut to either margin to increase exposure. While it is possible to extend the blade of the weighted speculum into the posterior cul-de-sac, this frequently puts lateral tension on the margins of the cul-de-sac and decreases exposure.

52

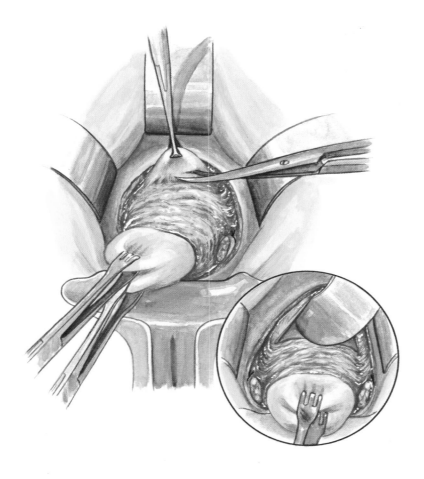

FIGURE 5.5.   If difficulty is encountered in isolating the anterior cul-de-sac, place a finger anterior to the uterus. Using the finger as a guide, dissect the bladder upward to avoid entering the bladder, which may be adherent from prior cesarean section or other surgery. The anterior cul-de-sac is best visualized by pulling up with Adson-Brown thumb forceps and entering in the midline. Inset: Insert a Deaver retractor between the bladder and uterus.

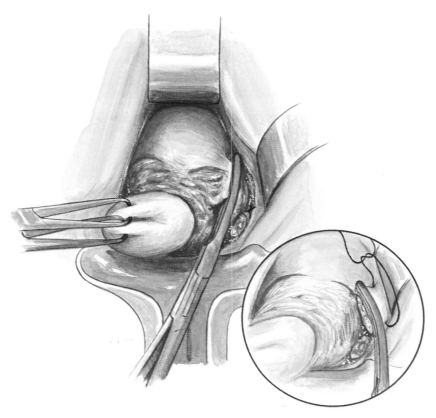

FIGURE 5.6.   Strong downward traction is applied on the uterus and the remaining part of the cardinal ligaments are singly clamped and cut with a knife. Inset: Tie the ligaments with 2-0 Vicryl or chromic catgut. Occasionally a difficult tie may require a large suture, in which case use 0 chromic. Single ties are adequate for these pedicles. Ties are carefully placed with the fingers in direct line, with tension being placed on the knot between the pads of the two index fingers. No sutures are tagged and the uterine arteries are also singly ligated.

53

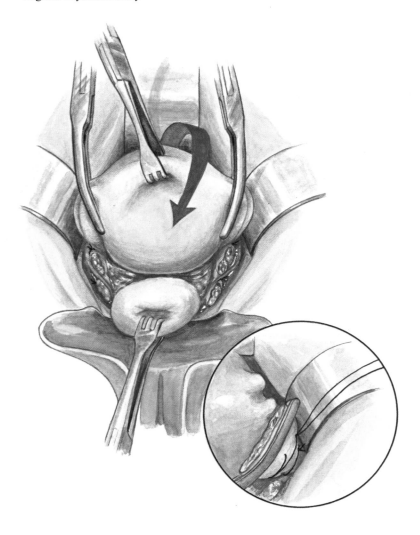

FIGURE 5.7. After ligating the uterosacrals, cardinal, and uterine arteries, place a thyroid clamp in the midline and pull the uterus downward. Inset: Place Masterson clamps laterally on the ovarian vessels and cut and doubly ligate them. The ovarian artery, which lies in the substance of the ovarian venous plexus, tends to retract and produce hematomas, and thus must be securely tied. The initial ligature is a single tie around the pedicle. Next a transfixation suture going through the middle of the pedicle is singly tied and then passed around the entire pedicle. The distal tie is held while the other is cut short.

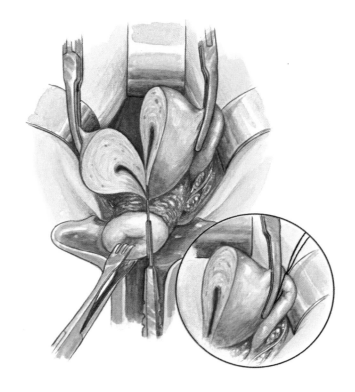

FIGURE 5.8. If visualization is difficult due to uterine size or a narrow arch, additional exposure can be obtained by dividing the uterus in the midline. No morcellation or division of the uterus is permissible unless the uterine malignancy has been ruled out by uterine sampling. Place the index and middle fingers behind the uterus, incise in the groove between the fingers, and divide the uterus in the midline, placing a thyroid clamp on each side of the cervix. Inset: By pulling one-half of the uterus into the operative site, good exposure is obtained for lateral placement of Masterson clamps on the tubovarian junctions. Each half of the uterus is then removed in this way with a significant increase in exposure.

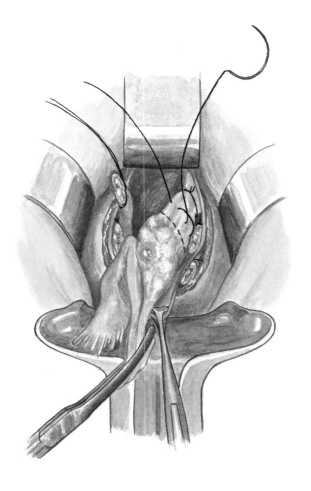

FIGURE 5.9. If the ovaries are to be removed, this is usually performed following uterine removal. Pull the utero-ovarian pedicle down, freeing up any adhesions with scissors. With good visualization, a free tie is placed about the ovarian vessels, followed by a transfixation suture. The ovaries are then cut while the transfixation suture is held. The same procedure is performed on the other side, completing ovarian removal. If good exposure is not obtained and ovarian removal is mandatory, then an abdominal incision is made. In this, as in other procedures, one does not compromise exposure.

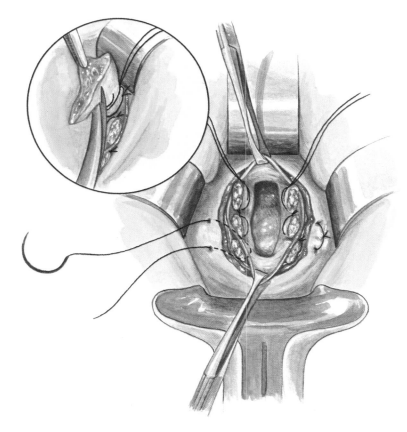

FIGURE 5.10. After any devitalized tissue is cut from the pedicles (inset), the uterine supports are sutured into the angles of the vagina with a simple stitch that encompasses all layers of the vaginal epithelium: it takes a full bite through the cardinal ligaments, comes back through the uterosacral ligament, and goes out again through the full thickness of the vagina. This will attach these structures firmly to the vaginal wall and produce good support. Vaginal vault prolapse is rare after the vault has been suspended in this fashion. It is important that these tissues be approximated and not strangulated so that they will heal, not necrose. The same procedure is performed on the opposite side.

55

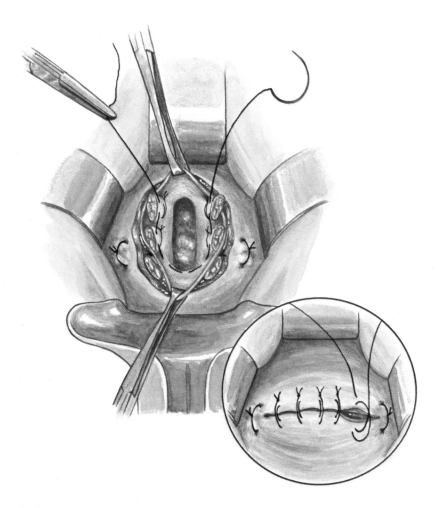

FIGURE 5.11. To close the peritoneal cavity, place a suture through the peritoneum from above and attach a small hemostat. Bring the suture down distal to the vascular ties and through the cardinal ligaments. If there is any excess peritoneum posteriorly, bring the suture well up on the peritoneum and excise the excess to prevent any tendency toward enterocele. Any additional reefing that is necessary may be done at this time by means of simple stitches imbricating the posterior cul-de-sac. Bring the suture up the opposite side and through the peritoneum again. Tying this down will produce an approximation of the peritoneum closing the peritoneal cavity. Inset: Close the vaginal vault with 3-0 Vicryl or chromic suture using a large round needle. Place the stitch deeply through all layers, taking care not to enter the bladder anteriorly. Bring the stitch back and direct it through the margins of the vaginal epithelium and then approximate it. This stitch will both obliterate the underlying dead space and produce an anatomical approximation of the vaginal epithelium, greatly decreasing the instance of postoperative granulations. It is important not to include the ovaries in the vaginal closure, and no attempt is made to pull the tubes in the closure; this would increase the incidence of tubal epithelial prolapse, which would require treatment in the postoperative period. The closure of the vagina is an anatomic closure. <u>Drains are not necessary</u>. The wound is usually dry prior to closure and no pack is required. In the absence of any associated repair, a catheter is not used.

use of fine suture material with a relatively dry pelvis at the time of closure is felt to be more satisfactory than the placement of a drain through a potentially infected wound, and its use is not recommended.

Postoperative Management and Complications

If vaginal hysterectomy without repair is performed, the patient is up the next day with regular diet as tolerated. Early ambulation is encouraged, as the patient has no abdominal wound. The patient is instructed to abstain from intercourse for 6 weeks and returns to the clinic in 2 to 6 weeks.

Byrd et al. have studied the use of long-term estrogen support after hysterectomy in 1,016 cases with 100% follow-up.[2] They noted that the general impact of long-term estrogen therapy following hysterectomy is favorable. While there is much controversy about estrogen usage, the absence of the uterus obviates its greatest single complication.

While ward service series are often reported with the comment that if the procedures were performed by more experienced surgeons the complication would be quite low, that is not necessarily the case. Harris reported 491 vaginal hysterectomies performed on private cases by Board Certified gynecologists.[6] The incidence of febrile morbidity was 37.8%; 75 patients received prophylactic antibiotics, and of these patients 21.4% had febrile morbidity. The average length of hospital stay was 11 days.

Copenhaver, in his excellent study of vaginal hysterectomy, reported febrile morbidity in 39% of patients, cystitis in 29%, excessive vaginal bleeding in 3%, and severe urinary retention and pelvic cellulitis in 2%; severe pyelonephritis, pelvic hematomas, thrombophlebitis, and pelvic abscess occurred in a smaller number.[3]

Bleeding

The principal complication of vaginal hysterectomy is bleeding. The average blood loss from vaginal hysterectomy with infiltration of a pressor agent is 305 ml with a range of 25 to 1,181 ml. When no pressor agents are used, the average operative blood loss is 755 ml. Operative transfusion is required in 35% of patients with infiltration and 80% of patients without infiltration. When pelvic repair is added to vaginal hysterectomy, 189 ml of additional blood loss is noted. When infiltrates are not used, an average of 305 ml is lost with associated repair.[7] Blood loss of this magnitude must be carefully monitored as it may approach 30% of the total blood volume of a small woman. Harris reports a 10.8% rate of hypovolemic shock in patients undergoing vaginal hysterectomy, with its attendant problems of increased infection rates and poor wound healing.[6]

To help reduce the blood loss, the author recommends the use of pressor agents such as a dilute solution of Neo-Synephrine, 1:200,000 not exceeding 30 ml or 1:400,000 if 60 ml of solution is used.

The sobering statistics of blood loss associated with vaginal hysterectomy makes meticulous attention to technique essential, which includes precise identification of vessels with careful isolation and ligature, careful closure of the vaginal cuff, and precise placement of closure sutures so they do not enter behind a hemostatic stitch, producing hematoma proximal to the tie.

A patient who has had a vaginal hysterectomy and has unusual post-

57

operative pain should be suspected of having concealed bleeding even though her initial hemoglobin level, blood pressure, and pulse may not indicate this. Any fall in blood pressure in association with severe abdominal pain is an indication that the patient should be re-explored. Prompt laparotomy is far preferable to the patient developing a large pelvic hematoma, sepsis, and multiple pelvic and abdominal abscesses with a prolonged postoperative recovery phase. There is approximately one laparotomy performed for postoperative bleeding for every 400 vaginal hysterectomies. The patient should be well aware that laparotomy is a realistic risk when vaginal hysterectomy is performed.[14]

Bladder Injuries

In Copenhaver's study, 1% of patients had bladder injuries from anterior colpotomy.[3] This injury is avoided through careful dissection with strong downward traction and the lifting upward of the bladder with thumb forceps. Often fluid may be present in the anterior cul-de-sac, producing some concern in the surgeon. If there is any confusion, a sound is placed in the bladder and the floor of the bladder is checked. If the bladder has been entered, close as described in Chapter 22.

Confining dissection upward to the midportion of the bladder obviates injury in an area where the ureter would be present, and ureteral injury is not of concern. If the surgeon feels there is any question of injury he should cystoscope the patient at the end of the operation following injection of intravenous indigo carmine and observe the dye from both ureters. The repair may also be checked at that time. Detection of the bladder injury and its repair will almost always result in satisfactory healing.

If the bladder is entered, place a Foley catheter in the patient for 7 days. Among 5,078 cases of vaginal hysterectomy at the Presbyterian Hospital in Chicago, only 7 vesicovaginal fistulas were recorded.[3]

Ureteral Injuries

Ureteral injuries are rare. In a review of 11,279 vaginal hysterectomies, only 4 ureteral injuries were noted by Copenhaver.[3] If one remains close to the body of the uterus and uses strong downward traction and lateral tension with well-placed narrowed Deaver retractors, ureteral injury is rare indeed. Should the uterine artery or vein bleed lateral to the uterus, the use of fine Adson artery forceps to isolate this bleeder and tying with a fine 3-0 or 4-0 ligature will be safe. The placing of a large clamp with suture ligature of large pedicles of tissue laterally is hazardous.

Rectal Injury

Rectal injuries are usually associated with pelvic inflammatory disease or endometriosis and some pelvic fixation. Such uteri are removed abdominally, where better exposure can be obtained. If one is unable to clearly enter the posterior cul-de-sac, then the vaginal route is abandoned. Early entrance into both the anterior and posterior cul-de-sac with well-placed retractors produces a smooth, safe, and relatively bloodless vaginal hysterectomy. The use of excessive traction in a fixed uterus and the inability to enter these two areas make vaginal hysterectomy unsafe and the procedure should be promptly abandoned.

Mortality

In a review of 13,441 vaginal hysterectomies by various authors, the incidence of death was 0.13%.[3] Those series of vaginal hysterectomies usually contained at least 1 death, often from embolic phenomena or associated vascular abnormalities; while there may have been no error in surgical technique, the patient did die during the postoperative course of her vaginal hysterectomy. Although the procedure may be accomplished with technical ease, associated death in the postoperative period makes the procedure, even in the most skilled hands, one that must be undertaken with the full realization that the patient may die as a result of operation.

References

1. Atkinson, S.M., and Chappell, S.M.: Sterilization by vaginal hysterectomy. *Obstet. Gynecol.* **39:**759–766, 1972.
2. Byrd, B.F., Burch, J.C., and Vaughn, W.K.: The impact of long term estrogen support after hysterectomy: A report of 1016 cases. *Ann. Surg.* **185:**574–580, 1977.
3. Copenhaver, E.H.: Vaginal hysterectomy: An analysis of indications and complications among 1000 operations. *Am. J. Obstet. Gynecol.* **84:**123–128, 1962.
4. Copenhaver, E.H.: Hysterectomy: Vaginal versus abdominal. *Surg. Clin. North Am.* **45:**751–763, 1965.
5. Coulam, C.B., and Pratt, J.H.: Vaginal hysterectomy: Is previous pelvic operation a contraindication? *Am. J. Obstet. Gynecol.* **116:**252–260, 1973.
6. Harris, B.A.: Vaginal hysterectomy in a community hospital. *N.Y. State J. Med.* **76:**1304–1307, 1976.
7. Lazar, M.R.: Blood loss prevention in vaginal surgery. *Surg. Clin. North Am.* **39:**1671–1677, 1959.
8. Ledger, W.J., Gee, C., and Lewis W.P.: Guidelines for antibiotic prophylaxis in gynecology. *Am. J. Obstet. Gynecol.* **121:**1038–1045, 1975.
9. Mayer, W., and Gordon, M.: Prophylactic antibiotics: Use in hysterectomy. *N.Y. State J. Med.* **76:**2144–2147, 1976.
10. Ohm, M.J., and Galask, R.P.: The effect of antibiotic prophylaxis on patients undergoing vaginal operations: The effect on morbidity. *Am. J. Obstet. Gynecol.* **123:**590–596, 1975.
11. Ory, H.W.: A review of the association between intrauterine devices and acute pelvic inflammatory disease. *J. Reprod. Med.* **20:**200–204, 1978.
12. Osborne, N.G., and Wright, R.C.: Effect of preoperative scrub on the bacterial flora of the endocervix and vagina. *Obstet. Gynecol.* **50:**148–150, 1977.
13. Pitkin, R.M.: Vaginal hysterectomy in obese women. *Obstet. Gynecol.* **49:**567–569, 1977.
14. Pratt, J.H.: Common complications of vaginal hysterectomy: Thoughts regarding their prevention and management. *Clin. Obstet. Gynecol.* **19:**645–659, 1976.
15. Pratt, J.H., and Gunnlaugsson, G.H.: Vaginal hysterectomy by morcellation. *Mayo Clin. Proc.* **45:**374–387, 1976.
16. Tasche, L.W.: 1700 vaginal hysterectomies. *Minn. Med.* **51:**1705–1711, 1968.

6 Pelvic Relaxation and Associated Conditions: Enterocele Repair

Historically, treatment of pelvic relaxation has varied from astringents, silver nitrate, tampons of okum and wool, pelvic massage, pessaries, red hot iron bars, or sulfuric acid, hanging by the heels to cervical amputation. Surgical attempts in the late 19th and early 20th century have included hysterectomy, round ligament uterine suspension, and Manchester and Watkins interposition operations. The LaForte operation is included in this group, although it too has generally been discarded.[10]

Enterocele, rectocele, cystocele, vaginal vault prolapse, and uterine prolapse will be presented as separate entities. In practice, one rarely sees these conditions as isolated occurrences, but rather in varying degrees or in combination with one another (Figures 6.1 through 6.3).

Pelvic relaxation has been associated with numerous etiologic factors. Holland reviewed the etiologic factors in genital prolapse and determined that the effect of childbirth was the most significant independent factor. Frequency of genital prolapse increases only slightly with rising parity, being most common in the para 2 to 3.[3] Age is an additional factor. Folsome et al. studied 680 females, 611 of whom were over 60 years of age.[1] They found rectoceles in 45%, cystoceles in 25%, uterine prolapse in 11%, and enterocele in 1 patient. Only 10% of the patients had symptoms referable to these findings.

Almost any condition associated with increasing intra-abdominal pressure will increase the incidence of genital prolapse. This includes chronic obstructive pulmonary disease with cough, chronic constipation requiring repeated Valsalva maneuver, obesity, visceroptosis, and large abdominal or pelvic tumors. Poor nutritional status has also been observed in this group of patients.

Preoperative Evaluation

The diagnosis of enterocele is considered when the patient presents with a bulge in the posterovaginal wall and complains of a feeling of pelvic heaviness, which is often accentuated by straining. Other symptoms include low back pain and, occasionally, with a large enterocele, some nausea with straining, protrusion, and constipation.

60

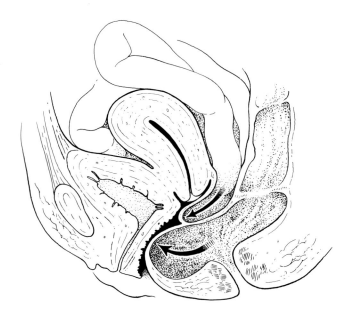

FIGURE 6.1.   An enterocele, which may or may not contain small bowel, may coexist with rectocele or exist independently. To identify an enterocele, place the third finger in the rectum and the index finger in the vagina and feel the enterocele between the two fingers.

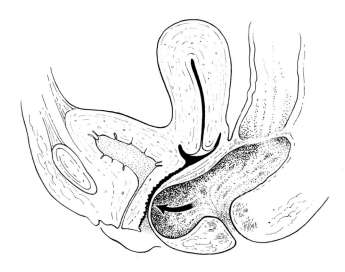

FIGURE 6.2.   With the patient straining downward, the rectocele is observed as a bulging from the posterior aspect into the vagina. The central portion of the rectocele may be quite thin and difficult to outline.

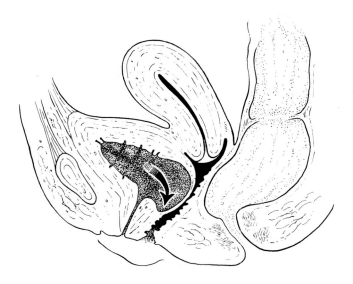

FIGURE 6.3.   The presence of a cystocele may initially be noted only when the patient is straining. As the supports of the bladder weaken, the downward bulge will increase. As the bladder moves downward, the urethrovesicovaginal angle increases, continuing continence; stress incontinence is therefore unusual with large cystoceles. Suburethral cysts and urethral diverticula, if large, may occasionally be confused with cystoceles but their diagnosis becomes apparent on closer inspection.

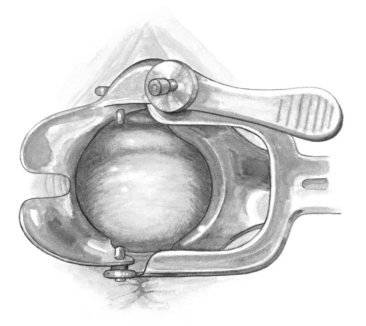

FIGURE 6.4. To differentiate enterocele and rectocele place a vaginal speculum transversely in the introitus. When opened, a secondary bulge will be seen below the cervix and between any rectocele present. Place the index finger in the introitus and identify the rectum; then, on removing the speculum, palpate the sac between the index and middle fingers. A small bowel series obtained with lateral films will show the bowel descending into the enterocele sac when a diagnostic problem arises.

Rectovaginal examination may reveal a thickening of the rectovaginal septum that varies with straining; the bowel may sometimes be palpated between the two fingers (Figure 6.4).

While there are numerous classifications of enteroceles, the classification used here is based on their relationship to other pelvic structures at the time the procedure is performed.

Operative Technique

Congenital Enterocele Repair

This particular type of enterocele may occur in the nulliparous patient, as did the first case reported by Marion in 1909.[11] The etiology of this interesting defect, which may occur without other observed abnormalities, is explained by the anatomic studies of Milley and Nichols.[6] These authors studied 143 anatomic specimens in their investigation of the existence of rectovaginal septum in the human female. They demonstrated that a definite rectovaginal septum exists in the human female and is well formed by the 14th fetal week. It consists of a vertical sheet of dense connective tissue that is translucent in the fresh state and parallels the sacral curvature. It also fuses posterolaterally with the parietal endopelvic fascia and extends inferiorly from the rectouterine perineal pouch to the peritoneal body. This structure is usually adherent to the posterior aspect of the vaginal connective tissue capsule. A bluish character to this septum was noted. Failure of fusion of this structure and its persistent connection to the rectal uterine pouch allows descent of small bowel into this cavity. Repair of this defect follows the basic principles of hernia repair: careful isolation of the sac, excision of the sac with high ligation of the neck of the defect, and its fixation to stronger surrounding tissues with obliteration of the prior space occupied by the hernia. Good results should be expected in this isolated defect where the remainder of the pelvic supporting structures have normal strength (Figures 6.5 through 6.7).

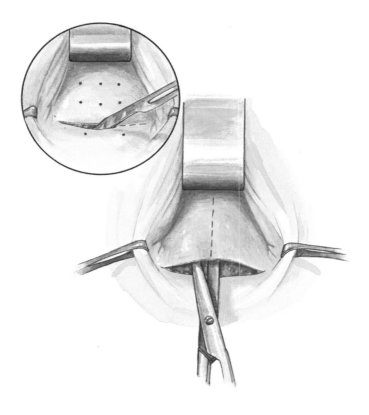

FIGURE 6.5.   Congenital enterocele repair. Infiltrate the vaginal epithelium with a dilute solution of Neo-Synephrine and make a transverse incision; traction is applied laying the field out as flat as possible (inset). Place the Deaver retractor upward and pull the vaginal epithelium anteriorly. Use sharp dissection and incise the vagina in the midline to establish the plane and carry the incision upward.

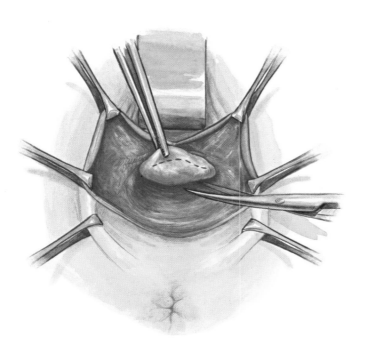

FIGURE 6.6.   The enterocele sac will be seen bulging downward between the rectovaginal septum and the posterior surface of the cervix. If the enterocele alone is to be repaired, dissect it from the surrounding tissues. The sac will contain small bowel or omentum, which may slide out of the sac when the patient is placed in the lithotomy position. Pulling upward with Adson-Brown thumb forceps, enter the sac in the midline and define the extent of the defect.

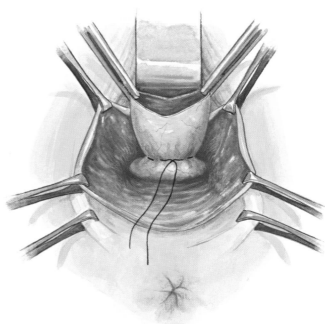

FIGURE 6.7.   Ligate the upper margin of the sac with 3-0 Nurolon or 2-0 chromic suture and place an additional stitch below it, transfixing the margins, and excise the sac. Place sufficient traction on the sac when it is ligated so that the sac will move slightly upward when released.

Prophylactic Repair for Enterocele

This is the most common enterocele repair performed and is associated with other vaginal and abdominal procedures such as vaginal hysterectomy for prolapse or abdominal hysterectomy when a very deep cul-de-sac is noted. With the vaginal approach the McCall uterosacral plication[5] (Figures 6.8 through 6.10) or Waters culdoplasty[11] is performed; abdominal re-

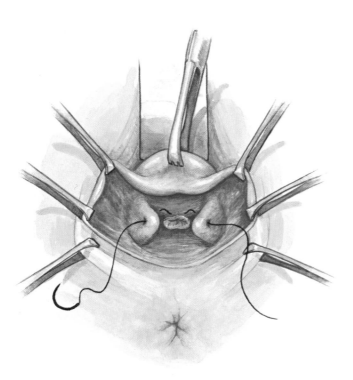

FIGURE 6.8. McCall uterosacral plication for prophylactic repair of enterocele. Identify the uterosacral ligaments by pulling the cervix upward with a tenaculum. Place a suture of 2-0 Vicryl or chromic catgut through the uterosacral ligament taking a lateral bite of peritoneum high in the cul-de-sac and continuing through to the opposite ligament.

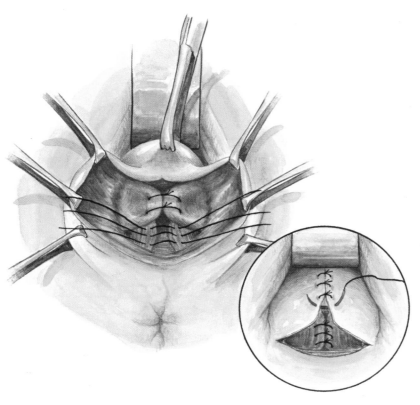

FIGURE 6.9. Imbricate the area below the uterosacral ligaments with interrupted sutures of 2-0 Vicryl or chromic catgut. Inset: Close the vagina with interrupted absorbable sutures.

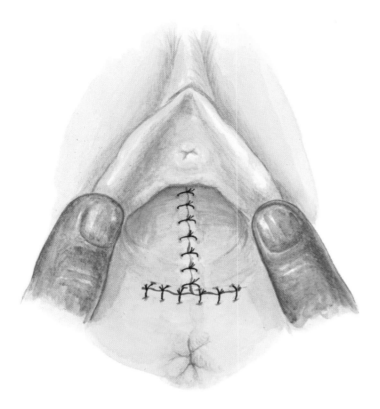

FIGURE 6.10.   Continue closure of the skin incision by approximating the vaginal epithlium. Be careful to avoid introital stricture. Close the skin with interrupted 3-0 nylon sutures or a subcuticular 3-0 absorbable suture.

pair is performed as in the Moschcowitz procedure[7] (Figure 6.11). All these procedures consist of reducing the area available for a bowel prolapse and strengthening the defect with available endopelvic fascia. Pratt[9] noted that 3% of patients develop enteroceles after vaginal hysterectomy and Hunter et al.,[4] in a review of the literature, found 15 cases of ruptured enterocele following a vaginal operation. In a review of 38 cases of vaginal evisceration, there were 3 deaths,[2] emphasizing the need for prophylactic repair to avoid this serious complication. The author advises including it whenever the anatomy of the cul-de-sac indicates it is worthwhile.

Combined Groups of Procedures

Enterocele exists in association with vaginal wall prolapse, uterine prolapse, and rectocele. The basic principles in this type of procedure, which must be modified when enterocele is associated with the other defects, consist of the excision of the enterocele sac, high ligation of its neck—minimizing the defect for subsequent herniation—and closure of the central defects. It is important to remember that cat gut, Vicryl, and Dexon lose almost all tissue strength by 21 days.[8] Silk likewise deteriorates, and the suture used for permanent repair of these defects should be polypropylene, Dacron, or nylon, which maintain their strength for some time and are not associated with fistula formation. Prolene has the disagreeable tendency to require a large number of knots, whose presence may be palpated in the vagina. Braided nylon such as Nurolon will hold with fewer knots and also involves only a low risk of sinus tract formation.

An important technical point in the surgery of any of these defects in which peritoneum alone is sutured is that good exposure is mandatory. In order to avoid bowel obstruction or fistula formation, be careful not to include small bowel in the peritoneal closure as small bowel and peritoneum resemble each other high in the vaginal repair.

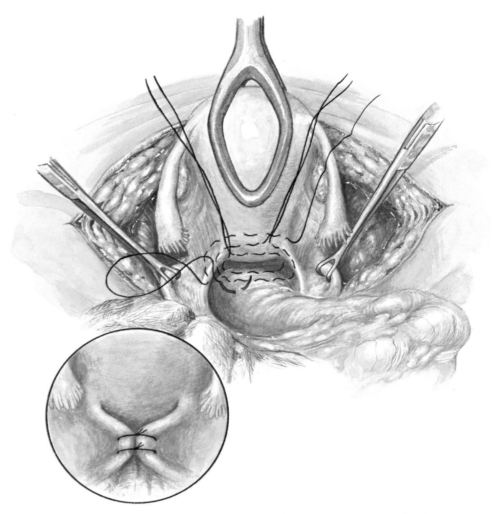

FIGURE 6.11.   The Moschcowitz procedure for prophylactic repair of enterocele is useful in those patients in whom the uterus is to remain in place and a deep cul-de-sac is present. A nonabsorbable suture such as Nurolon is placed in concentric circles beginning at the deepest portions of the cul-de-sac. Use a swedged-on round needle. As the upper portion of the cul-de-sac is approached, sutures should include a bite of the posterior uterus through the uterosacral ligaments, the anterior surface of the colon, and the opposite uterosacral ligament; tie the sutures in the midline. The ureters lie lateral to the uterosacral ligaments and must be carefully identified. A Babcock clamp is placed loosely about the ureters for additional safety. Inset: If the uterosacral ligaments are very mobile, bring them to the center of the midline to strengthen the repair.

Postoperative Management and Results

Postoperatively, patients are placed on long-term estrogens, particularly if the uterus is removed, to strengthen the endopelvic supportive structures and to produce a more pliable vaginal vault. While some authors[10] suggest that patients remain in bed for 1 week following surgery, the author has the patient out of bed the day after surgery. It makes little sense to keep a patient in bed when studies on hernia repair have clearly shown that the results are no worse with early ambulation.

There are no data in the recent literature comparing the different types of enterocele repair and their results. Note that evaluation of the results in pelvic defects requires at least a 5-year follow-up. Most of the repairs look good in the first 6 months following surgery, but the final success depends upon the ability of the patient to withstand the effects of aging and further pressure upon the operative site.

References

1. Folsome, C.E., Napp, E.E., and Tanz, A.: Pelvic findings in the elderly institutionalized female patient. *J.A.M.A.* **161**:1447–1454, 1956.
2. Fox, W.P.: Vaginal evisceration. *Obstet. Gynecol.* **50**:223–224, 1977.
3. Holland, J.B.: Enterocele and prolapse of the vaginal vault. *Clin. Obstet. Gynecol.* **15**:1145–1154, 1972.
4. Hunter, R.E., Jahadi, M.R., and Chandler, J.P.: Spontaneous rupture of enterocele: Report of a case. *Obstet. Gynecol.* **36**:835–839, 1970.
5. McCall, M.L.: Posterior culdoplasty: Surgical correction of enterocele during vaginal hysterectomy; a preliminary report. *Obstet. Gynecol.* **10**:595–602, 1957.
6. Milley, P.S., and Nichols, D.H.: Correlative investigation of the human rectovaginal septum. *Anat. Record* **163**:443–452, 1969.
7. Moschcowitz, A.V.: The pathogenesis, anatomy, and cure of prolapse of the rectum. *Surg. Gynecol. Obstet.* **15**:7–21, 1912.
8. Peacock, E.E., and Van Winkle, W.: Healing and repair of viscera. In: *Wound Repair.* Philadelphia, Saunders, 1976, ch. 12.
9. Pratt, J.H.: Operative and postoperative difficulties of vaginal hysterectomy. *Obstet. Gynecol.* **21**:221–226, 1963.
10. TeLinde, R.W.: Prolapse of the uterus and allied conditions. *Am. J. Obstet. Gynecol.* **94**:444–463, 1966.
11. Waters, E.G.: Enterocele: Cause, diagnosis, and treatment. *Clin. Obstet. Gynecol.* **4**:186–198, 1961.

7 Repair of Rectocele and Perineum

As a result of the increasing popularity of cosmetic surgery, gynecologists are sought for plastic repair of pelvic relaxation brought on by the aging process. Among the changes brought on are mild changes in perineal muscular tone, minimal degrees of pelvic relaxation, and minor changes in the appearance of the lower genital tract. A majority of the defects are best managed by observation.

Patients also present with specific sexual complaints that are rarely due to isolated changes in the perineum and are generally handled through sexual counseling. If the patient insists on a surgical repair, write a statement in the patient's record indicating that the patient understands that the surgical repair may not correct the sexual complaint.

Severe and symptomatic abnormalities in pelvic visceral support do merit operative intervention. This procedure must be carefully designed for the defect, incorporating existing structures into a new supporting framework.

Anatomy

The condensation of endopelvic fascia extends downward between the vagina and rectum. These tissues thicken laterally and extend upward to be continuous with the uterus and ligaments and lateral to the cardinal ligaments. Take care to avoid dissecting the hemorrhoidal plexus of veins, which may be quite large near the lateral rectum.

Rectoceles are described as high, mid, or low in location, but more frequently a varying combination of these defects is diagnosed. The rectoceles are classified as mild if they extend to the introitus on examination, moderate if they extend out the hymenal ring with straining, and severe if the defect extends through the hymen without straining.[4]

Preoperative Evaluation

A careful and precise clinical study by Gainey clearly documented the effect of childbirth in perineal relaxation and the effect of episiotomy in preventing pelvic defects.[1,2] Note that the defect is related more to the occurrence of childbirth than to the number of deliveries and is not necessarily cumulative in its effect.[5] Relaxed introitus has little effect on rectocele or uterine prolapse, nor does it prevent vault prolapse. Do not repair such defects by perineorrhaphy without a careful and thorough dissection involving repair of the perirectal fascia.[3]

The patient is evaluated in the office by means of a simple rectovaginal examination. The patient should not be anesthetized during the evaluation of perineal relaxation.

To diagnose the presence of associated enterocele and high rectocele, use a narrow speculum placed transversely during the rectovaginal examination. The introitus normally accommodates two fingers, the index and middle fingers, with the patient awake. When the patient contracts the vaginal muscles the fingers should fit snuggly in the introitus; however, an introitus that accommodates three fingers without symptoms needs no repair.

Avoid the plastic repair of nonsymptomatic pelvic relaxation as there is a high incidence of sexual dysfunction after vaginal plastic repairs. Jeffcoate reports that 30% of patients have sexual dysfunction after anterior and posterior colporrhaphy.[3] These procedures are a poor choice when the anatomic defect is minimal and the psychosexual element prominent.

If the patient is menopausal, preoperative oral estrogen (1.25 mg conjugated estrogens) for 6 weeks prior to surgery will increase the vaginal blood supply, the vaginal tone, and the strength of paravaginal supportive structures. If the patient has a combined prolapse with some inflammatory changes, a cream combining topical estrogens and sulfa is applied locally; the patient may mix commercially available preparations half and half.

A barium enema and proctoscopy are necessary to rule out gastrointestinal pathological abnormalities that produce straining at stool. Note that the number of carcinomas of the colon being found in the right colon is increasing and that barium enema is an integral part of evaluation of these patients. The presence of dysfunctional bowel syndrome has been associated with very poor results and may be a relative contraindication to this operation.[5] Patients have both a mechanical and an antibiotic bowel preparation according to Table 19.1 (page 220).

Operative Technique

Basic rectocele repair is illustrated in Figures 7.1 through 7.4. Patients who have a high rectocele repair in association with vaginal hysterectomy will have a continuous suture line from the hysterectomy site incorporating the uterosacral ligaments down to the perineal body. It is important to close any enterocele sac with fixation of the sac to the uterosacral ligament with permanent suture such as braided nylon. If the perirectal fascia is well formed, a second suture line may be used to bring it to the midline (Figure 7.3).

Midrectoceles may require imbrication (Figure 7.3), with the perirectal fascia pulled over the imbrication.

Low rectoceles are usually associated with significant perineal relaxation; close by approaching the rectocele through a transverse incision, inverting the mucosa, and pulling the perirectal fascia medially, including the levator muscles in a separate layer.

Take great care to avoid any rigid transverse scar tissue during perin-

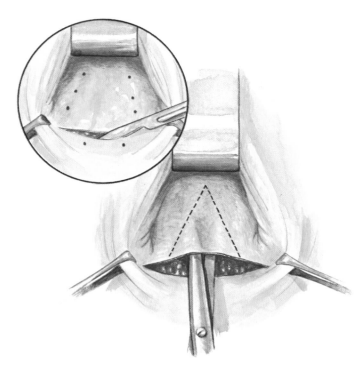

FIGURE 7.1. Inject the introitus and rectovaginal septum with a dilute solution of Neo-Synephrine; make a transverse incision at the introitus and carry it across to the opposite side of the vagina (inset). Do not incise up the vagina if the rectocele is low and the vaginal epithelium mobile. If, however, the vaginal epithelium is quite redundant, make a V-excision of epithelium.

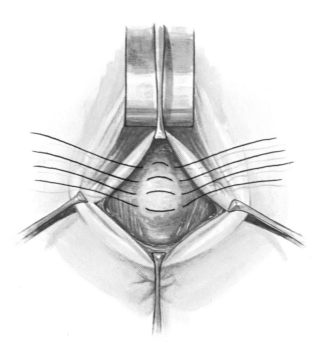

FIGURE 7.2. Dissect the vagina free of the rectum and extend the plane to the perirectal fascia. With a large rectocele the perirectal fascia may be absent in the midline and the lateral perirectal fascia must be approximated for effective repair. The hemorrhoidal veins are more prominent inferiorly and laterally; avoid them when possible. Imbricate the rectum with interrupted sutures of 2-0 or 3-0 absorbable suture. Approximate large portions of perirectal fascia to reinforce the repair.

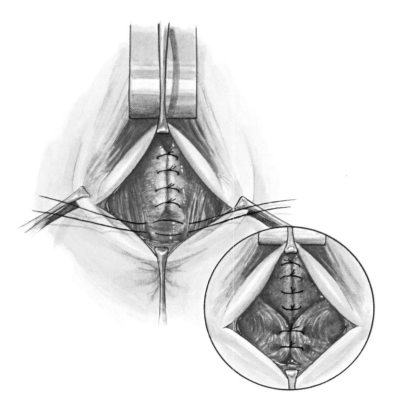

FIGURE 7.3. After reducing the rectocele and bringing the perirectal tissues to the midline, use the levator muscles to strengthen the incision. Pass a suture of 0 chromic catgut on a large general closure needle lateral into the lower portions of the levator muscles, bringing them to the midline. This procedure is reserved for the older patient with a large rectocele as introital stricture may result if one employs too aggressive a mobilization of the levators and their suture in the midline. Close the skin incision by approximating the vaginal epithelium with interrupted 3-0 absorbable suture. Drains and packs are not necessary. A Foley catheter is not necessary in rectocele repair alone.

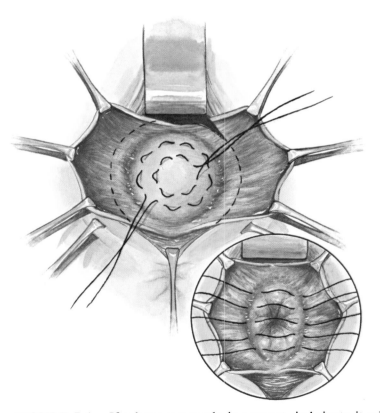

FIGURE 7.4. If a large rectocele is present, imbricate it with concentric rings of 2-0 Vicryl or chromic catgut. After bringing in the large central portion of the rectocele, imbricate the outer margins of the ring with interrupted sutures to include the perirectal fascia. Excise the redundant vaginal epithelium. Take care in the excision of any vaginal epithelium in the young, sexually active patient and avoid any introital stricture through careful planning of the rectocele incision.

71

eorrhaphy. Fashion a vaginal opening that easily admits two fingers. Remember that the patient is asleep, often with muscle relaxants, and has little of her normal perineal tone.

Postoperative Management

If the patient has a simple rectocele repair, vaginal packs and bladder catheters are not necessary. If the patient has associated pelvic repairs, use a vaginal pack for 24 hr and insert a Foley catheter for straight drainage. When the Foley is removed, place the patient on a urinary antiseptic such as sulfisoxazole (Gantrisin).

Owing to the healing curve of bowel fibrous tissue and fascia, rectocele patients require at least 6 weeks postoperatively to regain strength in the rectal area; thus stool softeners are ordered in the immediate postoperative period and are continued for 3 months.

Further postoperative measures include sitz baths and estrogen creams, supplemented with oral estrogens if the patient has an atrophic vaginal mucosa. Intercourse may be resumed in 6 weeks. A long-term change in diet and bowel habits is recommended for the prevention of future rectoceles and defects in the lower genital tract associated with straining.

References

1. Gainey, H.L.: Post-partum observation of pelvic tissue damage. *Am. J. Obstet. Gynecol.* **45:**457–466, 1943.
2. Gainey, H.L.: Postpartum observation of pelvic tissue damage: Further studies. *Am. J. Obstet. Gynecol.* **70:**800–807, 1955.
3. Jeffcoate, T.N.A.: Posterior colpoperineorrhaphy. *Am. J. Obstet. Gynecol.* **77:**490–502, 1959.
4. Porges, R.F.: A practical system of diagnosis and classification of pelvic relaxations. *Surg. Gynecol. Obstet.* **117:**769–773, 1963.
5. Pratt, J.H.: Surgical repair of rectocele and perineal lacerations. *Clin. Obstet. Gynecol.* **15:**1160–1172, 1972.

Anterior Colporraphy

8

Anterior colporraphy is a common operation in gynecologic surgery. While originally employed for stress incontinence alone, retropubic procedures are currently used to correct stress incontinence. In modern gynecologic surgery anterior colporraphy is performed primarily for prolapse of the anterior vaginal wall and secondarily for stress incontinence.

Anatomy

The anterior repair is an operation that utilizes as its plane of dissection the junction between the vaginal smooth muscle and the bladder muscularis. The anterior vaginal wall consists of vaginal mucosa, smooth muscle of the vagina, associated blood vessels, bladder muscularis, and transitional epithelium of the bladder. This plane is an artificial one and is made possible only through the effective use of strong traction on both sides of the dissecting field maintained in a planar fashion.

The anatomic relationships of significance are those of the arteries coursing laterally along the vagina and joining in arcades. The venous plexuses surrounding the bulbocavernosus muscle join near the pelvic floor and are continuous with those of the urethra and the venous plexus of the bladder. As these lie laterally, initial dissection is best conducted in the midline. A larger field is exposed before lateral dissection is performed so that hemostasis can be secured more easily. The precise histologic character of the tissue between the bladder and vagina has been subject to considerable debate. It appears to vary from predominantly smooth muscle in the younger patient to a more fibrous tissue in the elderly. These tissues are quite sensitive to estrogen; therefore, if the patient has atrophic vaginal tissues preoperative estrogen administration is recommended.

Preoperative Evaluation

The indication for anterior colporraphy is a large cystocele or moderate cystocele with stress incontinence. There is little indication in modern operative planning for anterior colporraphy as a prophylactic measure (as a

73

trial repair for stress incontinence, with an abdominal procedure planned later should failure occur) or as a procedure for stress incontinence when little relaxation exists.

The assessment of coexistent cystocele and stress incontinence includes the following: a detailed history and physical examination; laboratory studies to rule out neurological diseases; an evaluation of vesical neck support and anal and vaginal sphincter tone; the measurement of residual urine, urinalysis, and culture; the demonstration of incontinence with its relief by paraurethral compression; urethroscopic examination employing carbon dioxide urethroscopy; pressure measurements; and notations of urethral mobilization by manipulation such as the Q-tip test. Details of the evaluation of stress incontinence are found in Chapter 21.

While a vast number of abnormalities are associated with urinary incontinence, the following categories can be outlined: urge incontinence accompanying urethritis, trigonitis, or cystitis of infectious, atrophic, or psychosomatic origin; bladder neuropathy caused by lesions of the central or peripheral nerves, encompassing most of the disorders of the nervous system; congenital or acquired urinary tract anomalies such as ectopic ureters, urethral diverticula, postoperative scarring, and strictures and fistulas; and detrusor dyssynergia.[2] Careful study of the latter lesion by Hodgkinson and his colleagues revealed that increased intra-abdominal pressure may produce sudden uninhibited detrusor contractions, thereby producing actual voiding rather than a leaking type of anatomic incontinence.[3] This confuses the diagnosis as both events are precipitated by increased abdominal pressure.

Of all patients complaining of abnormal urinary leakage, 85% have a history of stress incontinence.[2] Of this group 90% to 95% have true anatomic stress incontinence while 5% to 10% suffer from a condition other than anatomic stress incontinence. A trial of anticholinergics may be worthwhile in the latter group of patients; most will respond, further documenting that surgery is not indicated. If the patient has true anatomic stress incontinence in the absence of marked anatomic defects of the vagina, the procedure of choice is the urethral suspension.

If the cystocele is of moderate size, anterior colporraphy is accomplished during hysterectomy, with the cystocele repair done as described in Chapter 13. Abdominal repair is adequate for small to moderate size cystoceles. When associated with urethral suspension, it produces good support of the defect in the anterior vaginal wall.[5] If undecided on which route to take, the surgeon should err on the side of suprapubic procedures. Low showed a failure rate of 42% in patients with minimal descensus when repaired vaginally.[4] Morgan noted that the 5-year success rate for anterior repair was 50% for stress incontinence, whereas suprapubic methods yielded an 80% success rate.[6]

Finally, remember that stress incontinence is not an emergency and that the presence of a cystocele does not rule out the simultaneous occurrence of one or more of the factors noted in stress incontinence. Careful preoperative evaluation with a therapeutic trial, if indicated, of anticholenergics, antibiotics to sterilize the urine, estrogens to relieve trigonitis, and office discussion and appropriate referral if psychosomatic symptoms exist is necessary. If the cystocele is symptomatic but other factors are present, the patient should be advised that the repair of her cystocele, when large enough to warrant independent surgery, may not necessarily relieve her other urinary symptoms.

Operative Technique

The patient is placed in the lithotomy position and prepared in the usual manner. The surgical procedure is illustrated in Figures 8.1 through 8.3.

Postoperative Management and Results

Patients with cystocele repair alone are promptly allowed to ambulate and are placed on a regular diet as tolerated. The vaginal pack placed during the procedure is removed on the second postoperative day.

While the author was an early advocate of the various suprapubic methods of draining the bladder, the disappearance of the ward nurse who personally took an interest in maintenance of such suprapubic devices has caused the author to return to the time-honored Foley catheter. The catheter is left in place for 4 days. Following removal of the catheter, the patient is allowed to void. If the residual urine is greater than 125 ml, the Foley is replaced and removed the following day. As soon as the catheter is removed, the patient is given sulfisoxazole or nitrofurantoin for 10 days. As soon as the patient is voiding properly, she is dismissed with instructions to void at no longer than 2-hr intervals during the day and to force

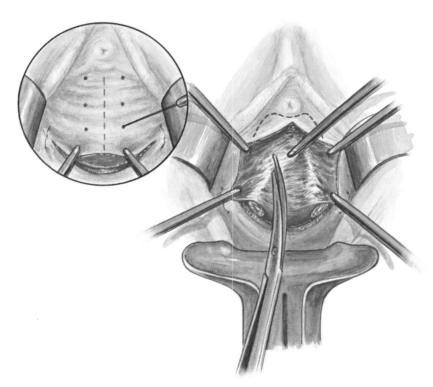

FIGURE 8.1. Anterior repair is performed independently or in conjunction with vaginal hysterectomy. Inject the space between the vagina and bladder muscularis with a dilute vasoconstrictor solution. Be sure to include the lateral paraurethral tissues and vagina. Using fine scissors with a very slightly rounded point and pulling downward on the vaginal mucosa, dissect between the bladder and vagina in a straight line toward the urethra. Using the scissors, follow the dotted line to where no cleavage plane exists between the urethra and vagina.

75

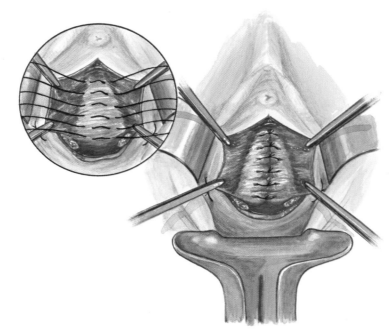

FIGURE 8.2. Have the assistant grasp the lateral vaginal margin with Allis Adair clamps or Adson-Brown thumb forceps and pull laterally and caudad. Grasp the tissue to be dissected with Adson-Brown thumb forceps and pull directly away from the vagina. Using fine sharp scissors, dissect between the bladder and vagina in the loose areolar tissue that lies in this area. Strong traction and countertraction will produce a plane that allows dissection upward. Continue the dissection upward and laterally near the urethra. Dissect the opposite side in a similar fashion. The bladder should be free of the vaginal wall in its mid and lateral portions. Small bleeders should be suture ligated with 3-0 or 4-0 absorbable suture.

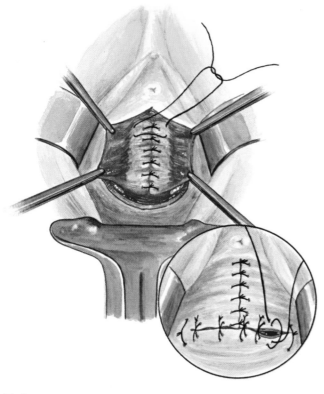

FIGURE 8.3. In older patients the central bladder may be quite atrophic and large, in which instance a single or double purse-string suture may be used to imbricate the large bulging central portion of the cystocele. When the defect is more modest, as illustrated, place 2-0 absorbable imbricating sutures to pull the midportion of the bladder upward. Place a layer of 2-0 absorbable suture at the lateral margins of the previous row and bring them together, tying them just lateral to the midline. Place an upward suture laterally at the margins where the dissection extended (dotted lines) and tie one or two of these sutures to support the urethra. Do not elevate the base of the bladder excessively where the urethral vesical neck cannot be well supported as incontinence results. Trim any redundant vaginal mucosa. Close the vagina with 3-0 absorbable suture using simple sutures in the vertical portion. Incorporate the anterior vaginal wall in the vaginal hysterectomy closure after the cardinal ligaments have been sutured to the angles of the vault with far-and-near 3-0 absorbable closure. Place a 2-inch Iodoform vaginal pack in the patient as well as a Foley catheter.

fluids. A urine culture is obtained when the patient is seen in the office after 6 weeks. Less than 5% of patients following this regimen have a positive urine culture. In addition, the patient is cautioned against intercourse and heavy lifting for 6 weeks.

Approximately 10% of patients have a recurrent cystocele; most are elderly patients with recurrence due to the general relaxation of pelvic tissues. For this reason more aggressive repair of cystocele is undertaken in the elderly. In the younger or premenopausal patient more moderate dissection is performed to avoid dyspareunia, and mucosa is rarely excised. Simmons has called attention to an increased incidence of dyspareunia following anterior vaginal prolapse repairs.[7] The success rate of anterior colporraphy, based on patients' subjective evaluations, is approximately 60%.[1]

References

1. Arnold, E.P., Webster, J.R., Loose, H., et al.: Urodynamics of female incontinence: Factors influencing the results of surgery. *Am. J. Obstet. Gynecol.* **117:**805–812, 1973.
2. Green, T.H.: Urinary stress incontinence: Differential diagnosis, pathophysiology, and management. *Am. J. Obstet. Gynecol.* **122:**368–400, 1975.
3. Hodgkinson, C.P.: Relationships of the female urethra and bladder in urinary stress incontinence. *Am. J. Obstet. Gynecol.* **65:**560–573, 1953.
4. Low, J.A.: Management of anatomic urinary incontinence by vaginal repair. *Am. J. Obstet. Gynecol.* **97:**308–315, 1967.
5. Macer, G.A.: Transabdominal repair of cystocele, a 20 year experience, compared with the traditional vaginal approach. *Am. J. Obstet. Gynecol.* **131:**203–207, 1978.
6. Morgan, J.E., and Farrow, G.A.: Recurrent stress urinary incontinence in the female. *Br. J. Urol.* **49:**37–42, 1977.
7. Simmons, S.C.: Dyspareunia following repair—"The skin bridge" and its prevention. *J. Obstet. Gynaecol. Br. Commonw.* **70:**476–478, 1963.

9 Vaginal Prolapse

There are at least 43 well-documented descriptions of surgical procedures designed to repair vaginal vault prolapse.[6] Vaginal vault prolapse is a result of an inherent weakness in the vaginal supporting structures (uterosacral and lower portion of the cardinal ligaments). Trauma from childbirth, obesity, postmenopausal atrophy, and unsatisfactory healing of the supporting structures following vaginal or abdominal hysterectomy are contributory factors.

Anatomy

At one time the suspension of the vagina to the anterior abdominal wall, round ligaments, or pubic symphysis was advocated; however, studies by Berglas and Rubin published in 1953 clarified the importance of the vaginal axis and its horizontal relationship to the ground with the patient in the erect position.[2] The long axis of the vagina points toward the hollow of the sacrum, not directly upward toward the symphysis nor toward the sacral promontory. Procedures that restore this more posterior axis of the vagina are therefore more likely to be effective over the long period of observation needed to determine the success rate of such procedures. While Beecham and Beecham and others have achieved good results with anterior fixation, their good results were more likely due to superior surgical technique and the use of a very strong fascial support rather than the inherent design of the procedure.[1] Langmade et al. described excellent results in 85 cases of vaginal vault suspension using Cooper's ligament.[4] The ligament was detached and the vault suspended in midposition. They noted no postoperative stress incontinence.

Preoperative Evaluation

The patient presents with complaints of vaginal protrusion, difficulty in voiding or defecating, unsatisfactory coitus, or complaints referable to ulceration of the vaginal mucosa. Preoperative diagnostic studies include very careful palpation of the protrusion with rectovaginal examination to determine the rectocele component of the mass, cytological study of the cervix and endometrium, cystoscopy, and intravenous pyelogram. Preoperative estrogen stimulation in the absence of any contraindications is begun to improve the quality and blood supply of the vaginal mucosa. Review the patient's sexual activity and anticipated results with the patient and her husband and note this discussion in the medical record.

Operative Technique

Vaginal vault suspension procedures are either vaginal or abdominal in approach. The vaginal procedures consist of Symmonds repair (Figure 9.1), transvaginal sacrospinous fixation (Figures 9.2 and 9.3),[5] and total vaginec-

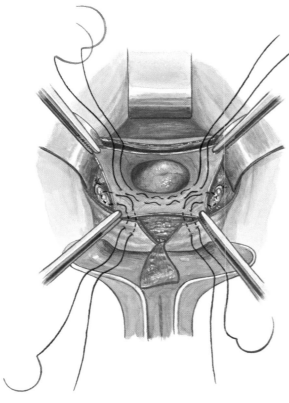

FIGURE 9.1. Symmonds vaginal vault prolapse repair after the completion of vaginal hysterectomy. If the uterus has previously been removed, isolate the associated enterocele sac (Chapter 6). Dissect the sac free and excise it. Excise a wide wedge of posterior vaginal wall as shown. Place a series of sutures of 2-0 absorbable suture through the vaginal wall, up over the sac and into the high uterosacral and cardinal ligaments. Bring these down and exit through the vaginal wall. Make certain the upper sutures are placed as high as possible in the uterosacral ligaments. Elevate the margin of the vault and tie the sutures from above downward. Close any defect left in the sac with 2-0 purse-string absorbable sutures. This will produce a solid wedge of tissue in the upper posterior vaginal wall. Close the vagina as in vaginal hysterectomy by securing the cardinals laterally and closing the vagina with far-and-near 3-0 sutures. Close any defect in the vaginal wedge with 3-0 far-and-near sutures. Any posterior repair should continue up to the wedge excision. Anterior repair can be performed in the usual fashion if indicated. Place a Foley catheter and Iodoform vaginal pack as in the usual vaginal repair.

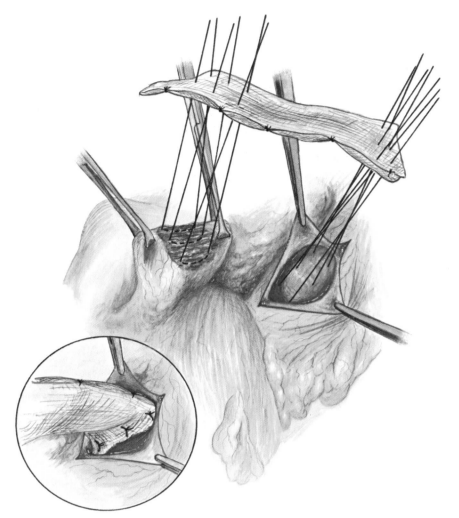

FIGURE 9.2. Sacrospinous fixation: the Birnbaum technique. Perform any needed vaginal repair of cystocele and rectocele. Place two long Allis clamps on the vaginal cuff. Prepare the abdomen and place the patient in the low lithotomy position. Open the abdomen with sufficient exposure to see the upper sacrum. Pack the abdomen and incise for 4 to 5 cm 5 cm below the sacrum. Stay medial to the ureter and avoid the gluteal vessels and the small sacral veins. Inset: Place three sutures through the double layer of Dacron mesh and through the presacral fascia and periosteum and out again through the graft. Use 3-0 Dacron in a non-traumatic needle. Identify the vaginal vault by manipulating and palpating the Allis clamps previously placed on the vaginal vault. Dissect the bladder off the vagina if it has been oversewn in prior surgery. Again lay the mesh over the vagina and adjust the tension by pulling the graft into its ultimate sacral position. Suture through one side of the mesh, into vaginal muscularis, and out again through the graft. Be certain not to enter the vaginal epithelium. Place three sutures approximately 1 cm apart and tie the vaginal sutures.

tomy. Abdominal procedures include posterior vaginal suture and Dacron graft suspension, and Moschcowitz-type excision and repair of the cul-de-sac.

Vaginectomy and colpectomy, while the most secure repair, renders intercourse impossible. Vaginectomy is the procedure of choice when the defects are large, the patient is elderly, and prior surgical repair has failed (Figures 9.4 through 9.7).

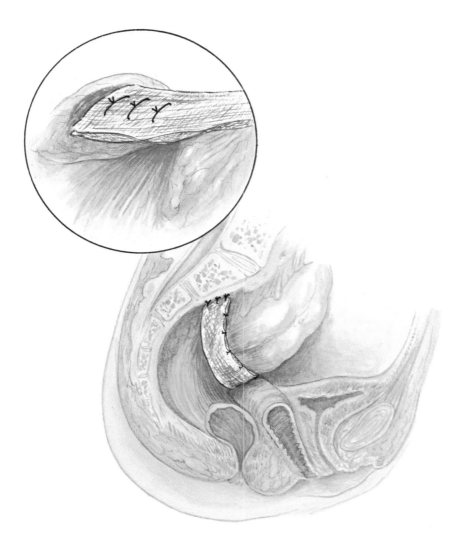

FIGURE 9.3. Tie the sacral sutures, pulling the vagina into position (inset). Suture the serosa over the mesh and approximate the serosa of the sigmoid to avoid internal hernia.

Jeffcoate[3] and Simmons[7] reported a 50% incidence of dyspareunia and apareunia following anterior and posterior repair; therefore, avoid the posterior repair and use an abdominal vault suspension to produce satisfactory sexual function.

For the patient undergoing vaginal suspension with Dacron graft, administer preoperative antibiotics prior to the placement of this prosthesis; advise the patient of the definite incidence of prosthesis sloughing and removal (Figure 9.2).

Many authors describe the use of silk suture with prostheses. Silk suture loses its strength in tissue; Dacron (which is the same substance as the graft) is much stronger and more permanent.

Postoperative Management and Results

Place a vaginal Iodoform pack and Foley catheter in the patient. The Foley catheter may be removed in 48 hr; antibiotics are administered while the Foley is in place and for 3 days following removal. The patient may be out of bed on the second postoperative day. Any rectocele or cystocele repair would require changes in procedure to accommodate postoperative care of those defects.

Sacrospinous ligament repair and, of course, colpectomy have the lowest incidence of recurrence. Vaginal repair has a failure rate of approxi-

81

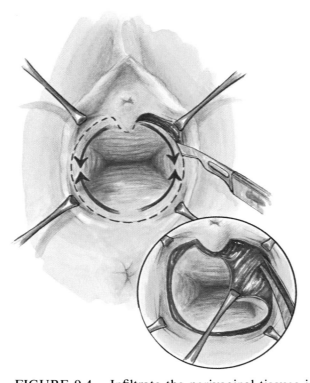

FIGURE 9.4. Infiltrate the perivaginal tissues in the area of the introitus with a dilute solution of Neo-Synephrine. Make a sharp incision about the introitus. If the excision is for carcinoma in situ, note the location of the lesion prior to excision. With sharp downward traction, begin the dissection in the anterior and posterior repair planes and carry it laterally; continue the dissection to the vaginal cuff. The area of the cuff and lateral margins of the vagina will then remain adherent with strong traction at each of the margins. Cut these sharply. Clamp and tie bleeders with 3-0 absorbable suture. Note the close approximation of the anterior portion of the lateral vagina to the ureter during dissection. Have a clear view when tying bleeders so that the ureters are not included in any of the ties. Isolate and clamp the vaginal supporting tissues, which extend downward from the upper portions of the cardinal ligaments. Cut the area of the old hysterectomy cuff as well.

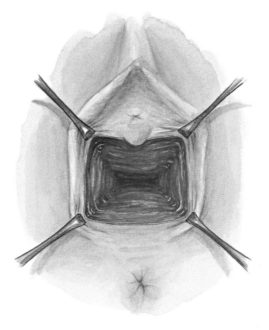

FIGURE 9.5. Following removal of the vaginal epithelium, spend a few minutes isolating and tying small vessels. It may be necessary to place a vaginal pack or use Avitene sheets in the areas that are oozing.

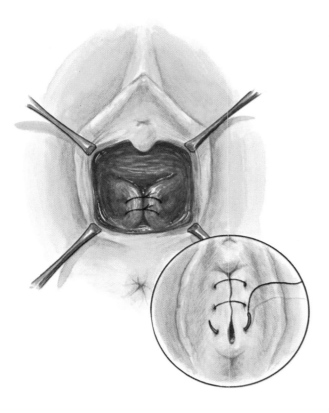

FIGURE 9.6.   If vaginal function is not to be preserved, the levator muscles are simply sutured in the midline with 0 chromic suture and the introital skin is closed with interrupted sutures of 3-0 Vicryl or chromic catgut. Any cystocele or rectocele of significance may be treated prior to the closure of the levator muscles in the absence of vaginal epithelium; however, recurrent prolapse is a rare problem. Cytoscope the patient immediately following the procedure and observe the passage of indigo carmine from each ureter.

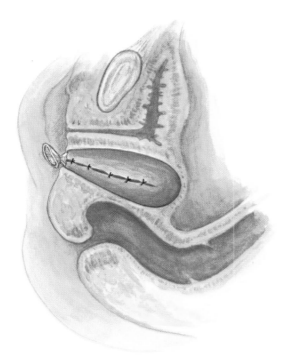

FIGURE 9.7.   If total vaginectomy is to be performed for a neoplastic process and vaginal function preserved, proceed as shown in Figures 9.4 and 9.5. Secure hemostasis and apply skin graft at this time. The graft is cut prior to the vaginectomy and is kept in saline-soaked sponges. The skin is cut with a Padget dermatome, which is excellent for this purpose. The epithelial surface is stretched over a foam rubber–filled condom, which is used to stint the skin in place in the vagina. The introitus is sutured over the stint. The stint is removed in 48 to 72 hour with a postoperative program of vaginal dilatation. When suturing the skin, be careful not to suture the skin to the condom as the skin will be pulled out when the condom is removed. The skin margins are sutured to the introitus and excess skin is trimmed.

83

mately 14%. The failure rate of abdominal prosthesis and vault suspension is approximately 5%. An equal number of patients have a prosthesis slough through the vagina requiring removal.

If one assumes that patients lost to follow-up are treatment failures, then approximately 20% to 30% of patients have recurrent prolapse.[8] Sacrospinous ligament fixation has good results and preserves sexual function; however, the author's best results have been with total vaginectomy.

References

1. Beecham, C.T., and Beecham, J.B.: Correction of prolapsed vagina or enterocele with fascia lata. *Obstet. Gynecol.* **42**:542–546, 1973.
2. Berglas, B., and Rubin, I.C.: Histologic study of the pelvic connective tissue. *Surg. Gynecol. Obstet.* **97**:277–289, 1953.
3. Jeffcoate, T.N.A.: Posterior colpoperineorrhaphy. *Am. J. Obstet. Gynecol.* **77**:490–502, 1959.
4. Langmade, C.F., Oliver, J.A., and White, J.S.: Cooper ligament repair of vaginal vault prolapse twenty-eight years later. *Am. J. Obstet. Gynecol.* **131**:134–142, 1978.
5. Randall, C.L., and Nichols, D.H.: Surgical treatment of vaginal inversion. *Obstet. Gynecol.* **38**:327–332, 1971.
6. Ridley, J.H.: A composite vaginal vault suspension using fascia lata. *Am. J. Obstet. Gynecol.* **126**:590–596, 1976.
7. Simmons, S.C.: Dyspareunia following repair—"The skin bridge" and its prevention. *J. Obstet. Gynaecol. Br. Commonw.* **20**:476–478, 1963.
8. Symmonds, R.E., and Sheldon, R.S.: Vaginal prolapse after hysterectomy. *Obstet. Gynecol.* **25**:61–67, 1965.

Rectovaginal Fistula and Anal Incontinence

10

Although improvement in the quality of obstetric care, radiation therapy, and surgery has decreased the incidence of rectovaginal fistula and anal incontinence, patients still present to the gynecologist for treatment of these problems.

Anatomy

Repair of both rectovaginal fistulas and surgical anal incontinence often requires division and later reestablishment of the anoperineal muscle complex. Remember this area is a functional unit. Successful repair reestablishes normal anatomic relationships rather than approximates a single muscle bundle.

The puborectalis muscle in the female is the thick and lower portion of the levator muscle, which forms a sling about the rectum. Contracting, this muscle pulls the rectum vertically and compresses the anal canal from side to side. This striated muscle continues downward to form the external sphincter, which closes the anal canal. While it is often described as having multiple portions, the surgeon will find one elliptical muscle band, indistinguishable from the puborectalis above, attached anteriorly to the central perineal tendon and posteriorly to the anococcygeal ligament.[1] The transverse perineal muscles that insert into the central tendon and proceed laterally to the ischial ramus are important in perineal tone and anal incontinence.[8]

The internal sphincter is the distal thickening of the circular smooth muscle of the bowel which is approximately 3 cm in length and palpable as the superior margin of the intersphincteric groove. While involved in defecation, it plays only a small role in anal continence. The internal and external sphincters are separated by the conjoint longitudinal muscle, which becomes increasingly fibrous as it extends distally and ultimately attaches to the perianal skin. The anal canal is closed by the puborectalis pulling upward and the reflex tone of the external sphincter. The latter is assisted by points of fixation to the anococcygeal ligament and the central perineal tendon, which has attachments to the transverse perineal muscles and perineal membrane. The lower space between the rectal and vaginal mucosa contains some fine areolar tissue and blood vessels, the azygous system of the vagina.

Pathology

Rectal sphincter and anal perineal muscular division may occur with extension of episiotomy, an uncontrolled delivery, or as an unrecognized event in anorectal surgery. When sphincter division occurs as a result of a midline episiotomy, successful repair is expected.[7] If unattended, the perineum may heal with the muscles retracted laterally, with a resultant complete perineal laceration. Patients may maintain continence with hypertrophy of the lower levator muscle in some instances.

Unrecognized surgical division of perineal muscles with retraction may occur as well. This is observed as a small lateral dimple in the perianal skin. When injury extends through the lower vagina into the rectum and the surrounding tissues are normal, spontaneous healing may still occur. If the defect is larger than 1 cm, with associated hematoma, excess suture, or other unrecognized injury, rectovaginal fistula may occur. This is seen most commonly in the obstetric injury due to unobserved entry into the rectum or improper repair at the time of a third-degree injury to the rectum. This group of obstetric fistulas occur in the lower third of the vagina; they comprise the majority of most modern series of rectovaginal fistulas and have an excellent prognosis.

Radiation injury produces particularly difficult fistulas, which occur most commonly in the middle third of the vagina. The basic etiology of radiation-induced fistula is obliteration of the small vessels with resultant ischemic necrosis. Radium or cesium application may produce a localized reaction, whereas whole-pelvis irradiation affects the entire pelvic vasculature; consequently, to promote healing one must bring blood from some nonirradiated site. While improved results occur with labial fat pad transplant and omental lengthening, permanent sigmoid colostomy is often the final result of such fistulas.[2]

Fistulas in the upper third of the vagina are usually postsurgical or result from recurrent cancer of the cervix or colon. For example, in pelvic surgery for endometriosis, in which difficult dissection between the rectum and vagina is common, undetected rectal perforation may occur. Abscess will usually result, which then ruptures through the vagina, and a fistula soon becomes apparent by the character of the drainage. If the injury is small, spontaneous closure is anticipated, whereas a larger defect may persist. Recurrent cancer of the cervix or colon may also produce fistulas in the upper third of the vagina. Biopsy the margins of the fistula to rule out recurrent cancer in those patients with prior pelvic malignancy even though the fistula occurs years later. The author has seen a patient with a small vaginal fistula due to recurrent cancer of the cervix 30 years after treatment.

Preoperative Evaluation

In patients with anal incontinence following obstetric injury, study of the perineal musculature is important. Look for other defects in the puborectalis and transverse perineal muscles and plan their repair, as well as external sphincter approximation. Do a neurological examination to detect underlying neurological disease and note the perineal muscle tone of the uninjured portion of the levator. If the rectovaginal fistula is small and difficult to visualize, instill methylene blue in the rectum and observe its appearance in the vagina. If it cannot be detected, pack the vagina with white gauze and recheck after the patient has been ambulatory; blue stain will confirm the presence of this fistula.

If the vaginal mucosa is atrophic, prescribe topical and systemic estrogens for 60 days, which will produce a stronger mucosa more tolerant of suture. If local infection is present, begin a regimen of sitz baths and systemic and local antibiotics.

Order anoscopic and proctoscopic, upper and lower gastrointestinal, and small bowel barium studies to detect associated gastrointestinal fistulas or primary gut disease. The patient may have an ileal fistula, particularly when severe radiation injury has occurred, as well as a slough of the upper rectum or proctosigmoiditis with stricture.

Patients with various types of colitis, such as ulcerative colitis, have a high incidence of rectovaginal fistula, and these fistulas may initially present in the postpartum period. Spontaneous healing of these fistulas is rare. Conservative surgery usually fails and most of these patients undergo total proctocolectomy and ileostomy.[3]

While some authors have advised delay in the repair of postpartum fistulas for long periods of time, excellent results are obtained with surgery after inflammatory and vascular changes of pregnancy have subsided. Hibbard reports excellent results in series of patients whose surgery was performed within 3 months of the development of the postpartum fistula.[6] When irradiation fistula occurs repair is delayed for at least 6 months. Remember that the changes in radiation arteritis continue for many months and that the full extent of the pelvic injury may not be known at the time of the original rectovaginal fistula. Vesicovaginal fistula, ileovaginal fistula, and ureterovaginal fistula, or external fistula, may be the next clinical event.

In contrast to the other types of rectovaginal fistulas, repair of irradiated rectovaginal fistula requires colostomy. This colostomy is not closed until the fistula appears healed and the barium study is negative for 2 months following repair.

Operative Technique

Careful mechanical bowel preparation, as described in Chapter 19, will reduce the infection rate associated with rectovaginal fistula repair. Additionally, Betadine douches and enemas the night before surgery will aid in reducing intraoperative contamination.

Basic principles of fistula repair are similar in any site (Figures 10.1 through 10.5). Excise the fistula so that normal tissues are present. Separate the mucosal layers at least 2 cm from the edge of the fistula and close the mucosa without tension. Bring a layer of well-vascularized tissue between the two layers. When this is not available, one must provide tissues containing a good blood supply, such as the omentum, labial fat pad, gracilis, or gluteus muscle, for successful repair.[9] Inversion of mucosa or through-and-through closure are equally successful if the layers are well separated.[4,6] When the patient has had a failed repair or associated irradiation injury, diverting colostomy is indicated. Finally, repair of the entire muscular unit is recommended for associated anorectal incontinence. While some use a paradoxical incision in the external sphincter, the author has not found this necessary, and in Hibbard's recent series this procedure was used in only 1 of 27 cases.[6] Although rectal pressure may reach 85 cm H_2O[5] this does not pose a threat to the usual fistula repair as such pressure is reduced by maintaining the patient on an elemental diet following surgery, thereby eliminating the need for a paradoxical incision.

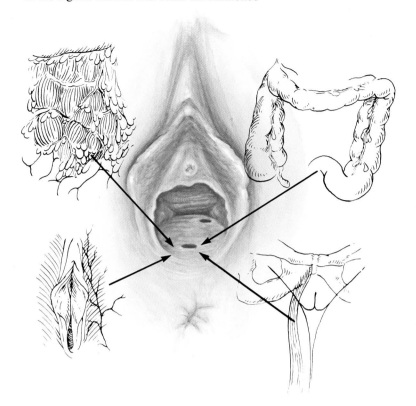

FIGURE 10.1. A rectovaginal fistula may occur in the lower third of the vagina associated with obstetric injury, the middle third of the vagina associated with irradiation therapy or cancer management, and in the upper third of the vagina following abdominal hysterectomy. When the blood supply is poor or irradiation injury contributes to fistula formation, an accessory blood supply must be brought in by means of a labial fat pad transplant, insertion of a tunnel of omentum between the rectum and vagina, resection and mobilization of the normal sigmoid down to normal tissue, or a gracilias muscle transplant.

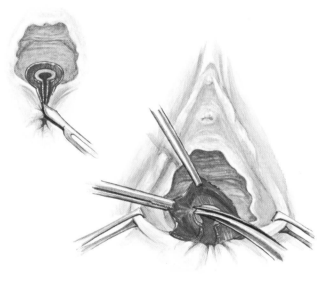

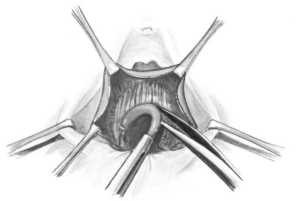

FIGURE 10.2. Surgery of fistula in the lower third of the vagina. Trim the margins of the fistula and incise sharply into the rectum, converting the fistula to a third-degree injury. Using sharp dissection, free up the margins 2 cm about the fistula. Excise the fistula so that the margins have good blood supply.

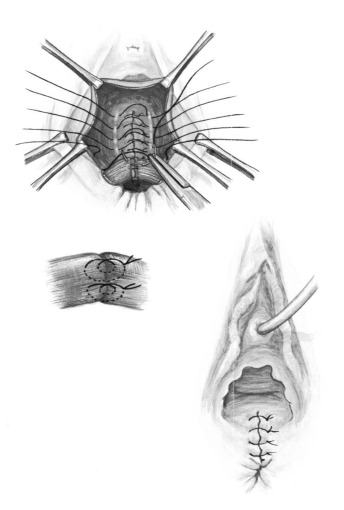

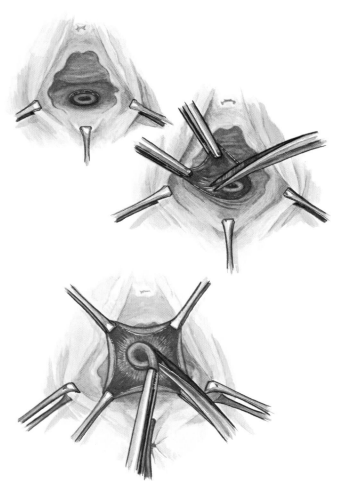

FIGURE 10.3.   Close the rectal mucosa in a vertical fashion, employing wedge-type sutures which pull more submucosa together than rectal mucosa. Place a second layer of fine 4-0 Vicryl sutures above this and imbricate the second layer over the suture line. There should be no compromise in the mucosal blood supply and all mucosa must be covered. Use 2-0 Vicryl in the lower margins of this incision to secure the lateral distal portion of the levator ani muscle as it courses downward to insert in the central perineal tendon. Bring the lower part of this suture through the anterior portion of the capsule of the rectal sphincter. Isolate the rectal sphincter and close it with far-and-near sutures of 2-0 Vicryl. Close the vaginal wound with interrupted sutures of 3-0 nylon.

FIGURE 10.4.   Surgery of fistula in the middle third of the vagina. Isolate the fistula from the surrounding structures, insert a Foley catheter to improve visibility, pull directly upward, and incise sharply around the margins of the fistula. Using fine thumb forceps and sharp scissors, dissect 2 cm away from the fistula margin. Excise the margins of the fistula back to normal appearing tissue.

89

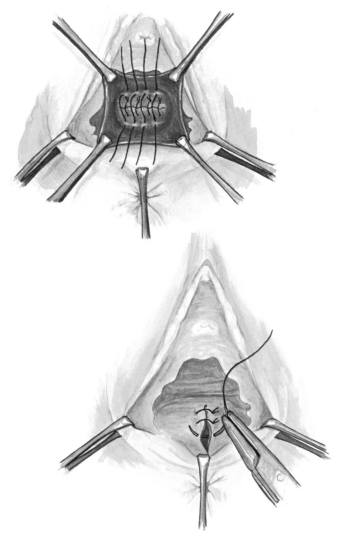

FIGURE 10.5. Close the rectal mucosa, employing a wedge-type suture containing larger amounts of submucosa than epithelium. Imbricate the perirectal tissues and muscle over this in a transverse fashion. Close the defect produced with interrupted sutures of 3-0 monofilament nylon or Vicryl.

Postoperative Management and Results

The postoperative hospital stay for simple sphincter repair and small obstetrical fistula repair is usually 3 to 4 days. Remove the patient's catheter as soon as she is awake and alert and begin sitz baths. Place the patient on a liquid diet for 3 days and prescribe stool softeners. The patient may continue using estrogen and local antibiotic creams in the vagina if postmenopausal. Remove the monofilament nylon sutures in the vaginal epithelium 7 to 10 days postoperatively. Continue the stool softeners and sitz baths for 3 weeks.

The patient is instructed not to have an enema for 2 weeks and to resume intercourse in 6 weeks. If the patient has a colostomy, she is instructed in routine colostomy care. In cases of abdominal closure for high fistula, postlaparotomy care is sufficient.

When anorectal incontinence is due to the failure to approximate the muscles following surgery or vaginal delivery, 92% of patients improve following repair.[8] The initial repair of a low rectovaginal fistula due to obstetric trauma is successful in 95% of patients.[6] The results in midlevel rectovaginal fistula due to irradiation vary greatly with the severity of other associated injuries to the bladder or small bowel and associated rectal stricture. If rectovaginal fistula alone exists, the use of accessory blood supply and diverting colostomy is usually successful.

If severe injury extends throughout the anorectum with proctitis and stricture, colostomy is recommended. Associated urinary or small bowel fistula indicates widespread damage and makes colostomy advisable.

References

1. Anson, B. (ed.): *Morris' Human Anatomy*, 12th ed. New York, McGraw-Hill, 1966.
2. Boronow, R.C.: Management of radiation-induced vaginal fistulas. *Am. J. Obstet. Gynecol.* **110:**1–7, 1971.
3. Falconer, H.W., and Muldoon, J.P.: Rectovaginal fistula in patients with colitis: Review and report of a case. *Dis. Colon Rectum* **18:**413–415, 1975.
4. Given, F.T.: Rectovaginal fistula. *Am. J. Obstet. Gynecol.* **108:**41–45, 1970.
5. Greenwald, J.C., and Hoexter, B.: Repair of rectovaginal fistulas. *Surg. Gynecol. Obstet.* **146:**443–445, 1978.
6. Hibbard, L.T.: Surgical management of rectovaginal fistulas and complete perineal tears. *Am. J. Obstet. Gynecol.* **130:**139–141, 1978.
7. Kaltreider, F.D., and Dixon, D.M.: A study of 710 complete lacerations following central episiotomy. *South. Med. J.* **41:**814–819, 1948.
8. Moore, F.A.: Anal incontinence: A reappraisal. *Obstet. Gynecol.* **41:**483–493, 1973.
9. Stirnemann, H.: Treatment of recurrent rectovaginal fistula. *Am. J. Proctol.* **20:**52–54, 1969.

11 Vesicovaginal Fistula

Kermit E. Krantz

The obstetric vesicovaginal fistula was described in the Hindu medical literature as early as 800 BC. The mummy of Egyptian Queen Henheit dating from 2050 BC had a vesicovaginal fistula of probable obstetric origin.[5] A high percentage of fistulas still occur in the underdeveloped and emerging nations due to obstetric causes; Naidu recently reported 208 cases from Hyderabad, India.[9] Hamlin and Nicholson collected more than 2,000 cases in Ethiopia by 1972. In the United States, however, as in most developed countries, a majority of fistulas are due to gynecologic surgery. Abdominal hysterectomy alone accounts for 75% of cases seen; vaginal hysterectomy and anterior repair account for another 15%.[4]

Most fistulas resulting from abdominal hysterectomy are due to the failure to adequately dissect the bladder well down off the cervix and anterior vagina. A portion of the bladder is then included in either the clamp used or the sutures placed, with resultant necrosis and fistula. Urine usually appears in the vagina 1 to 2 weeks after surgery in these patients. If the bladder has been incised and not closed, urine appears promptly through the vaginal cuff. Fistulas appearing later are usually associated with a hematoma and infection.

Preoperative Evaluation

Initial studies should include an evaluation of the upper urinary tracts. Lagundoye et al. studied 216 cases of vesicovaginal fistula and noted that 105 patients had calyceal blunting, 75 had hydroureter, and 10 had kidneys that did not function at all.[5] While some of these were chronic fistulas, this study serves to emphasize the importance of an investigation of the upper urinary tract in studying vesicovaginal fistula. An injury that involves the bladder may well obstruct the ureter, or the patient may have multiple injuries.

To evaluate the patient, a Foley catheter is placed into the bladder and a solution of methylene blue is injected. If the patient has a vesicovaginal fistula, it will of course appear promptly in the vagina. If the fistula is a large one, little difficulty will be encountered in isolating it. Very small fistulas, particularly those in a recent postoperative site, may be hard to de-

92

tect and may require the placing of a vaginal tampon in the vagina. The patient is then placed in bed with the Foley catheter clamped. If the tampon is stained blue on removal, a vesicovaginal fistula is documented. If the tampon is urine soaked but colorless, the patient most likely has a ureterovaginal fistula.

Wesolowski and Meaney recommend insertion of a vaginal tampon prior to the administration of a contrast medium for excretory urography in patients in whom a small fistula is suspected but has not been documented.[11] The tampon is left in place until the bladder is distended; it is then removed and placed alongside an unused tampon and a film is taken. Opacification of the tampon confirms the presence of these small fistulas.

Most gynecologic fistulas are in the midline and are well away from the ureters; however, if there is any question, cystoscopy and injection of indigo carmine for identification are recommended. The author routinely has a cystoscope available in the operating room so that the fistula may be observed prior to and following its repair.

Ureteral catheters are usually unnecessary. If the ureteral orifices are near the edges of the fistula, however, a catheter is placed prior to the repair to avoid incorporating the ureter in the fistula repair. If the ureter is in the edge of the fistula, it is best cut and reimplanted into the bladder (Chapter 22).

Keettel suggests waiting 3 to 4 months to repair a vesicovaginal fistula; however, the long delay in fistula repair is useful only if the fistula is surrounded by intense inflammatory reaction and necrosis.[4] If the fistula is observed in the immediate postoperative period, the patient can be taken promptly to the operating room and the fistula can be repaired before any significant collagen formation has a chance to occur. The fistula is easily exposed and repaired, and the edema, which is one of the initial responses of inflammation, increases the ease of dissection. The formation of collagen does not begin until after the fifth day of wound healing, so that repair prior to this time is uncomplicated by scar formation.[10]

During the preoperative evaluation the patient is placed on local antibiotics and, if postmenopausal, estrogens. The estrogens will increase the blood supply to the vagina, making it much easier to work with the vaginal epithelium. If the inflammatory changes are acute, the patient is placed on systemic antibiotics. If there are significant changes in the surrounding skin due to urine irritation, zinc oxide applied locally on a tampon will aid healing and decrease maceration.

Operative Technique

Postoperative Fistula

The great majority of postoperative fistulas can be repaired through the vagina (Figures 11.1 through 11.5). The author of this technique has not had a failure in an uncomplicated postoperative fistula in 18 years.

Transitional epithelium is remarkable in its ability to seal when approximated and to be watertight within 24 hr. Peacock and Van Winkle have demonstrated the prompt healing of bladder muscle in less than 14 days with a significant and appreciable percentage of original tissue strength regained by that time.[10] For this reason, and because stones may form if a permanent suture is placed in the transitional epithelium, repair of bladder muscle is accomplished with absorbable suture (such as 3-0 or 4-0 chromic catgut or Vicryl placed in bladder muscle).

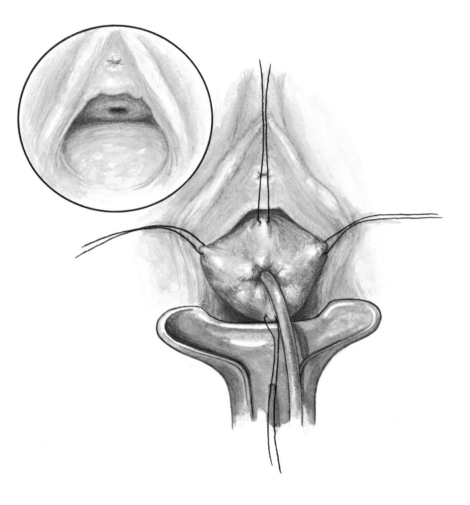

FIGURE 11.1. Place the patient in the lithotomy position and expose the fistula. If the patient has a very stenotic introitus and the fistula cannot be visualized, make a midline episiotomy, or if the perineum is moderately scarred and stenotic, make a Schuchardt-type incision up to the apex of the vagina exposing the fistula.

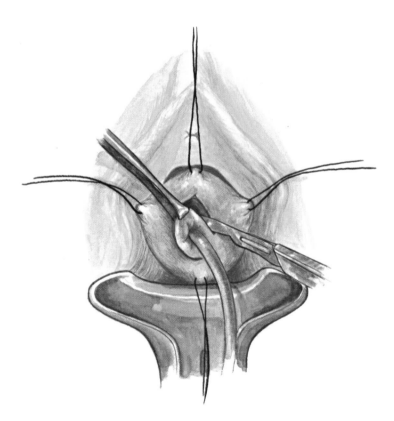

FIGURE 11.2. Place a small Foley catheter in the fistula and inflate the bulb, pulling the fistula downward. Place four traction sutures at each margin of the exposed vagina, pulling laterally. Using a small sharp blade, make an incision about the fistulous tract through all layers and into the bladder.

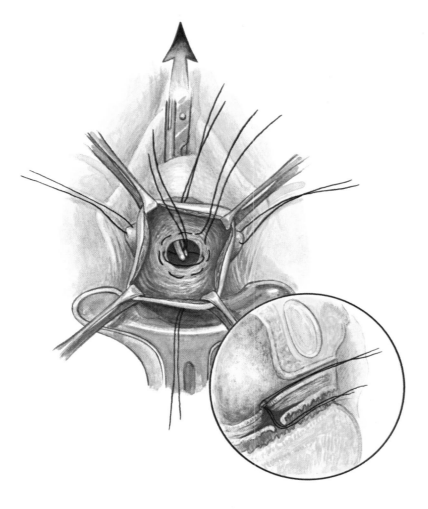

FIGURE 11.3. Dissect the bladder muscularis free of the vagina for a distance of 2 cm on each side and trim any remaining fibrous tissue in the bladder wall and excise any remaining fistulous tract. Place a 2-0 chromic suture through the margins of the fistula. Pass a long hemostat through the urethra and grasp the suture, tenting the fistulous tract into the bladder. Place the 4-0 purse-string suture around the tract, avoiding the suture perforating the transitional epithelium of the bladder. Tie the purse-string.

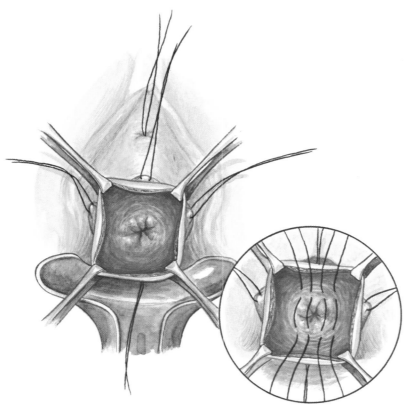

FIGURE 11.4. After the purse-string suture has been tied, place vertical imbricating sutures of 3-0 or 4-0 chromic through the bladder muscularis, imbricating adequate margins of bladder muscle. Have no epithelium visible in the muscularis closure and use great care not to enter the bladder mucosa with the stitches. While placing and tying the muscularis suture, tension on the traction suture through the urethra minimizes the chance of epithelial involvement.

95

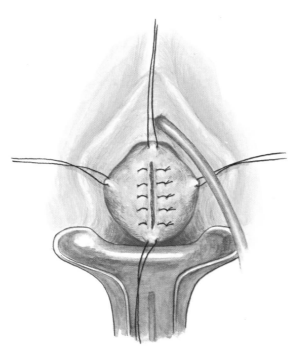

FIGURE 11.5.   Pull one end of the 2-0 margin suture so that it is removed from the bladder through the urethra. Close the vaginal epithelium with vertical mattress sutures of 2-0 chromic catgut. Remove the traction sutures.

Following closure, triple sulfa cream containing estrogen is placed in the vagina along with a vaginal pack. A Foley (No. 24) catheter is placed in the urethra. The catheter is removed as soon as there are not more than four red cells per high-power field in the urine. Most patients have clear urine in 3 to 5 days. Patients are allowed to ambulate immediately and are discharged as soon as the Foley catheter is removed. The patient is managed essentially as a patient who has undergone a vaginal hysterectomy except that she is cautioned not to resume intercourse for 6 weeks. There is no increased incidence of stress incontinence nor should significant sexual dysfunction result after this type of repair.

One might question whether a bladder that has not been distended for a period of years could resume normal function. Moir notes that bladder capacity returned to normal after repairs of fistulas that had existed for as long as 32 years.[7]

Obstetric Fistula

Whereas the gynecologic fistula is brought on by crushing injury, misplaced suture, or undiagnosed laceration, the obstetric fistula is usually due to ischemic necrosis caused by obstructed labor. Tissue loss may be much greater in these patients. Naidu reported 201 cases of fistula due to obstetric trauma.[9] Most of these were managed by separating the bladder from the vagina and inverting the bladder mucosa. Sixty-nine of the large fistulas were repaired by mobilization of the bladder downward with fixation to the lower remainder of the bladder as described by Thomas. Hassim and Lucas noted an increasing incidence of postoperative stress incontinence if the fistula involves the bladder neck; consequently, they found better postoperative results when closing the fistula in the long axis of the vagina and reinforcing the bladder neck.[3] Where the repair was under tension, labial fat pad grafts were used to assist closure. Where there was extensive destruction of the bladder and urethra, the Hamlon-Nicholson gracilis muscle transplant produced the best final result. Of their 150 patients with obstetric fistula, 11 (7%) showed residual stress incontinence. Of these 11 patients, 8 were treated with the Marchall-Marchetti-Krantz procedure and 4 improved. Three patients were treated with ureterosigmoidostomy.

In patients with recurrent fistula, the reason the original repair failed must be considered. If the vagina is so badly scarred and strictured that exposure is difficult, transvesical repair may be considered. The Schuchardt incision may also be used for exposure. Recurrent fistula with any question of sufficient blood supply should have a labial fat pad transplant for additional blood supply.

Irradiation-Induced Vesicovaginal Fistula

Surgery of vesicovaginal fistula associated with irradiation therapy requires great experience and proper timing for success. Fistulas occurring after radiation therapy are due to obliterative endarteritis. The basic abnormality in irradiation is endothelial injury in the small vessels with an ischemic necrosis. Additional blood supply must be brought from an unirradiated area to restore the blood supply necessary to heal the suture line. The inability of the irradiated tissue to produce fibroblasts as rapidly as unirradiated tissue must be taken into account in the postoperative period.[2]

The incidence of fistulas usually increases as the total dose of irradiation increases. If the blood supply to the bladder is compromised, additional injury is probably present in the rest of the pelvic viscera as well. The vesicovaginal fistula may be the first of a line of fistulas including ureterovaginal, rectovaginal, and ileovaginal fistulas. The presence of a cystocele increases the irradiation-induced complication rate in the urinary tract as well.[6] The patient must understand this prior to surgical repair or she may feel that the subsequent fistulas are a complication of the original procedure. Additionally, the fistula may be due to recurrent pelvic cancer which requires a biopsy at the fistula margin and a workup for metastatic disease.

The attendant fibrosis in radiation therapy makes mobilization of tissues difficult and associated vaginal stenosis and mucosal atrophy may render the fistula difficult to expose. If the fistula is associated with cervical cancer treatment, estrogens may be used without risk. If prior malignancy was endometrial cancer, of course, estrogens are not used unless the date of original tumor treatment makes recurrence unlikely. Careful study of the patient's intravenous pyelogram must be made as the ureters may be injured as well and obstructive uropathy may promote deterioration of renal function.[1] Where the fistula can be exposed vaginally, the gracilis muscle or labial fat pad are additional sources of blood supply in the lower portion of the bladder. Where the fistula is at that apex of the vagina, the omental pedicle may be used to separate the bladder mucosa from the vagina. Inversion of the mucosa, separate muscular layer suture lines in both bladder and vagina, and placement of accessory blood supply between bladder and vagina are essential for a satisfactory result. Unfortunately, the underlying vascular damage and tissue loss may be so great as to preclude successful repair.

Approximately 50% of patients with irradiation-induced vesicovaginal fistula will best be initially managed by or ultimately require an ileal or colon conduit for urinary control.

References

1. Boronow, R.C., and Rutledge, F.: Vesicovaginal fistula, radiation, and gynecologic cancer. *Am. J. Obstet. Gynecol.* **111**:85–90, 1971.
2. Grillo, H.C., and Potsaid, M.A.: Studies in wound healing: IV. Retardation of contraction by local x-irradiation and observations relating to the origin of fibroblasts in repair. *Ann. Surg.* **154**:741–750, 1961.
3. Hassim, A.M., and Lucas, C.: Reduction in the incidence of stress incontinence complicating fistula repair. *Br. J. Surg.* **61**:461–465, 1974.
4. Keettel, W.C.: Vesicovaginal and urethrovaginal fistulas. In: *Gynecologic and Obstetric Urology.* Philadelphia, Saunders, 1978, ch. 17.
5. Lagundoye, S.B., Bell, D., Gill, G., et al.: Urinary tract changes in obstetric vesico-vaginal fistulae: A report of 216 cases studied by intravenous urography. *Clin. Radiol.* **27**:531–539, 1976.
6. Masterson, B.J., and Rutledge, F.: Irradiation ulcer of the urinary bladder. *Obstet. Gynecol.* **30**:23–27, 1967.
7. Moir, J.C.: Personal experiences in the treatment of vesicovaginal fistulas. *Am. J. Obstet. Gynecol.* **71**:476–491, 1956.
8. Moir, J.C.: Vesico-vaginal fistulae as seen in Britain. *J. Obstet. Gynaecol. Br. Commonw.* **80**:598–602, 1973.
9. Naidu, P.M.: Vesico-vaginal fistulae: An experience with 208 cases. *J. Obstet. Gynaecol. Br. Commonw.* **69**:311–316, 1962.
10. Peacock, E.E., Jr., and Van Winkle, W., Jr.: Healing and repair of viscera. In: *Wound Repair.* Philadelphia, Saunders, 1976, ch. 12.
11. Wesolowski, D.P., and Meaney, T.F.: Use of a vaginal tampon in the diagnosis of vesicovaginal fistulae. *Radiology* **122**:262, 1977.

Surgery of the Vulva

12

Ernest W. Franklin, III

Modern surgical therapy for vulvar disease consists of diagnostic studies, excisional procedures, and reconstructive operations. The cornerstone of diagnosis is the vulvar biopsy, which is described in detail in Chapter 1. Except for those lesions of an infectious etiology such as *Trichomonas vaginalis* or *Candida albicans,* most other chronic vulvar conditions will require biopsy for definitive diagnosis. Use of the nomenclature of the International Society for the Study of Vulvar Disease is recommended.[11] Note that this is a histologic classification; hence, accurate diagnosis is only possible after appropriate biopsy material has been obtained (Table 12.1).

Anatomy

The blood supply of the vulva consists of labial branches of the pudendal artery coursing from the lateral margin of the vulva medially, as well as a small transverse perineal artery. A small branch of the femoral artery, the external pudendal, enters the vulva anteriorly and laterally. The veins

TABLE 12.1. New Nomenclature for Vulvar Disease (International Society for the Study of Vulvar Disease)

I.	Vulvar dystrophies	
	A.	Hyperplastic dystrophy
		1. Without atypia
		2. With atypia
	B.	Lichen sclerosus
	C.	Mixed dystrophy (lichen sclerosis with foci of epithelial hyperplasia)
		1. Without atypia
		2. With atypia
II.	Vulvar atypia	
	A.	Without dystrophy
	B.	With dystrophy
III.	Paget's disease of the vulva	
IV.	Squamous cell carcinoma in situ	

drain laterally and up into the iliac system. The sensory nerves supplying the vulva enter laterally with the vessels and branch out into the labial cutaneous nerves.

The lymphatics of the vulva have recently been studied by Jones.[7] He observed that the lymphatics have a discrete margin at the labial crural fold and drain upward to the medial group of the superficial groin nodes. While there are lymphatic pathways demonstrable to the urethra and clitoris, direct metastasis to the deep pelvic nodes, omitting the groin nodes, is a rare clinical occurrence.[4] The superficial groin nodes drain upward, join the lymph channels from the leg, and collect around the great vessels in the thigh and in the lymph nodes situated there. They course medially to enter the node of Cloquet, which is the highest groin node, usually located in the space next to the femoral vein. The lymph drainage is upward, continuous with the external iliac system and, hence, to the periaortic nodes.

Preoperative Evaluation

As noted, a representative biopsy is the basis for the planning of both medical and surgical therapy of vulvar disease. Where moderate or severe vulvar cellular atypia is found, colposcopic examination of the cervix and endometrial suction curettage are in order. Both intraepithelial and invasive carcinoma of the vulva are frequently associated with prior, concurrent, or subsequent neoplasia of the vagina and cervix. In the author's experience, associated malignancies of the lower reproductive tract may be seen in as many as 40% of patients with vulvar neoplasia. Staining of the vulva with 1% toluidine blue to detect nuclear activity and application of 3% acetic acid to accent hyperkeratosis are useful to find multicentric foci. Vulvar colposcopy is of limited benefit for biopsy site selection as the overlying keratin obscures the vascular patterns.

Complete physical examination, admission blood screens, chest x-ray, cystoscopy, proctoscopy, intravenous pyelograms, and barium enema complete the preoperative evaluation of these patients.

Operative Strategy

The vulvar dystrophies without atypia require no surgical therapy. Progesterone or topical cortisone creams are useful in controlling distressing pruritus, which often accompanies these disorders.[6] Condyloma may be treated with podophyllin or laser. Where increasing cellular atypia is noted on biopsy, local excision and close observation are in order because of the multifocal nature in as many as 35% of these lesions.[5] Local excision is adequate for small areas of carcinoma in situ as well; when multifocal, superficial vulvectomy is needed. Remember that it is the entire anogenital tract including the cervix, vagina, vulva, perineum, anus, and intergluteal crease which is at risk where vulvar precancerous lesions occur.

Vulvectomy does not remove all of this epithelium and may be an excessive procedure for a lesion of low malignant potential. Forney et al. reported that of 25 patients with carcinoma in situ of the vulva managed conservatively, none progressed to invasive cancer.[3] Japaze et al. noted no deaths due to invasive cancer in a 5-year follow-up of conservative management of 71 cases of carcinoma in situ of the vulva.[5] It is imperative when superficial vulvectomy is employed that invasive cancer be ruled out by biopsy of any thickened or ulcerated areas. Due to the looseness of the vulvar skin, the margins can usually be mobilized and approximated to cover the defect in this superficial excision (Figure 12.1).

If a split-thickness graft is required, preservation of the labial fat pads will produce a more normal appearing external genitalia. Split-thickness skin grafting may be extended to the anal verge without colostomy if preoperative bowel preparation and postoperative liquid diet of 1 week are ordered.

Fibrosis due to chronic trauma or postoperative scarring may produce an introital stricture (Figures 12.2 and 12.3). The use of preoperative estrogens and a carefully performed vaginal wall advancement or Z-plasty will increase introital size and relieve sexual discomfort.

Chronic vulvar pruritis may be associated with psychosexual difficulties and the patient must be carefully evaluated prior to any surgical procedure for the purpose of improving sexual function.

Basal cell carcinoma occurs in 1.4% of vulvar neoplasms; granular cell myoblastoma appears much less frequently.[12] While prone to local recurrence if inadequately excised, these lesions rarely metastasize to lymph nodes. Adequate wide local excision will usually suffice; the frequent use of frozen sections and the changing of instruments should a suspicious tissue be encountered will reduce the local recurrence rate to a minimum.

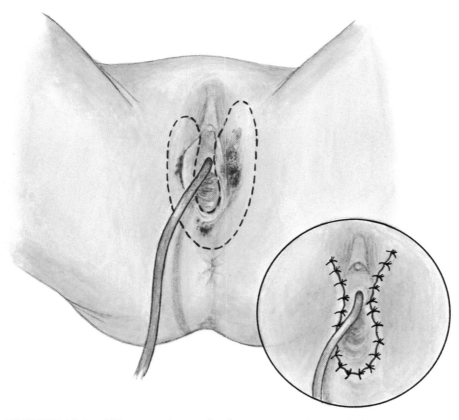

FIGURE 12.1.   When carcinoma in situ or severe dysplasia is multifocal, perform a simple vulvectomy. Be certain that no invasion exists by means of a prior biopsy. Preserve the clitoris if uninvolved. Incise the area using hooks to elevate the skin; undermine and free up the full thickness of the vagina and vulvar skin. Secure bleeders with 4-0 absorbable suture and skin edges with 3-0 monofilament nylon. If too much tension exists, use full-thickness flaps for coverage. Although a split-thickness graft covers the defect nicely, it produces a poorer functional result.

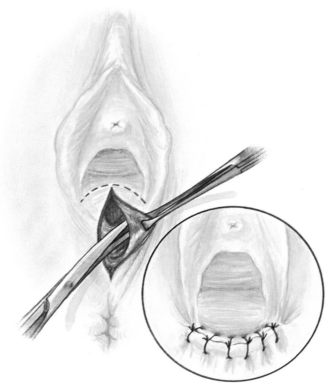

FIGURE 12.2.   Use a posterior vaginal wall advancement when an introital stricture is present and adequate posterior vagina is available. Free up the posterior vagina widely after incising in the midline. Advance the posterior vagina and close in a transverse fashion with monofilament nylon.

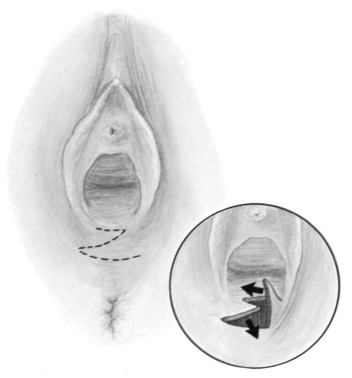

FIGURE 12.3.   Use a Z-plasty for introital stricture when a transverse scar is present. Outline the flaps with a marking pen. Cut sharply to underlying fascia and transpose with skin hooks. Suture with monofilament 3-0 sutures.

102

A few primary soft tissue sarcomas of the vulva have been reported with varying results. Wide local excision is needed for these lesions.[2]

Paget's disease is a rare skin lesion that occurs in the vulva and is associated with skin adnexal tumors or other malignancies in approximately 20% of cases. Complete thorough preoperative evaluation as outlined is necessary in these lesions, which appear grossly as exematoid weeping skin disease. Paget's cells often extend beyond the gross margins of the lesion and frequent frozen sections are needed. Toluidine blue is of no value in demonstrating the margins of these lesions; frozen sections are required for excision of this lesion. If an adnexal cancer is associated with the cutaneous lesion, radical vulvectomy and superficial node dissection is required. While excision of deep nodes is often recommended, there appear to be no survivors with positive deep pelvic nodes.[1] As this disease often occurs in elderly patients, excision of deep nodes may be omitted without significantly affecting long-term survival.

As the excision of vulvar skin is often extensive, additional coverage may be required. Single or bilateral rotational thigh flaps are very useful in covering these defects (Figure 12.4).[8]

Malignant melanoma is the second most common lesion of the vulva and accounts for 4.8% of vulvar neoplasms.[12] Vulvar pigmented nevi are often precursors of melanomas and should be routinely excised. Therapy for malignant melanoma varies with the level of the penetration of the skin. Histologic interpretation of pigmented vulvar lesions, particularly those that are chronically inflamed or infected, is fraught with hazard and expert opinion should be obtained. Where definite invasive malignant melanoma

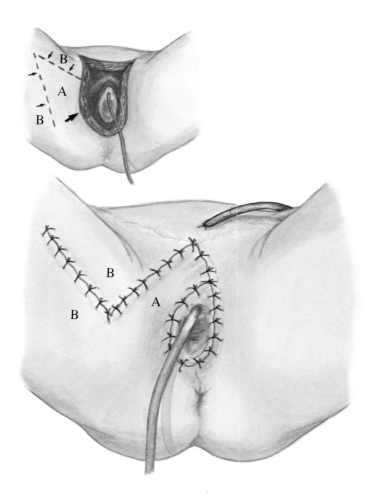

FIGURE 12.4. Woodruff's group has described the management of extensive vulvar defects by means of local flap grafts. The author has utilized this procedure with good results and recommends its use. When vulvectomy procedures produce too large an excision of vulvar skin for primary closure, as in the excision of local recurrence as illustrated, Paget's disease, or carcinoma in situ, skin flaps are useful. Outline the flap with a marking pen and carefully measure the area of placement. Make certain the base is as wide as the flap is long. Use a template cut from a disposable drape. Cut the flap directly downward to the fascia and free the flap along the fascial plane. Handle the flap gently with hooks. Secure hemostasis with fine mosquito clamps and 4-0 Vicryl. Transpose the graft and attach it as it lies loosely in the defect. Absolutely no tension is permitted. Mobilize the margin of the flap site, taking care not to injure the blood supply at the base. Insert a small suction catheter through the mons and carry it downward beneath the flap. Attach the flap with 3-0 monofilament nylon. Mobilize the margin of the flap site and close with 3-0 nylon. No dressings are required and the sutures are removed in 2 weeks.

103

exists, exploratory laparotomy with evaluation of the liver and periaortic nodes is in order. When the liver is negative for metastatic disease, retroperitoneal and pelvic node dissection followed by groin dissection and vulvectomy is recommended. The use of immunotherapy is under investigation and current data suggest it is useful in level II melanomas.

Invasive Carcinoma of the Vulva

Approximately 86% of vulvar malignancies occur as squamous cell cancer in elderly patients presenting with vulvar itching and a lesion of long duration.[12] These cancers are usually low grade and metastasize late in their clinical course through predictable pathways via the inguinal lymph nodes.

TABLE 12.2.   Clinical Staging of Carcinoma of the Vulva (International Federation of Gynecologists and Obstetricians, April 12, 1970)

T: Primary tumor
   T1. Tumor confined to the vulva—2 cm or less in largest diameter
   T2. Tumor confined to the vulva—more than 2 cm in diameter
   T3. Tumor or any size with adjacent spread to the urethra and/or vagina and/or perineum and/or anus
   T4. Tumor of any size infiltrating the bladder mucosa and/or the rectal mucosa, including the upper part of the urethral mucosa and/or fixed to the bone

N: Regional lymph nodes
   N0. No nodes palpable
   N1. Nodes palpable in either groin, not enlarged, mobile (not clinically suspicious of neoplasm)
   N2. Nodes palpable in either or both groins, enlarged, firm, and mobile (clinically suspicious of neoplasm)
   N3. Fixed, confluent, or ulcerated nodes

M: Distant metastases
   M0.   No clinical metastases
   M1A. Palpable deep pelvic lymph nodes
   M1B. Other distant metastases

Stage	Classification	Characteristics
I	T1 N0 M0 T1 N1 M0	All lesions confined to the vulva with a maximum diameter of 2 cm or less and no suspicious groin nodes
II	T2 N0 M0 T2 N1 M0	All lesions confined to the vulva with a diameter greater than 2 cm and no suspicious groin nodes
III	T3 N0 M0 T3 N1 M0 T3 N2 M0	Lesions extending beyond the vulva but without grossly positive groin nodes
	T1 N2 M0 T2 N2 M0	Lesions of any size confined to the vulva and having suspicious groin nodes
IV	T1 N3 M0 T2 N3 M0 T3 N3 M0 T4 N3 M0	Lesions with grossly positive groin nodes regardless of extent of primary
	T4 N0 M0 T4 N1 M0 T4 N2 M0	Lesions involving mucosa of rectum, bladder, or urethra, or involving bone
	M1A M1B	All cases with distant or palpable deep pelvic metastases

The classification of vulvar cancers developed by the International Federation of Gynecologists and Obstetricians is presented in Table 12.2.

While Wharton et al. have reported a series of patients with no positive groin nodes when invasion was less than 5 mm,[14] Magrina et al. recently reported 96 patients with microinvasive cancer with 5 mm or less invasion and a 10% incidence of positive groin nodes.[9] If the lesion is anaplastic or invades lymphatics or vessels, groin dissection is still recommended in microinvasive cancer of more than 2 mm invasion at the present time.

Planning the therapy for invasive squamous cell carcinoma of the vulva involves excision of the primary, management of the groin nodes, and therapy for pelvic lymph nodes (Figures 12.5 through 12.18).

Excision of the Primary

In all invasive vulvar cancers perform a radical vulvectomy extending from the skin of the labial crural folds inward and include sufficient skin and soft tissues to allow free margin about the tumor. While most vulvar cancers arise laterally on the labium majora, some advanced lesions involve the bladder or rectum. Vulvectomy with proctectomy or exenteration may be needed. Although in the older literature Boronow noted only 16% survivors with stage III and IV vulvar cancers, more recent reports suggest improved survival.[13] Increasing the amount of irradiation therapy and reducing the amount of tissue surgically excised has produced better 5-year survival rates as well.[12] Although the advisability of lymph node dissec-

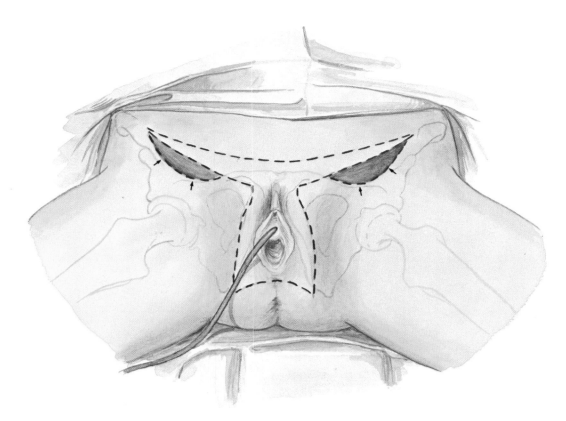

FIGURE 12.5. Planning of excision of the primary lesion and regional nodes begins with evaluation of the clinical extent of the disease to assure its complete excision as well as closure of the primary incision. The incision for inguinal lymphadenectomy begins 2 cm inferior and medial to the anterior superior iliac spine.

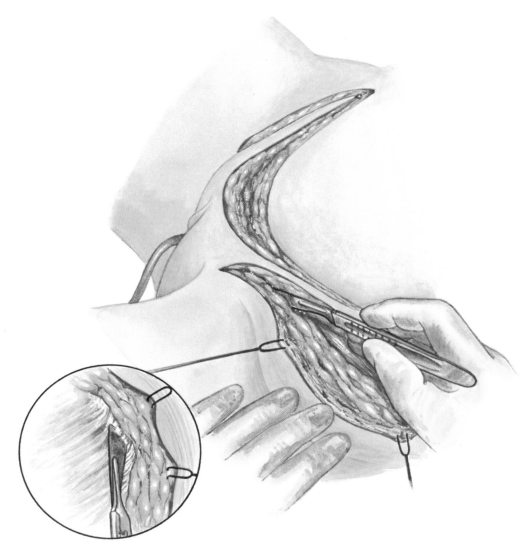

FIGURE 12.6.   Place the patient in the supine position with the legs slightly flexed and the hips rotated outward. Drape the patient with multiple sterile half-sheets, allowing for repositioning of the patient for the vulvectomy. Prepare the perineal field last, and place sterile sheets under the patient. Begin the skin incision 2 cm inferior and medial to the anterior superior iliac spine and curve it down to a point 2 to 3 cm above the symphysis. Make the lower incision outlined in Figure 12.5 parallel to and curving downward slightly toward the vulva. When N2 or N3 nodes are present, excise the overlying skin in continuity and cover it with a flap or graft. For lesions of the posterior vulva, bring the crescentic incision quite low over the mons to a point just superior to the base of the clitoris but retreat to the superior margin of the mons pubis for clitoral and anterior vulvar lesions. Similarly, the posterior limit of excision may advance to the lowest margin of the vagina with sparing of the perineal body and skin for an anterior vulvar lesion, while a posterior lesion may require excision of the perineal body or, on occasion, proctectomy. Inset: The plane of dissection is in the fine areolar tissue just anterior to the aponeurosis of the external oblique muscle and is entered with strong upward traction on the overlying tissues with skin hooks. Avoid unnecessary trauma to the flap edges and moisten them with saline intermittently. Ligate any bleeding perforators in the anterior abdominal wall and clamp the round ligament where it exits the ring of the abdominal wall.

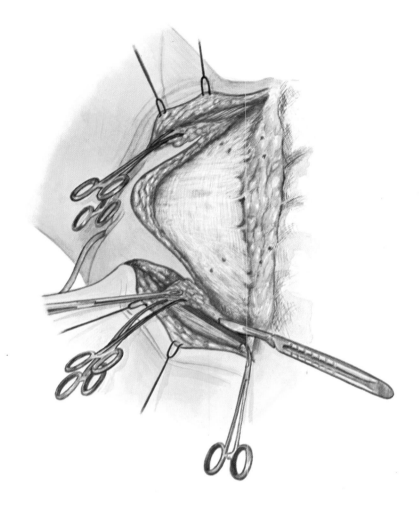

FIGURE 12.7. Extend the transverse crescentic incision to the rectus sheath and external oblique fascia, mobilized by the sharp dissection, avoiding trauma to skin edges. Palpate the course of the sartorius muscle laterally within the groin incision. Incise down to the medial margin of the sartorius muscle through its fascia to allow entrance to the plane of dissection deep to the femoral fascia across the femoral vessels. Carefully dissect at the upper lateral aspect of the incision medial and inferior to the anterior superior iliac spine to define the superficial circumflex iliac vessels, which are clamped, divided, and sutured. The medial pedicle of these vessels provides a point of traction as the sharp scalpel dissection proceeds medial to the sartorius muscle and across the femoral nerve. The origin of the circumflex iliac vessels must be identified on the lateral aspect of the femoral artery when this is reached.

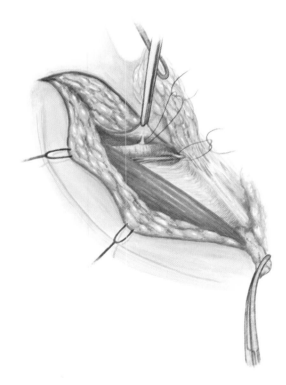

FIGURE 12.8. Palpate and identify the femoral artery. Dissect with the scalpel medially across the femoral artery as the deep femoral fascia is reflected medially. The superficial external pudendal artery is secured and its location is noted as the origin of the saphenous vein passing through the fossa ovalis is immediately adjacent. Isolate, secure, and divide both vessels.

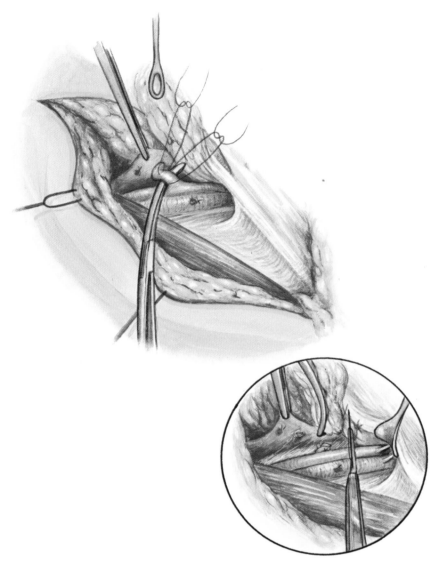

FIGURE 12.9. Suture the saphenous vein pedicle in such a fashion as to leave it flush with the wall of the vein to avoid the formation of a thrombus or turbulance, which would predispose to embolism. Incise the inferior margin of the specimen to expose the saphenous and possibly the accessory saphenous vein. Palpate the surrounding tissues to identify the induration of the accompanying lymphatics. Clamp, divide, and ligate both vein and lymphatics with 2-0 braided nylon in order to prevent persistent lymphatic drainage into the groin dissection, resulting in a lymphocutaneous fistula or lymphocele. Medial traction on the specimen allows sharp dissection across the pectinius fascia and medial branches from the femoral artery and vein to the pectineus muscle may be identified and preserved. After clamping and division of the round ligament, the specimen is advanced by sharp dissection across the fascia covering the pubis, and the specimen hangs dependent over the vulva. Carefully explore the femoral canal, placing the inguinal ligament on anterior traction to expose the inferior epigastric vessels arising from the most inferior limit of the external iliac vessels. Inset: The femoral lymphatics enter the femoral canal medial to the vein. Careful palpation will identify the lymphatic fat pad containing Cloquet's node. Extract the lymphatics, which are clipped at their upper limit and divided. Cloquet's node and any palpable and suspicious lymph nodes within the groin dissection are submitted for frozen section. In the absence of metastasis to either site, pelvic lymphadenectomy may be omitted.

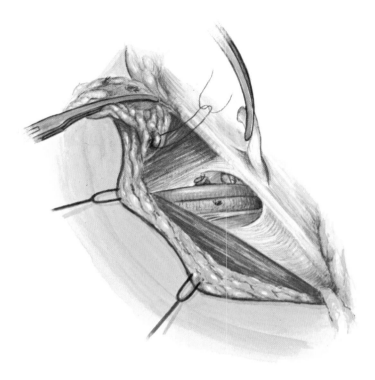

FIGURE 12.10. Continue the medial dissection in the pectineus fascia, then proceed to the medial inferior margin of the adductor longus, where the saphenous vein exits the femoral triangle. Ligate and transfix this vessel with 2-0 braided nylon and reflect the specimen medially.

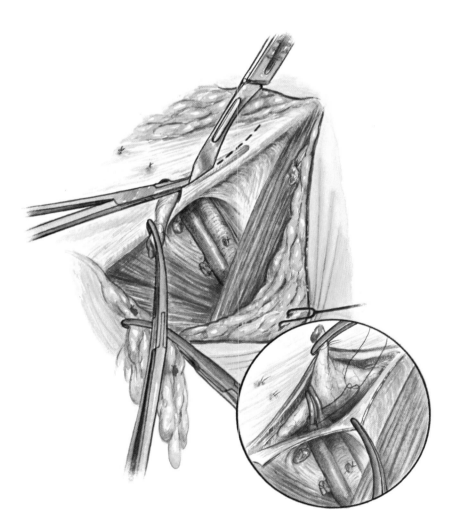

FIGURE 12.11. Extraperitoneal node dissection is indicated when metastasis to the groin or Cloquet's node is present. Initiate this dissection by placing the round ligament in traction. Insert a Coller clamp into the inguinal canal and incise the overlying muscle and fascia. Place the inferior fascial margin and round ligament in traction while identifying the origin of the inferior epigastric vessels from the external iliac artery and vein. Inset: Ligate and divide these vessels with 3-0 braided nylon. Traction on the round ligament results in medial traction on the peritoneum, exposing the extraperitoneal space.

109

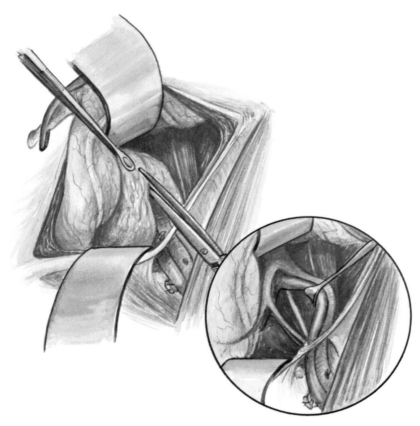

FIGURE 12.12.   Blunt dissection separates the peritoneum medially
This measure, plus traction of the bladder, allows exposure of the
course of the external iliac vessels and of the obturator fossae to the
level of the common iliac artery and vein. Place a fiberoptic light
source into the wound. Begin the lymph node dissection laterally
on the illiacus fascia medial to the genitofemoral nerve. Reflect the
lymph node specimen medially across the vessels with care to preserve the origin of the deep circumflex iliac artery and vein just
superior to the inguinal ligament and note the possibility of an
aberrant obturator vein on the medial aspect of the external iliac
vein just superior to the inguinal ligament. Inset: Lift the external
iliac upward with a vein retractor. Identify the site of transection
of the lymphatics passing through the femoral canal and reflect this
medially and superiorly as the specimen is removed from the obturator
fossae. Identify the obturator nerve and the artery and vein lying
deep to the nerve. Identify the ureter on the peritoneal reflection
retracted medially as the lymphatic specimen is dissected from the
obturator fossae and up the course of the iliac vessels to the bifurcation. Be alert for an anomalous iliac vein. Further traction superiorly
will allow for extensive palpation and dissection lateral to the common iliac vessels, but this is not usually indicated. Secure hemostasis
with 4-0 braided nylon or clips. Place a sump suction drain into the
bed of dissection via a stab incision superior to the surgical incision
in order to ensure adequate dependent drainage. All nodal tissue
from the common iliac to the distal margin of the femoral triangle
should now be excised close to the incision in the external oblique
with 2-0 braided nylon.

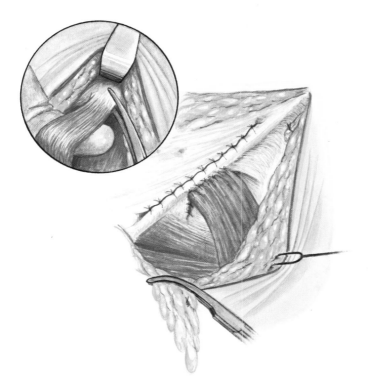

FIGURE 12.13.   Unless a myocutaneous flap is to be used for closure of the groin defect, the transposition of the sartorius muscle to cover the femoral vessels should be carried out following closure of the incision along the course of the inguinal canal. Insert a finger beneath the sartorius muscle and incise the fascia lata on the lateral aspect of this muscle. With retraction to expose the easily palpable anterior superior iliac spine, the sartorius muscle may be traced to its tendinous insertion to this spine; transect the tendon from the bone. Inset: Place the muscle in gentle medial traction and incise the fascial attachments laterally with care to preserve the blood supply that enters on the medial deep surface of the muscle. Mobilize the muscle until its tendinous insertion reaches the inguinal ligament overlying the femoral vessels. Close the femoral canal to prevent postoperative femoral herniation with 2-0 braided nylon and suture the tendinous insertion of the sartorius muscle to the inferior margin of the inguinal ligament with braided nylon or absorbable suture.

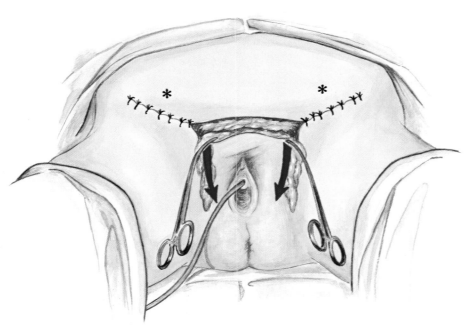

FIGURE 12.14.   Initiate closure of the groin incisions by suturing of the superficial fascia of superior and inferior skin flaps to the underlying muscle and fascia in such a fashion as to oppose skin edges as closely as possible while obliterating underlying dead space. Avoid suturing margins of skin and fascia directly to one another as this creates a "bridge" with underlying dead space in which fluid accumulation may occur. Bring all suction catheters out the upper abdominal wall, never through the lower flap. Prior to fascial closure, underlying suction drains are placed through stab incisions. Following the wide excision of skin overlying the groin, as will be necessary in the presence of clinically suspicious or positive nodes or following preoperative irradiation, the use of myocutaneous flaps or primary skin grafts is necessary for closure of the wound defect.

111

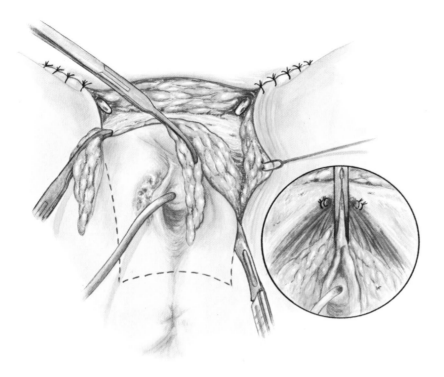

FIGURE 12.15. Planning of the vulvar incision has allowed for adequate margins of excision of the primary lesion as well as skin, adipose tissue, and lymphatics medial to the labiocrural fold to encompass pathways of metastasis. Blunt digital dissection beneath the labiocrural folds along the pectineus and adductor fascia undermines and mobilizes the lateral extent of the vulvectomy specimen. Scalpel incision of the skin completes definition of the line of excision. Use the cautery to significantly decrease blood loss in dissection of the underlying tissues directly down to the level of the fascia. Reflect the specimen inferiorly by sharp dissection across the pubis to identify the base of the clitoris and insertions of the bulbocavernosis muscles lateral to this structure. Inset: Each vessel is clamped, divided, and sutured. Take particular care to secure the dorsal vein of the clitoris passing beneath the pubic symphysis.

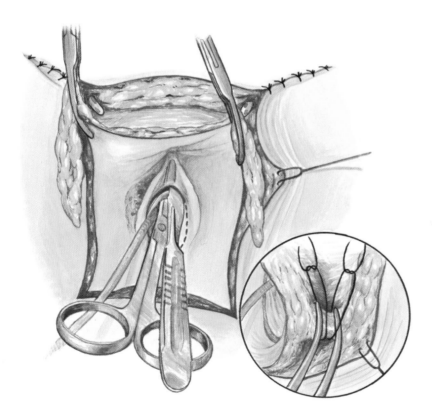

FIGURE 12.16. Sacrifice the distal third of the urethra for lesions in proximity to this structure. Otherwise, preserve the urethra by incising approximately 1 cm anterior to the meatus. Define a plane of dissection at this point to the deep fascia and pubic symphysis. Incise and mobilize the lateral margins of the vulvectomy specimen. Inset: Identify the perineal branches of the external pudendal artery on the posterior lateral and deep aspect of the vulvectomy specimen and secure these with 2-0 braided nylon. Proceed from the anterior point of vulvectomy incision anterior to the urethral meatus to incise along the introitus or vagina. The initial incision line should be contralateral to the malignant lesion in order that the vulvectomy specimen may be mobilized and the vaginal margin adjacent to the vulvar lesion clearly visualized.

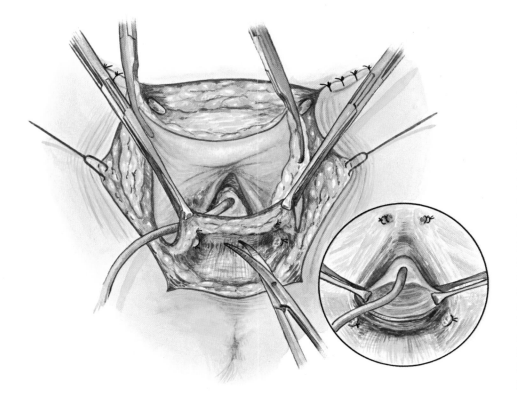

FIGURE 12.17. Incise the posterior line of excision to the transverse perineus muscle and fascia while reflecting the specimen anteriorly. Mobilize the vagina from the rectum for an adequate margin for incision of the lesion and for utilization of some of the posterior vagina for closure of the perineal defect. Inset: Following excision of the specimen, mobilization of the vaginal margins fascilitates subsequent closure. Have the pathologist examine the specimen for adequacy of deep margins. Secure hemostasis with 3-0 absorbable suture ligatures and cautery. Suture the levator muscle into the midline to strengthen the perineum.

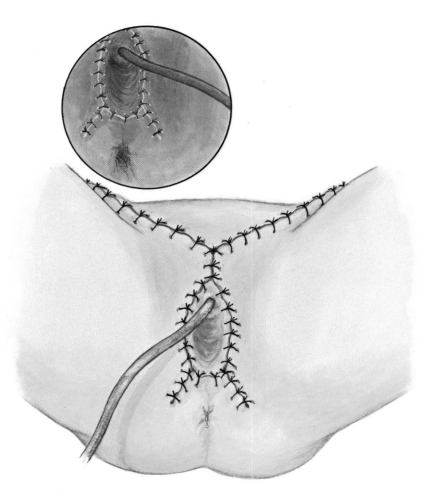

FIGURE 12.18. Assure hemostasis and place suction tubes beneath lateral skin flaps mobilized from the medial aspect of the thigh. Closure of the wound defect should avoid undue tension on the suture lines, which may necessitate primary or delayed split-thickness skin graft, use of relaxing incisions, pedicle skin grafts, or myocutaneous flaps for closure in more extended cases. Use interrupted 3-0 monofilament nylon sutures. Inset: Inject the patient with 3 to 5 ml of fluorescein on completion of skin closure and observe under Wood's light. Areas of nonviability which fail to fluoresce should be excised, revised, or grafted. Do not use pressure on delicate wound edges. Instead, rely on suction drains to remove fluid and obliterate dead space.

tions is a controversial issue, all authors agree that complete excision of the primary vulvar lesion is mandatory if therapy is to be successful. It makes little sense to spend 2 to 4 hr on bilateral groin and pelvic lymph node dissections for sites where disease might possibly be, and then expend only a few minutes on the most important phase of treatment where disease is most assuredly present. The local control of the primary cancer is essential for successful vulvar cancer treatment.

Inguinal Lymphadenectomy

On the basis of a large collected series of cases, 13% of clinically palpable, but not suspicious, lymph nodes (NoNl) contain occult cancer.[4] Large firm mobile nodes (N2) contain metastatic cancer 70% of the time, and 90% of fixed confluent or ulcerated nodes (N3) contain metastatic cancer. Fundamental treatment of invasive cancer of the vulva therefore includes resection of the inguinal nodes. This resection is rarely omitted, and then only in those patients in whom the added operating time is a serious threat to life.

As lymph nodes fill with cancer the collateral lymphatics fill and widespread retrograde metastases occur. While unsuspicious nodes (NoNl) are rarely associated with recurrence in the operative site, in patients with N2 or N3 nodes cancer recurs in the groin incision 40% or more of the time.[4] Therefore, if a large suspicious node is present, obtain a percutaneous needle biopsy. If the results are positive, the author prefers to perform an extraperitoneal exploration (Schellhas technique), as well as an examination of the peritoneal cavity and abdominal organs.

In the absence of abdominal disease, begin an extensive course of radiation therapy that includes 5,000 rads midplane to the pelvis and 5,000 rads at a depth of 0.5 cm in the groin. Vulvectomy and groin dissection with compound myocutaneous flaps based on the gracilis or tensor fascia lata are then performed (Figures 12.19 through 12.23). Improved control of disease and wound healing have been observed with this technique. These pedicle flaps bring an intact blood supply to a vascular bed compromised by irradiation and are integral to the healing of the groin wounds.

It is sometimes suggested that in poor-risk patients groin dissection should be delayed awaiting the clinical appearance of metastasis. Morley showed absolute 5-year survival rates of 60% with radical vulvectomy alone, as compared to 85% with radical vulvectomy and groin dissection.[10] Furthermore, there is a 20% higher rate of incisional recurrence when metastasis becomes clinically overt. In addition, the 80% to 90% 5-year survival with occult nodal metastasis drops to less than 50% after removal of clinically suspicious or positive lymph nodes. Finally, the risk of positive pelvic nodes is minimal with N0 or Nl nodes, but where nodal metastasis is larger, the possiblity of spread to distant sites outside the planned treatment field is greatly increased.

Pelvic Lymphadenectomy

Pelvic lymphadenectomy is selectively employed in vulvar cancer where a significant probability of pelvic nodal metastasis exists. Metastasis to the pelvic lymph nodes bypassing the inguinal lymphatics occurs in less than 3% of patients, so that the clinical status of the inguinal nodes accurately reflects the probability of pelvic lymph node metastasis. Of 85 patients who underwent pelvic lymphadenectomy, 10 of 11 patients with positive pelvic lymph nodes had clinically suspicious N2 or positive N3 inguinal nodes prior to surgery.[4] The remaining patient had a metastasis to Cloquet's node within the femoral canal. Of the 50 patients with negative Cloquet's nodes none had pelvic metastasis at lymphadenectomy or at subsequent follow-up. Of 5 patients with positive Cloquet's nodes (the highest of the groin nodes medial to the femoral vein), 2 had pelvic lymph node metastasis.

Additional information is obtained at the time of inguinal lymphadenectomy. The presence or absence of enlarged nodes within the specimen is valuable information in determining the risk of pelvic metastasis. Obtain frozen sections of any enlarged nodes in the specimen as well as both Cloquet's nodes. If any are positive the patient should have a pelvic lymphadenectomy. The absolute survival rate after positive pelvic lymphadenectomy is 12.5% to 25%.[4]

As surgery cures only 20% of the 16% of patients who have pelvic metastasis, very few patients benefit from routine pelvic lymphadenectomy.[15] Recognition of the factors that increase the risk of metastasis to pelvic lymph nodes and selective pelvic lymphadenectomy is a better approach to treatment.

Success in surgical management of vulvar abnormalities depends on precise diagnosis, study of the anatomic pathways of spread, careful design of the excisional procedure, and the use of the newer reconstructive techniques to minimize the disabilities produced by the surgical excision.

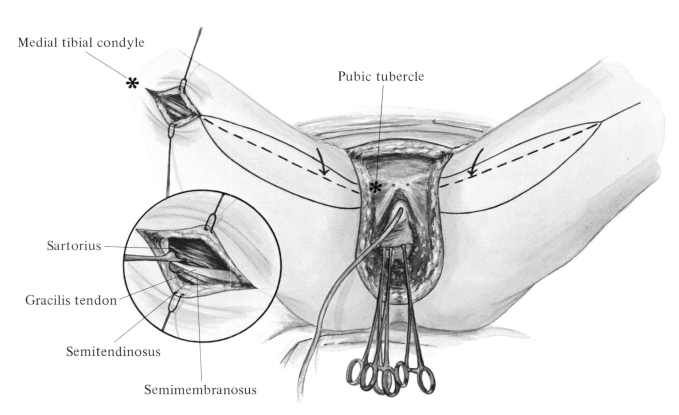

FIGURE 12.19. The gracilis muscle flap technique as performed by Dr. Foad Nahai, Assistant Professor of Plastic Surgery, Emory University Clinic. The gracilis muscle lies below a line drawn from the pubic tubercle to the medial tibial condyle.* The associated myocutaneous unit is outlined. The blood supply enters from the ascending branch of the medial femoral circumflex branch of the profunda femoris artery (arrow). Inset: Incise above the knee and identify the tendon of the gracilis between the sartorius anteriorly and the fascia of the semimembranosus posteriorly. Pull downward on the tendon, identify the overlying skin island, and outline it with a marking pen.

115

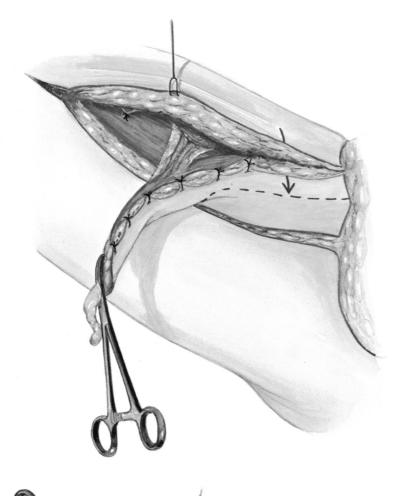

FIGURE 12.20. Cut the gracilis tendon, begin to elevate the flap distally, and incise inferiorly along the outline of the unit through the skin and fascia. Identify and ligate the two inferior vascular pedicles, which are branches of the superficial femoral artery. Preserve the vessels indicated at the arrow. Suture the skin to the underlying muscle with absorbable suture.

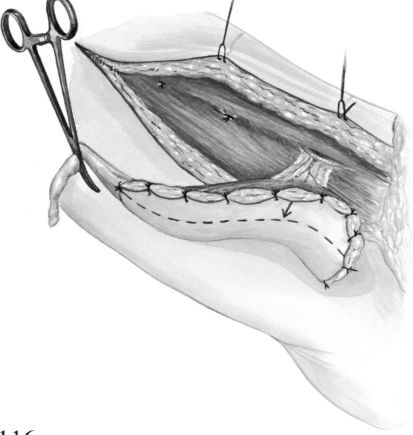

FIGURE 12.21. Carry the dissection sharply to the major vascular pedicle, which emerges deep to the adductor longus and enters the gracilis on its medial surface. Preserve this artery and its accompanying vein, the ascending branch of the medial circumflex. Complete the dissection. The flap is now free to close large defects of the vulva and groin. Approximate the thigh incision with 3-0 absorbable and 3-0 nylon sutures in the skin. Suture the flap in position, avoiding excess tension or injury to the vascular pedicle.

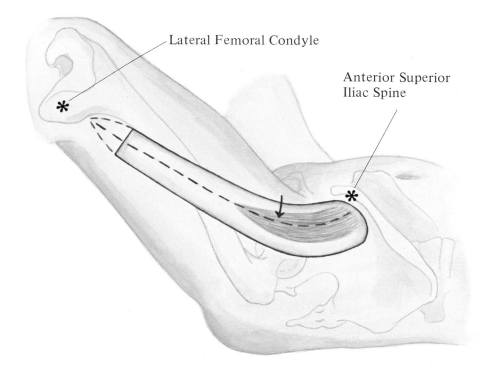

Lateral Femoral Condyle

Anterior Superior
Iliac Spine

FIGURE 12.22. When lateral coverage is needed, the tensor fascia lata flap may be chosen. While mostly tendon, this small muscle has an excellent blood supply to the skin from the profunda femoris (arrow) along the entire length of the flap. Identify the anterior superior iliac spine and the lateral femoral condyle. Identify the tendon and clamp it. Mark the skin margin with a pen and, beginning distally, incise through skin and fascia and elevate the flap, which will be 6 to 10 cm in width along its entire length.

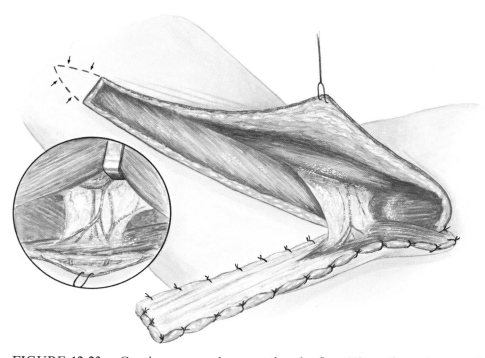

FIGURE 12.23. Continue upward, separating the flap. Blunt dissection may be used as there are no perforators. Dissect the muscle sharply from the gluteus minimus and suture the skin edges to the fascia. Inset: The vascular pedicle lies deep to the rectus femoris and enters the tensor fascia lata on the medial aspect. The lateral femoral circumflex artery supplies the tensor fascia lata and divides into three branches before entering the muscle. Note the skin hook exposing the abundant perforation providing excellent blood supply to the skin. If this flap is to be rotated under an existing skin bridge, excise skin and leave subcutaneous tissue to preserve perforators. Rotate the flap at the pedicle to cover large groin or vulvar defects. Trim the distal end and close with 3-0 absorbable suture and 3-0 nylon in the skin approximating the defect.

References

1. Boehm, F., and Morris, McL. J.: Paget's disease and apocrine gland carcinoma of the vulva. *Obstet. Gynecol.* **38**:185–192, 1971.
2. DiSaia, P.H., Rutledge, F., and Smith, J.P.: Sarcoma of the vulva—Report of 12 patients. *Obstet. Gynecol.* **38**:180–184, 1971.
3. Forney, J.P., Morrow, C.P., Townsend, D.E., et al.: Management of carcinoma in situ of the vulva. *Am. J. Obstet. Gynecol.* **127**:801–806, 1977.
4. Franklin, E.W., and Rutledge, F.D.: Prognostic factors in epidermoid carcinoma of the vulva. *Obstet. Gynecol.* **37**:892–901, 1971.
5. Japaze, H., Garcia-Bunnuel, R., and Woodruff, J.D.: Primary vulvar neoplasia—A review of in situ and invasive carcinoma. *Obstet. Gynecol.* **49**:404–411, 1977.
6. Jasionowski, E.A., and Jasionowski, P.: Topical progesterone in treatment of vulvar dystrophy. *Am. J. Obstet. Gynecol.* **127**:667–670, 1977.
7. Jones, D.P.: Lymphatics of the vulva. *J. Obstet. Gynaecol. Br. Commonw.* **70**:751–765, 1963.
8. Julian, C.G., Callison, J., and Woodruff, J.D.: Plastic management of extensive vulvar defects. *Obstet. Gynecol.* **38**:193–198, 1971.
9. Magrina, J.F., Webb, M.J, Gaffey, T.A., et al.: Stage I squamous cell cancer of the vulva—Prognostic factors and treatment. Central Association Meeting, Kansas City, Missouri, 1978.
10. Morley, G.W.: Infiltrative carcinoma of the vulva: Results of surgical treatment. *Am. J. Obstet. Gynecol.* **124**:874–888, 1976.
11. Report of the Committee on Terminology: New nomenclature for vulvar disease. Proposal of the International Society for the Study of Vulvar Disease. *Obstet. Gynecol.* **47**:122–124, 1976.
12. Rutledge, F., Boronow, R.C., and Wharton, J.T.: *Gynecologic Oncology.* New York, Wiley, 1976.
13. Thornton, W.N., and Flanagan, W.C.: Pelvic exenteration in the treatment of advanced malignancy of the vulva. *Am. J. Obstet. Gynecol.* **117**:774–781, 1973.
14. Wharton, T.J., Gallager, S., and Rutledge, F.N.: Microinvasive carcinoma of the vulva. *Am. J. Obstet. Gynecol.* **118**:159–162, 1974.
15. Yazigi, R., Piver, M.S., and Tsukada, Y.: Microinvasive carcinoma of the vulva. *Obstet. Gynecol.* **51**:368–370, 1978.

Selected Bibliography

Chung, A.F., Woodruff, J.N., and Lewis, J.L.: Malignant melanoma of the vulva: A report of 44 cases. *Obstet. Gynecol.* **45**:638, 1975.

Green, T.H., Ulfelder, H., and Meigs, J.V.: Epidermoid carcinoma of the vulva: An analysis of 238 cases. Part I, Etiology and diagnosis. Part II, Therapy and end results. *Am. J. Obstet. Gynecol.* **75**:848–864, 1958.

Julian, C.G., Callison, J., and Woodruff, J.D.: Plastic management of extensive vulvar defects. *Obstet. Gynecol.* **38**:193–198, 1971.

McAdams, A.J., and Kistner, R.W.: The relationship of chronic vulvar disease, leukoplakia, and carcinoma in situ to carcinoma of the vulva. *Cancer* **11**:740–757, 1958.

Merrill, J.A., and Ross, N.L.: Cancer of the vulva. *Cancer* **14**:13–20, 1961.

Piver, M.S., and Xynos, F.P.: Pelvic lymphadenectomy in women with carcinoma of the clitoris. *Obstet. Gynecol.* **49**:592, 1977.

Rutledge, F., Smith, J.P., and Franklin, E.W.: Carcinoma of the vulva. *Am. J. Obstet. Gynecol.* **124**:874, 1976.

Schellhas, H.F.: Extra peritoneal periaortic nodes dissection through an upper abdominal incision. *Obstet. Gynecol.* **46**:444–447, 1975.

Shingleton, H.M., Fowler, W.C., Palumbo, L., et al.: Carcinoma of the vulva: influence of radical operation on cure rate. *Obstet. Gynecol.* **35**:106, 1970.

Way, S.A.: *Malignant Disease of the Female Genital Tract*. Philadelphia, Blakiston, 1951.

Way, S.A.: Carcinoma of the vulva. Guest lecture, Society of Gynecologic Oncologists, Jan. 1974.

Abdominal Surgery

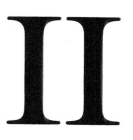

Total Abdominal Hysterectomy 13

Hysterectomy is one of the most common operations performed in the United States. The Commission on Professional and Hospital Activities estimates that 787,000 hysterectomies were performed in 1975; 1,700 women died in association with this procedure and approximately 80,000 women were morbid postoperatively.[12] Attention to specific detail greatly decreases the morbidity from this operation and this chapter will outline precise measures to minimize injury to the adjacent structures and tissue trauma during total abdominal hysterectomy (Figure 13.1).

Blood Supply

Arteries

The primary blood supply to the uterus is the uterine artery, which arises either as a separate branch of the internal iliac or more likely as a branch of the superior vesical artery (Figure 13.2). The uterine artery runs anteriorly and medially across the top of the cardinal ligament over the ureter, to which it gives a small branch and then divides into cervical, vaginal, and coporal branches. A lesser but important source of blood supply to the uterus are the ovarian arteries, which arise from the anterior surface of the aorta and travel down through the infundibulopelvic ligaments along with the ovarian veins. The superior vesical artery, which arises at the termination of the anterior segment of the hypogastric system, is the primary blood supply to the bladder. As mentioned above, the uterine vessel is frequently a branch of this vessel. The superior vesical artery gives branches to the vagina, and several vesical branches leave it medially as it courses along the lateral side of the bladder to become the umbilical ligament. An easy way to demonstrate this vessel is to grasp the corner of the bladder peritoneum with an Allis clamp and hold it anteriorly on tension; the artery will be seen as a fold in the peritoneum. Once this anterior peritoneum is opened, the area lateral to the superior vesical artery is the paravesical space and the tissue medial to it includes the bladder.

The common iliac artery runs diagonally across the pelvic brim and ends as the internal iliac system and external iliac artery. The latter vessel has no branches in the pelvis, except perhaps muscular branches to the

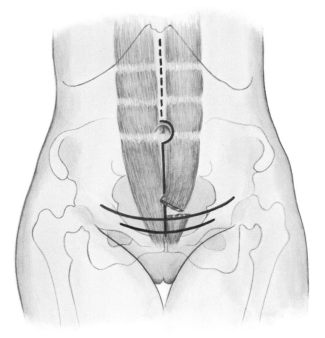

FIGURE 13.1. Basic bony landmarks for the usual incisions in gynecologic surgery.

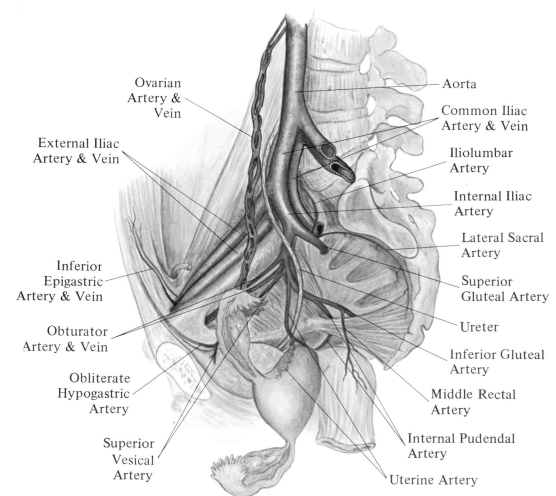

Ovarian Artery & Vein

External Iliac Artery & Vein

Inferior Epigastric Artery & Vein

Obturator Artery & Vein

Obliterate Hypogastric Artery

Superior Vesical Artery

Aorta

Common Iliac Artery & Vein

Iliolumbar Artery

Internal Iliac Artery

Lateral Sacral Artery

Superior Gluteal Artery

Ureter

Inferior Gluteal Artery

Middle Rectal Artery

Internal Pudendal Artery

Uterine Artery

FIGURE 13.2. Common pattern of arterial blood supply to the pelvis. Great variability exists, however, and many major and minor variations have been observed. Observe that all pelvic arteries arise from the internal iliac with the exception of the superior rectal, which arises from the inferior mesenteric and the ovarian and median sacral arteries from the aorta.

124

psoas muscle, until the distal portion of the artery is reached, where the circumflex iliac artery arises and goes laterally. Just as the vessel exits under the inguinal ligament the inferior epigastric artery arises from the anterior medial surface and runs medially and superiorly over the anterior abdominal wall peritoneum.

The pelvic ureter receives branches from the ovarian artery and a branch from the internal iliac. This small vessel arises approximately 2 cm from the origin of the internal iliac artery and leaves the artery on its medial anterior surface. It is important to recognize this vessel and preserve it as it is the major source of blood supply to the pelvic ureter. The uterine artery gives a small branch to the ureter as it crosses over and this may be sacrificed. The ureter also receives several branches as it nears the bladder from the vesical system and these likewise may be sacrificed. Occasionally, in older patients, the arteries may lose their elasticity and the vessel lengthens. This occurs occasionally in the pelvis as serpiginous common, external, and internal iliac arteries.

Collaterals

The collateral vessels of the pelvis are extensive and of diffuse origin. The anterior division of the internal iliac artery anastomoses with its counterpart from the opposite side, except for the inconstant middle rectal artery; it anastomoses with the superior rectal from the inferior mesenteric and the inferior rectal from the internal pudendal artery. More sizable anastomoses occur with the posterior division of the internal iliac artery; the superior gluteal anastomoses with the circumflex branch of the femoral artery, the lateral sacral anastomoses with the middle sacral from the aorta, and the iliolumbar anastomoses with the lumbar artery from the aorta. With these rich collateral blood supplies, simple internal iliac artery ligation will fail to control pelvic hemorrhage, as illustrated when one ligates both anterior divisions and cuts the uterine artery and then observes the extensive blood flow that remains through the pelvis. Obviously, internal iliac artery ligation is no substitute for careful identification, isolation, and ligation of a bleeding pelvic vessel.

Veins

The uterine veins leave the uterus laterally and may surround the uterine artery. They travel along the surface and through the substance of the cardinal ligament to enter the pelvic wall plexus and eventually the internal iliac venous system. The ovarian, tubal, and part of the uterine venous blood drains out the infundibulopelvic ligament through multiple veins that ultimately unite and drain into the vena cava on the right and the renal vein on the left. The common iliac vein is formed by the external iliac vein and the internal iliac venous system, which is very variable. The major branch lies lateral and below the artery and drains the cardinal ligament. The circumflex iliac vein generally goes over the external iliac artery but occasionally may go under that vessel. In approximately one-third of cases the obturator vein, instead of following the course of the obturator nerve and artery, turns superiorly just after it enters through the obturator foramen and enters the inferior medial side of the external iliac vein. Watch for this vein during obturator node dissection. Part of the venous drainage from the bladder is included in the lateral cervicovesical ligament, which arises from the corner of the bladder base and enters into the lateral third of the cardinal ligament.

The most difficult bleeding to control in pelvic surgery is venous, and it is probable that most operative deaths from hemorrhage are from venous sources. Most venous bleeders can be isolated and either clamped, clipped, or sutured with adequate exposure and suction. Some, however, will require pelvic packs. Packing of a diffuse venous bleed and proceeding to the opposite side will save significant operating time and produce surprisingly good hemostasis.

One area where pelvic bleeding may be impossible to control with conventional methods is the junction of the gluteal veins and the internal iliac vein. These veins, if torn, may produce bleeding of sizable proportions and may be almost impossible to isolate. In some instances, suture of the adjoining structures, including the sciatic nerve, may be necessary to prevent exsanguination.

Nerves

The sympathetic system descends lateral to the great vessels in the abdomen and forms a plexus over the area of bifurcation of the vena cava, courses over the sacral promontory, divides and follows the uterosacral ligaments to enter the uterus, and continues anteriorly to enter the bladder. The parasympathetic nerves on both sides arise from the upper sacral foramina and transverse the deep portion of the uterosacral ligament on both sides of the rectum to enter the uterus, penetrate through the cardinal ligament, and enter the bladder through the lateral cervicovesical ligament. The genitofemoral nerve runs along the surface of the psoas muscle adjacent and parallel to the lateral surface of the external iliac artery and should be preserved during the lymphadenectomy. Remember that the femoral nerve runs through the substance of the psoas muscle in its pelvic portion; therefore, avoid placing self-retaining retractors laterally on this muscle as they may produce pressure and femoral nerve paralysis.

The obturator nerve appears from the area lateral to the hypogastric vein and artery, transverses the lateral pelvis through the lateral paravesical fossa, and exits through the obturator foramen. It is accompanied by the obturator vessels. The nerve is several millimeters in diameter and easily identified.

Ligaments

Uterosacral
The uterosacral ligaments are broad structures containing primarily fibrous tissue, some smooth muscle, autonomic nerves, and, in their lower portions, small arterioles from the hemorrhoidal vessels. They encircle the lateral rectum to enter the upper vagina and cervix medially, while the lateral fibers join the posterior sweep of the cardinal ligaments. Until one dissects the entire system of uterosacral ligaments, it is difficult to appreciate their broad superior–inferior attachment to the sacrum and uterus–vagina.

Cardinal
The cardinal ligaments arise from the cervix and upper third of the vagina —actually more of the cardinal ligament is attached to the vagina than to the cervix. They sweep laterally and posteriorly to attach to the fascia that covers the sciatic plexus. Keep this in mind if there is bleeding at the base of the cardinal ligaments as deep sutures may injure the sciatic plexus.

The cardinal ligaments are made up of condensed bands of fibrous tissue, uterine and vaginal veins, lymphatics, and autonomic nerves. The cervix and vagina are covered anteriorly and posteriorly by a rather dense fascia, which cancer usually only penetrates late in its course. However, the fascia is incomplete laterally at the attachment of the uterosacral and cardinal ligaments; thus the tumor finds its way laterally into the parametria. The parametria is made up of the uterosacral and cardinal ligaments and their attachments. The cardinal ligament divides the paravesical space from the pararectal space.

Bladder Pillars

The medial bladder pillar runs from the anterior surface of the cervix across the upper vagina onto the base of the bladder and contains a small artery.

The lateral bladder pillar (lateral cervical vaginal ligament) is a lateral extension of the medial bladder pillar and arises from the lateral corner of the base of the bladder and swings laterally to join the outer third of the cardinal ligament. In this structure are a large plexus of vesical veins as well as the entrance and exit of the autonomic nervous system of the bladder along with some ganglia.

Spaces

There are two important spaces that must be developed to adequately dissect the lateral pelvic wall, the paravesical space anteriorly and the pararectal space posteriorly. The paravesical space is bound medially by the bladder, anteriorly by the obturator foramen and superior ramus of the pubis, laterally by the obturator internus muscle and the pelvic wall vessels, and posteriorly by the cardinal ligament. Its floor is the junction of the obturator internus muscle and levator ani. Approach it by separating the superior vesical artery from the external iliac vein and artery just anterior to the round ligament and then dissect it inferiorly down toward the pelvic floor, where there is loose areolar tissue (Figure 13.3). Once this space is

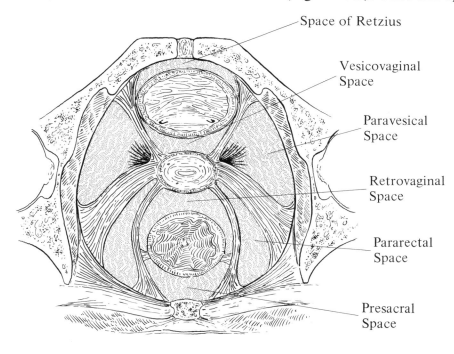

Space of Retzius

Vesicovaginal Space

Paravesical Space

Retrovaginal Space

Pararectal Space

Presacral Space

FIGURE 13.3. The pelvic spaces are filled with areolar tissue, as shown by the stippling; they are exposed through traction and the deep placement of retractors.

127

opened, the bladder is pushed medially and the space is well developed. The area anteriorly and laterally is called the obturator fossa.

The pararectal space is bound medially by the rectum. It is bound laterally by the connective tissue and fascia overlying the sciatic nerve and its divisions, and the venous system of the hypogastric vein. Posteriorly it is bound by the sacral hollow and anteriorly by the cardinal ligament. Its floor is the levator ani muscle and the hollow of the sacrum. Enter the space by dissecting medially along the hypogastric artery and pushing the rectum medially, being careful not to sever the artery to the ureter from the hypogastric artery. The uterosacral ligaments will be on its medial wall.

The alterations in the intraperitoneal space caused by pelvic inflammatory disease, endometriosis, and irradiation of malignant disease may distort the anatomical findings. The surgeon may usually depend, however, on a standard anatomical relationship in the extraperitoneal space and the author recommends this basic approach in gynecologic surgery. As a result of the embryonic development of the female genitalia, round ligaments are a constant structure and are easily found. On dividing the round ligaments and proceeding initially to the extraperitoneal space in abdominal hysterectomy, a ready reference with easy landmarks will be found even in a patient with severe endometriosis with intense distortion of the intrapelvic findings. The peritoneal dissection should be lateral to the ovarian vessels as they enter the pelvis; they will be superior at all times to the ureter, which is easily isolated from them both by palpation and direct visualization. A small vessel extends below the round ligament, which on some patients requires brief cauterization to avoid staining the extraperitoneal space, and the dissection is made infinitely more simple by the avoidance of any staining through blood loss. Light, fine areolar tissue is an excellent surgical medium but blood-stained extraperitoneal tissue is of little advantage as an operative plane.

Remember that the only vessel in the pelvis that is spiral in its course is the uterine artery, aiding its easy identification. With traction anterior and cephalad on the uterus, the plane between the bladder and the uterus is easily found. Strong traction produces the planes in the pelvis and is an essential factor in any well done pelvic surgical procedure. Such tension should be planar in type, laying tissues out by layers in a flat surface so that they may be divided with a knife or scissors. Study of a well done radical neck dissection will aid in visualizing this vital maneuver as the structures are much easier to see in this procedure. On dissecting the bladder from the vagina, the plane will be found in the midline by dissecting down sharply toward the vagina. A few white fibers will be seen in this area, which is relatively avascular. Using this as a reference point, dissection may be carried downward in this plane with very little blood loss. There is another plane of equal use directly in front of the uterine arteries.

While many descriptions of hysterectomy techniques show dissection of the posterior pelvic peritoneum free of the vagina and cervix to achieve better mobilization of the ureters, a study of the ureters at the time of this dissection will show that they are little affected by this maneuver and all one achieves is additional bleeding. The ureters are best protected by direct visualization and palpation with the uterine arteries divided above the branch to the cervix. If the next clamp is placed medial to this tie, the ureters are free of the field. Uterosacral ligaments may be included in clamps as the procedure continues down the uterine side wall without their separate dissection. The plane between the rectum and the vagina is likewise avascular and is best entered with sharp dissection in the midline. Strong traction upward as well as directly downward on the rectum is useful. The avascular plane extends down the posterior vagina, allowing easy visualization of the anterior rectum.

Preoperative Evaluation

Major indications for abdominal hysterectomy include dysfunctional uterine bleeding, leiomyomas, pelvic inflammatory disease, adenocarcinoma of the endometrium, atypical adenomatous endometrial hyperplasia. carcinoma in situ of the endometrium, and uterine removal associated with adnexal or other pathology or urinary system surgery.

If dysfunctional uterine bleeding persists after diagnostic studies, endometrial biopsy and curettage, and the use of progesterone (the author prefers progesterone in oil), hysterectomy is often sought if the family is completed. While this can frequently be accomplished with ease by the vaginal approach, it may on occasion be desirable to perform the procedure abdominally. Leiomyomas may be present or the patient may have associated adnexal pathology, rendering abdominal excision a more satisfactory technique. Adenomyosis with associated bleeding may also be found. Removal of the ovaries is also recommended in the majority of these patients over 35.

Leiomyomas of the uterus greater than 8 weeks in size are best managed abdominally. Simple leiomyomas may be removed with myomectomy; however, if childbearing is complete, hysterectomy is the preferred procedure. The incidence of malignancy in leiomyomas is less than 1%[2]; however, the symptoms of pressure, increasing abdominal size, ureteral obstruction, or urinary pressure, or the association of menorrhagia may make hysterectomy the most reasonable method of handling this particular abnormality.

The uterus is usually removed with associated pelvic inflammatory disease as both tubes and ovaries are usually involved. Likewise, if both adnexae are removed for benign or malignant ovarian tumors, the uterus should be removed as well.

An additional indication for uterine removal is surgery for stress incontinence. Patients have better long-term results if the uterus is removed,[7] which should pose no problem if childbearing has been completed.

Adenocarcinoma of the endometrium is a common indication for uterine and ovarian removal. The treatment for endometrial cancer is biphasic, and radiation therapy is an integral part of it. In stage I endometrial cancer the author prefers to first remove the uterus and then, following surgical staging, treat the patient with radiation therapy. Therapy may be irradiation of either the total pelvis or vaginal ovoids, depending on the findings.

Diagnosis of the abnormalities is usually obtained with careful pelvic examination, vaginal cytology, and a well done endometrial suction curettage. Patients with abnormal bleeding must be carefully studied prior to abdominal hysterectomy to make certain that they do not have an undetected cervical, endocervical, or endometrial cancer. Biopsy any cervix of abnormal appearance and always obtain endometrial tissue as endometrial cytology is misleading.

There is little rationale for simple hysterectomy in the management of invasive carcinoma of the cervix; however, early microinvasive cancer of the cervix is well managed with simple abdominal hysterectomy. Christopherson et al. reported 111 patients with microinvasive carcinoma of the cervix with unequivocal invasion to a depth of up to 5 mm.[4] The majority were followed 10 years or longer; 1 patient was lost to follow-up. Of these 110 patients, including 79 treated by simple hysterectomy, none died of cancer of the cervix. Lymphatic or vascular-like space invasion did not affect prognosis. Intense pathological study of adequate amounts of tissue is essential to arrive at an accurate preoperative diagnosis. There is little justification for unexpected extensive invasive carcinoma in the hysterectomy specimen.

Operative Strategy

Place a Foley catheter in the patient and prepare the patient with a Betadine vaginal and abdominal preparation. Exposure is obtained in most instances with traction upward from the true pelvis.

Venous bleeding is greatly decreased through the use of appropriate traction, properly chosen instruments, and suture material as described in Chapter 3. The author prefers the Masterson clamp for use in the paracervical tissues and for grasping the pelvic tissues. This clamp has fine nontraumatic teeth that hold tissue quite satisfactorily. The usual clamps available, such as the Heaney, Ochsner, and Kocher clamps, are needlessly traumatic and produce an unnecessary amount of dead devitalized tissue, as discussed in Chapter 3. Suture material needs to only be as strong as the situation requires and should promote the least tissue reaction. The author recommends fine 3-0 Vicryl in the pelvis on the medium size nontraumatic needle, 2-0 and 3-0 chromic catgut, or 2-0 or 3-0 braided nylon for suture material inside the pelvis. Absorbable suture should be used to close the vagina and in the cardinal ligaments; the remainder of the sutures may be 3-0 braided nylon without significant risk of suture extrusion to the vaginal cuff.

Bleeding from the bladder may be controlled with cauterization or fine ties of 3-0 Vicryl or gut. Avitene is a most useful adjunct if numerous small bleeders are present deep in the pelvis, but the areas should be relatively dry before it is placed. It is best placed with an open 4 × 4 sponge directly over it and pressure is applied for 2 min after its application. Remove any excess Avitene before closure.

Another useful instrument is the flexible fiberoptic light source that may be placed directly in the wound. It significantly illuminates the deep recesses of the pelvis without constant manipulation of overhead lights.

Operative Technique

The abdominal incision is chosen on the basis of the patient's weight, the disease process involved, and the height of the pubic symphysis. If the symphysis is very high, a low transverse incision may lend much more exposure to the distal pelvis than a midline incision, and all factors should be carefully evaluated before the incision is made.

The author prefers to stand on the patient's left side with his assistant on the patient's right, second assistant to the surgeon's left side, and scrub nurse to the right of the first assistant. The surgeon proceeds with the incision and follows the procedure illustrated in Figures 13.4 through 13.21.

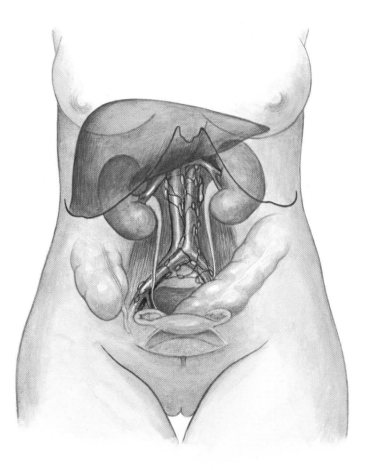

FIGURE 13.4. Observe, explore, palpate, and later record the status of the peritoneum, omentum, liver, gallbladder, stomach, small and large bowel, kidneys, ureters, para-aortic and pelvic lymph nodes, uterus, tubes, and ovaries.

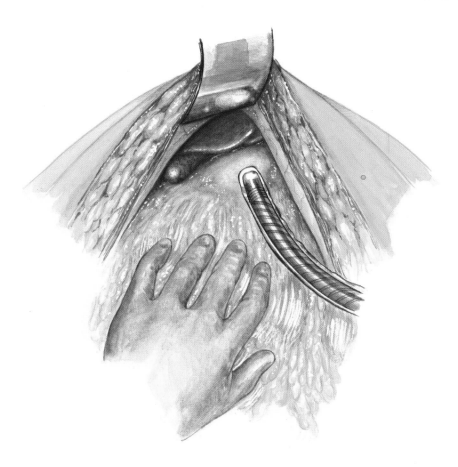

FIGURE 13.5. Enter the abdomen with a knife, incising to the fascia. Make the skin incision longer than the fascial incision, and the fascial incision longer than the peritoneal incision. Make the entire incision with a knife, laying the tissues out in a planar fashion. There is no need for scissors. Do not dissect laterally between the fascial planes. Keep the incision margin smooth to avoid dead spaces in the wound. With the aid of a long Deaver retractor, strong upward traction, and a fiberoptic light source placed well into the wound, carefully inspect the abdominal and pelvic structures. This is a vital part of any laparotomy. A surgical specialist is not excused from recording a thorough exploration of the entire abdominal and pelvic viscera.

131

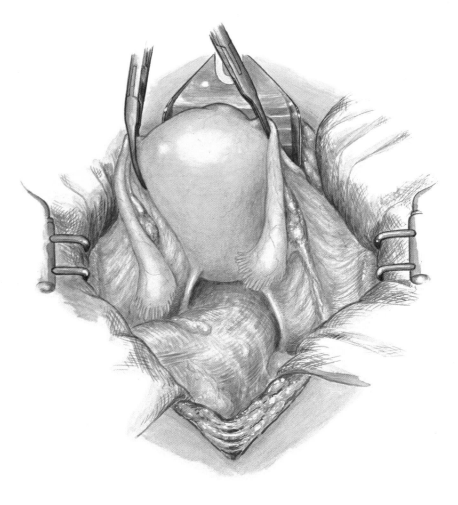

FIGURE 13.6. Following exploration, place damp laparotomy tapes over the wound margin and install a self-retaining retractor over the wound edges. Take care to use the appropriate blade lengths and to correctly position the retractor so as to avoid pressure deep on the lateral pelvic wall with possible subsequent femoral nerve palsy. Grasp the uterus with two Masterson clamps, pull upward, and pack the abdominal viscera out of the wound. Pack the cecum with one laparotomy tape on the right. Place folded tape over the small bowel and push upward. The remaining tape packs the let gutter and fixes the sigmoid in place. Place a wide pelvic Deaver retractor on the upper part of the wound to aid in exposure.

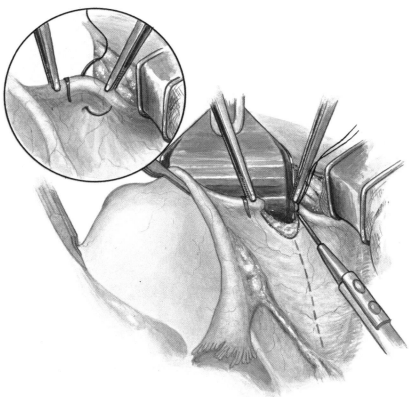

FIGURE 13.7. Pull the uterus upward; place a clip on the proximal round ligament and a 3-0 Nurolon suture beneath the round ligament; divide the ligament with a knife. Inset: Cauterize the small, rather constant artery running in the areolar tissue below the round ligament. Pull the uterus upward to the left using delicate 10-inch Nelson scissors and Adson-Brown forceps, carrying the dissection lateral to the ovarian vessels and being careful to avoid the external iliac artery.

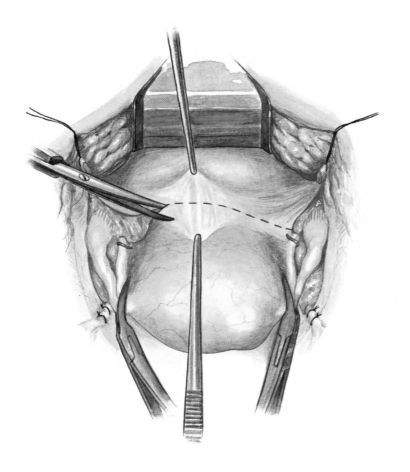

FIGURE 13.8. Using strong upward traction and tension between long Adson-Brown thumb forceps, dissect between the two round ligaments.

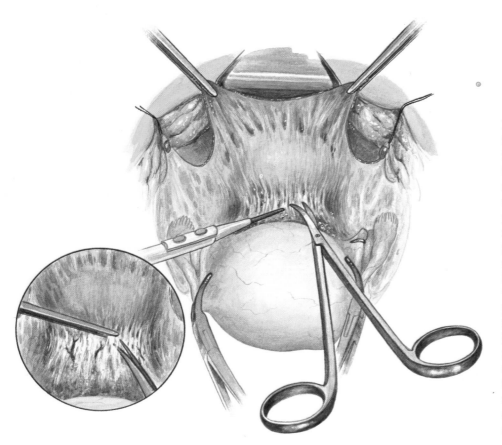

FIGURE 13.9. Grasp the peritoneum and upper surface of the bladder with Adson-Brown thumb forceps and pull strongly upward and anteriorly. Pull the uterus backward, exposing the plane between the bladder and cervix. Precise entrance of this plane is vital to the safety and ease of conduct of this operation. Pushing a laparotomy tape downward is a poor substitute for precise dissection. Use the cautery for small venous bleeders in this area. Constant planar traction on the field makes the dissection much easier. Inset: Observe the specific nature of this plane. Its white, rather avascular nature is an aid in this dissection.

133

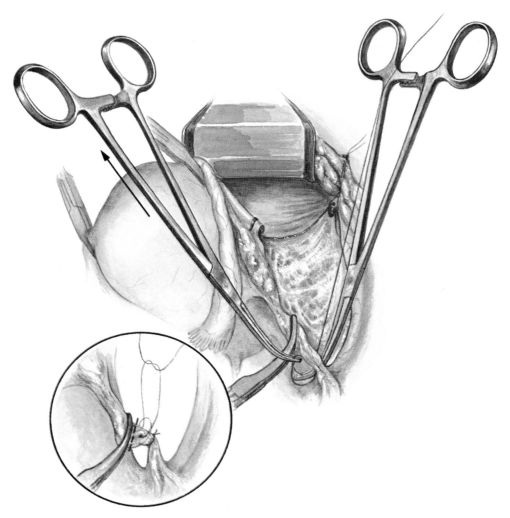

FIGURE 13.10. If the bladder dissection produces bleeding, place a dry laparotomy sponge anterior to the uterus, which will exert some pressure on this
bleeding during this phase of the ligation of the ovarian vessels. Isolate the ovarian
vessels, identify the ureter as it lies below the ovarian vessels, and ligate them with
2-0 or 3-0 braided nylon suture. Place the proximal tie around the ovarian vessels
and tie. Inset: Pass the next suture through the structure to fix it. Place a single
throw using a Gemini clamp; grasp the opposite end, pull upward, and ligate. Cut
the distal sections, pull upward, and either clip or leave them within the clamp.
There should be no question as to the strength of these ligatures; always adhere
to the policy of double ligation of the ovarian vessels due to the tendency of these
vessels to retract, particularly the ovarian artery, which lies in the center of these
venous structures. If hematoma occurs, the peritoneal dissection is continued
laterally above the area of hematoma and the procedure is performed again, obtaining secure hemostasis.

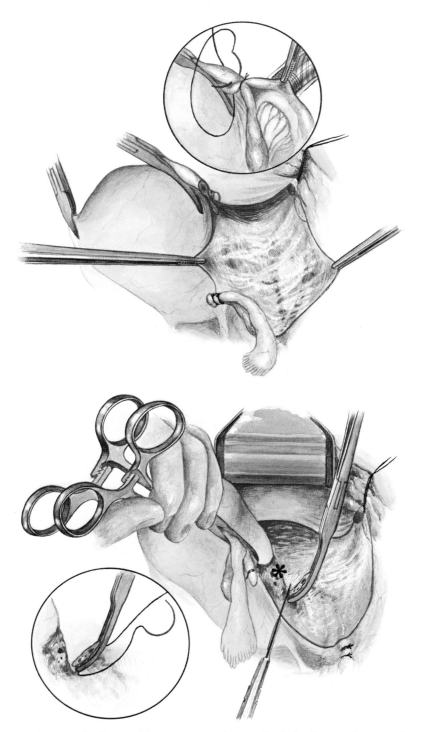

FIGURE 13.11. When the ovaries are to be left, perform the procedure as described in Figure 13.8, with the double ligation below the tube and ovary. Inset: Carry the incision down alongside the Masterson clamp along the fundus. Cauterize any small peritoneal bleeders.

FIGURE 13.12.   With strong traction to the left, the uterine arteries will be visible in the lower end of the dissection. Dissect them using long Nelson scissors and Adson-Brown forceps. Determine the position of the ureter lateral to the uterine arteries both by observation and palpation; as these structures course upward along the uterus they may be angled slightly anterior. One may observe the uterine artery arising from the obliterated hypogastric assuming a slightly spiral course as it nears the uterus. After these vessels have been identified, place a curved Masterson clamp at the cervouterine junction with the tip directly on the uterus. The uterine portion may be handled in a variety of ways. If the vessels are small, brief pressure or a clip will control the bleeding. Asterisk: If the uterus is large and vascular, straight Masterson clamps are placed in the proximal side. Inset: Divide the artery and place a suture of 3-0 Nurolon at the tip of the clamp with three secure square knots. Cut the sutures along the knot.

135

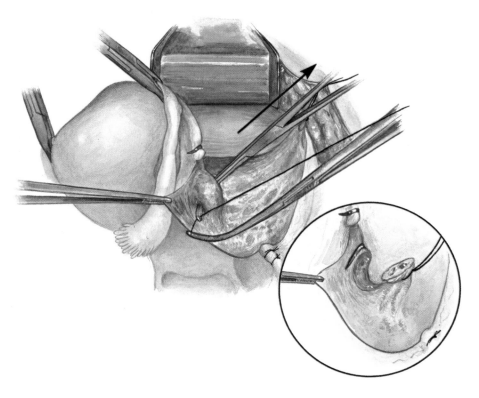

FIGURE 13.13. Another method of handling the uterine arteries when they are small and venous congestion is minimal is to place a Gemini artery forceps between the vascular bundle lying alongside the uterus. Pass a 3-0 Nurolon suture with a similar clamp, pull through, and ligate. Inset: If the vessels are small, place a clip above them for better visibility; if not, use a small hemostat to secure them proximally.

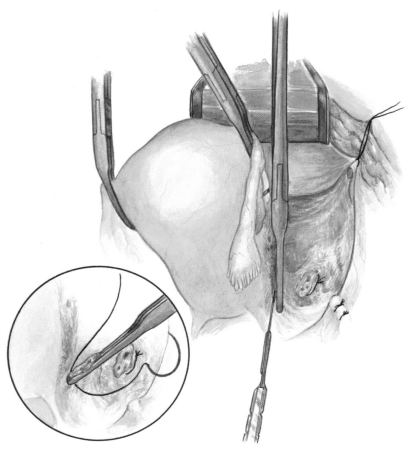

FIGURE 13.14. Once the uterine arteries are secured bilaterally, the uterine supports are seen. Vital to the remaining dissection is the adequacy of the original bladder dissection. If the bladder is well down, the white fibers of the vagina may be seen, with the upper portion of the cardinal ligaments visualized. Place straight Masterson clamps along the cervix, making a sharp division of tissues with a knife. When necessary, take two small bites of tissue and do not attempt to secure too large a portion of tissue in a clamp. Close the clamp only tightly enough to hold the tissue for suture approximation. Inset: Ligate the pedicle with 2-0 or 3-0 Vicryl or 0 or 2-0 chromic catgut. While many complex sutures have been described for use in the pelvis, a single simple tie with three square knots will hold these tissues most satisfactorily.

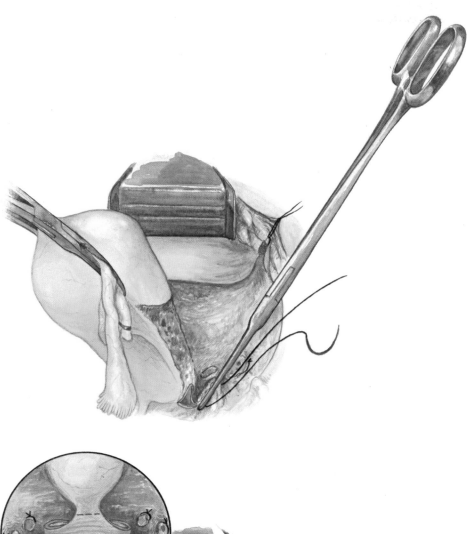

FIGURE 13.15. The anatomy of the vaginal fornix varies considerably. When small, one purchase after the cardinal ligament will enter the vagina: secure with 2-0 or 3-0 absorbable suture. In other patients, two bites will be needed. Place the next clamp medial to the tissues just ligated.

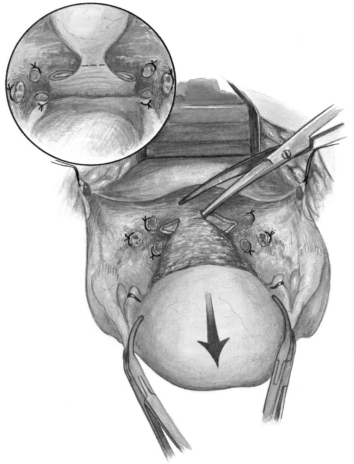

FIGURE 13.16. Following the bilateral entry into the vaginal fornix, the specimen is ready for removal. Use a knife or a heavy scissor with a blade sharply angled for this purpose. Do not use fine dissecting scissors as they will lose their preciseness in cutting heavy vaginal tissues. Inset: Pull the uterus upward. Note the position of the three supporting and vascular pedicles as one looks at the pelvic floor. The uterine arteries will be the uppermost pedicle, the cardinal pedicle will be directly at the angle of the vagina, and the uterosacral and posterior vagina will lie slightly posterior.

137

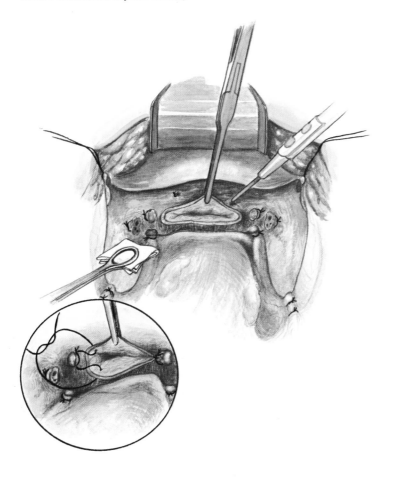

FIGURE 13.17.   After removing the specimen, obtain careful hemostasis. Use the cautery on small bleeders and suture the arterial bleeders with 3-0 Vicryl or chromic catgut. If bleeding persists following vaginal closure, a small portion of Avitene may be placed laterally. Inset: After hemostasis is secured, the vagina is supported with a suture that passes from the anterior vagina through to the interior, up into the cardinal ligament, back to the interior of the vagina, and out again. Tying this suture provides adequate support for the vagina. If nearby, the uterosacral may be included, but it is not necessary. The use of taper needles will minimize the bleeding associated with passage of this particular suture.

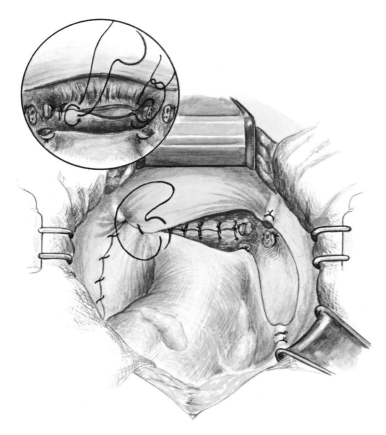

FIGURE 13.18.   Suture the opposite cardinal ligament to the vagina and close the vagina by passing a 3-0 Vicryl or chromic catgut suture through the vagina approximately 6 to 8 mm from its edge; then bring the suture over, catching the margins and tying them. Inset: This modified far-and-near suture provides sufficient strength with small suture, obliterates dead space, and accurately approximates the epithelial margins. This prevents granulations in the vaginal cuff and provides additional vaginal strength. If the ovaries have been removed, the pelvis may then be peritonealized using a running 3-0 absorbable suture. Dead spaces should be obliterated by passing the needle through the upper part of the vagina in one or two areas. If no peritoneum is available or the quality of the peritoneal coverings are insufficient due to inflammatory changes, allow the sigmoid to cover the wound.

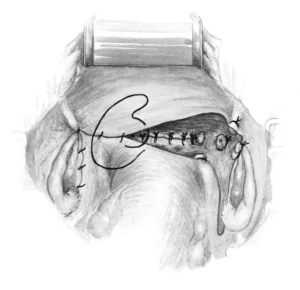

FIGURE 13.19. When the ovaries are to remain in place, take care that they are well into the intraperitoneal space, particularly the left ovary. On closing, the ovary should be sutured well up on the lateral wall to prevent it from becoming enmeshed in healing peritoneum. When this occurs, a seroma-like tumor will form, creating a subsequent need for exploration 6 months to 1 year following this procedure. Pay particular attention to the location of the ureters during closure, always visualizing them carefully when suturing next to them and using long Adson-Brown thumb forceps for peritoneal traction.

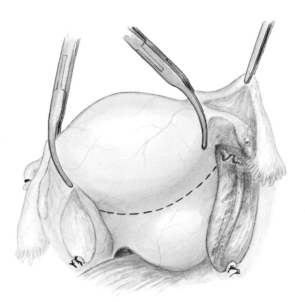

FIGURE 13.20. Identify and ligate the ovarian vessels and round ligaments as in total abdominal hysterectomy. Isolate the ureters and uterine arteries with sharp and blunt dissection. Ligate the uterine arteries under direct vision with 3-0 braided nylon. Transect the uterus above the uterine arteries as shown by the dotted line.

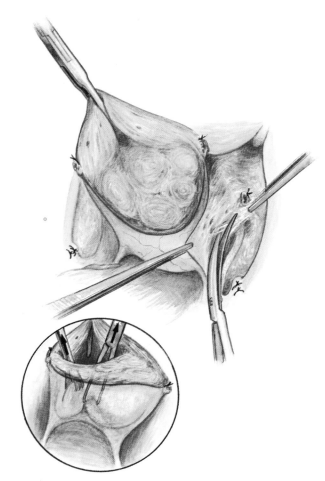

FIGURE 13.21. Pull strongly upward on the remaining cervix and the stump of the uterine artery. Free the ureter. Inset: Place thyroid clamps, pulling the cervix upward, and open the cervical canal. Enter the vagina and excise the remaining cervix. Secure hemostasis and close the vagina in the usual fashion.

139

Endometriosis

Although 17% of abdominal surgical patients have pelvic endometriosis, less than one-half of these patients have symptoms referable to this disease. Some patients with extensive masses may be relatively asymptomatic, while other patients with a small amount of endometriosis more strategically located have severe symptoms.

Carter has outlined information necessary to determine appropriate therapy in pelvic endometriosis: the desire for children, age of the patient, duration of infertility, severity of symptoms, and associated pelvic pathology must all be considered as well as the extent of endometriosis.[3] Hammond's modification of Acosta's classification of endometriosis is useful (Table 13.1).

Most patients with mild endometriosis are evaluated with the laparoscope and do not initially come to laparotomy. If the patient is young and children are desired, conservative therapy with Danazol is recommended. Dmowski and Cohen report a clinical improvement rate of 88% in patients with mild and moderate endometriosis and 69% in patients with severe endometriosis; of the 84 infertile women who desired pregnancy, 46.4% conceived following Danazol therapy.[5]

When the above program does not produce the desired result or more extensive endometriosis is found, conservative surgery is in order. Sharp excision of the endometriomas and implants in the cul-de-sac, bladder, and bowel are indicated.

Careful peritonealization as well as suspension of the uterus and fixation of the tubes to the parietal peritoneum are worthwhile. An important point is to prevent the uterus and adnexae from again becoming adherent in the cul-de-sac. Depending on the initial severity of the endometriosis from 40% to 87% of such patients may achieve pregnancy but as high as 25% of these patients will require reoperation.[8]

While presacral neurectomy is often suggested, the author is aware of no prospective study documenting its effectiveness and does not recommend it for routine use.

Several studies have shown that combination of pseudopregnancy

TABLE 13.1. Classification of Endometriosis

Extent of Disease	Findings
Mild	Scattered, superficial implants on structures other than uterus, tubes, or ovaries; no scarring
	Rare, superficial implants on ovaries
	No significant adhesions
Moderate	Involvement of one or both ovaries with multiple implants or small endometriomas (<2 cm)
	Minimal peritubular or periovarian adhesions
	Scattered, scarred implants on other structures
Severe	Large ovarian endometriomas (>2 cm)
	Significant tubal or ovarian adhesions
	Tubal obstruction
	Obliteration of cul-de-sac, major uterosacral involvement
	Significant bowel or urinary tract disease

From Hammond, C. B., Rock, J. A., and Parker, R. T.: *Fertil. Steril.* 27(7):756–766, 1976. (Adapted from Acosta et al.) Acosta, A. A., Buttram, V. C., Besch, P. K. et al.: A proposed classification of pelvic endometriosis. *Obstet. Gynecol.* 42:19, 1973.

and surgery is less productive than conservative surgery alone, and post-opertive progestational therapy is not beneficial.[1] The more extensive and severe forms of endometriosis have a low pregnancy rate and the reoperation rate when managed conservatively may approach 85%. In such patients the initial procedure of total abdominal hysterectomy and bilateral salpingo-oophorectomy with the excision of implants in the bladder, cul-de-sac, and any constricting lesions of the small bowel and colon is recommended. While there are proponents of ovarian conservation, there is an associated 10% to 12% reoperation rate.[16] It seems unwise to leave one of the most common sites of endometriosis in a patient who requires hysterectomy for control of her disease, and the author advises total abdominal hysterectomy and bilateral salpingo-oophorectomy in these patients.

Estrogen replacement therapy may be given, particularly if the patient is young, without undue risk of recurrence of disease. If symptoms such as dyspareunia recur, which is rare in the author's experience, estrogen may be stopped for a few weeks and resumed at a later date. If extensive gastrointestinal endometriosis is left in situ, begin estrogen therapy 3 weeks after surgery. Resect severe rectosigmoid endometriosis as well as extensive endometriomas of the small bowel and bladder if they compromise the lumen or deeply invade these structures.

Finally, the presence of cul-de-sac nodules in a fixed ovarian mass in a young patient, while very suggestive of endometriosis, is not an indication for a therapeutic trial of progestational agents. A 20-year-old female presented on the author's service with these findings but her underlying disease process was that of a stage III serous cystadenocarcinoma of the ovary. Such patients should have laparoscopic documentation and laparotomy as indicated.

As endometriosis often involves the cul-de-sac and uterosacral ligaments and destroys the intraperitoneal planes by fixation of large endometriomas into the cul-de-sac, the usual surgical planes are often lost; therefore, approach these lesions in a peripheral fashion, working in the extraperitoneal spaces. Trace the ureters downward after ligating the ovarian blood supply. As soon as the ureters are dissected well into the pelvis, mobilize the ovarian masses medially and free the uterus upward. Stay extremely close to the uterus in this particular disease process as the ureters do not mobilize in the usual fashion because the uterosacral ligaments and the areas near the ureters are often primarily involved with this disease. As the posterior peritoneum and cul-de-sac may be completely obliterated with endometriosis, enter the vaginal vault anteriorly in the midline. Pull the vault upward with traction on two Masterson clamps near the cervix after dissecting the bladder downward. Enter the vault in the midline with a knife and carry the dissection laterally close to the uterus. Place the thumb in the vault and direct the index finger toward the adherent colon, making posterior dissection of the uterus much safer. Grasp the vault with Masterson clamps, pull upward, and suture. Place 3-0 Vicryl or chromic catgut near the vaginal margins as mobilization of the bladder and ureters is often quite limited. Do not worry about vaginal cuff suspension in patients with severe endometriosis as marked fibrosis makes prolapse uncommon. If there is marked destruction of the pelvic peritoneum and the sigmoid fails to cover the defect, fashion an omental carpet by bringing the omentum along the left side of the pelvis.

Depending on how carefully one looks, endometriosis of the bowel may be found in 15% to 50% of patients. Gray reported 179 cases of endometriosis of the bowel occurring in 1500 patients operated on for endome-

141

triosis: 81 patients had simple excision of the endometriosis, 61 patients had incomplete excision, and 37 patients had bowel resection for extensive lesions with either end-to-end anastomosis (10 cases) or excision of the full thickness of the anterior bowel wall (27 cases).[6] Of the 81 patients who had surface excision of the bowel, 79 received estrogens postoperatively, and approximately 20% developed some recurrent symptoms that were relieved by cessation of estrogens. Note that in none of these cases was the mucosa of the gut perforated and proctosigmoidoscopy always revealed a normal mucosa. While some bowel lesions responded to castration, those patients with marked intestinal symptoms and severe lesions required excision of the bowel endometriosis, and this was the preferred approach in this group of patients. Colostomy was rarely necessary. Pratt in discussing Gray's paper recommended bowel resection if endometriosis diminishes the lumen of the gut to 50% of its size or if the lesion completely surrounds the bowel. Furthermore, if the patient is young, her need for estrogens or the possibility of conservative surgery would point toward resection in these patients.[6]

Leiomyoma

Prior to hysterectomy obtain a suction biopsy of the endometrial cavity or perform gross examination of curettings with frozen section where indicated.

Often the surgery of large leiomyomas is limited by their size. Once the ovarian vessels have been ligated, exposure can be gained by excision of the larger leiomyomas and suturing of their base. Hysterectomy can then proceed in a more orderly fashion. It is absolutely vital that the surgeon be certain that there is no malignancy in the uterus in the course of such maneuvers, as operating through an area of cancer would prove disastrous for the patient.

Cervical leiomyomas can pose a difficult problem in pelvic surgery, particularly if the lesion has been allowed to expand and trap itself inside the pelvis. The ability to mobilize such lesions may be severely limited and exposure may be greatly compromised. Very careful examination under anesthesia preceding the operation is helpful in delineating the lesion. Although ureteral catheters are often advised in such patients, if the lesion is really large the trigone will be so distorted that insertion of ureteral catheters will be quite difficult. Abdominal insertion of a plain or illuminated ureteral catheter through a longitudinal incision in the ureter is an alternative route in these patients (Figures 13.20 and 13.21).

Pelvic Inflammatory Disease

Large pelvic abscesses and pelvic inflammatory disease greatly complicate uterine removal but the uterus should be removed with the diseased adnexae almost without exception. It is most useful to remove the abscesses first, if possible, and then proceed to hysterectomy. The abscesses are most easily removed by entering the retroperitoneal space, mobilizing the abscesses medially, indentifying the ureters, and dividing the ovarian vessels from above, sharply dissecting the lesions off the ureters under direct vision. Avoid blunt mobilization of these abscesses as clamping of their blood supply with large clamps is an invitation to ureteral injury. The ovarian vessels and blood supply to these abscesses should not be divided until the ureter has been carefully identified visually coursing below and lateral to the inferior portion of these abscesses.

Stress Incontinence Surgery

The removal of the uterus with urethral suspension has been shown to improve long-term incontinence cure rates.[7] It produces no difficulties nor compromise of the blood supply to the bladder. The retropubic space is not usually entered until the peritoneal cavity is closed, although no increase in morbidity has been noted in performing the procedures jointly.

A cystocele may be repaired through the transabdominal approach (Figure 13.22).

Associated Vaginectomy

Colposcopy has replaced the use of routine vaginal cuff resection with hysterectomy in carcinoma in situ. Occasionally, however, the colposcope reveals that the lesion extends onto the vaginal cuff and partial vaginectomy is performed with hysterectomy (Figure 13.23). Note the lack of correlation of intraepithelial neoplasia and Schiller's stain; do not use this stain for guidance on the limits of excision.[14]

Adenocarcinoma of the Endometrium

The author believes that it is important not to unduly manipulate adenocarcinoma of the endometrium due to the demonstration of increased numbers of cells in the draining venous blood in the manipulated cancer; therefore, place no tenaculum on the fundus in endometrial cancer. Hemisection for exposure or subtotal excision of the uterus is also unacceptable. The standard technique recommended has the blood supply to the upper uterus immediately clamped. The ovarian vessels are tied and dissection proceeds with ligation of the uterine blood supply. Long et al. recommend the use of a vaginal occlusive clamp and washing of the vagina with a dilute solution of vaginal formalin or other intravaginal cytotoxic agent,[10] and some recommend an intravaginal plug or suturing of the cervix.

A classification of endometrial carcinoma is presented in Table 13.2. The author routinely recommends the use of irradiation therapy in almost all endometrial cancers in association with surgery; the vaginal cuff recurrence rate of stage I endometrial cancer approximates 1% or less with this combination. Such local measures are not necessary with combination

TABLE 13.2. Classification of Endometrial Carcinoma (International Federation of Gynecologists and Obstetricians, 1976)

Stage		Characteristics
0		Carcinoma in situ; histologic findings suspicious of malignancy (cases in stage 0 should not be included in any therapeutic statistics)
I		Carcinoma confined to the corpus, including the isthmus
	a	Length of uterine cavity is 8 cm or less
	b	Length of uterine cavity is over 8 cm
		Stage I cases should be subgrouped with regard to the histologic type of the adenocarcinoma as follows:
	G1	Highly differentiated adenomatous carcinoma
	G2	Differentiated adenomatous carcinoma with partly solid areas
	G3	Predominantly solid or entirely undifferentiated carcinoma
II		Carcinoma has involved the corpus and the cervix, but has not extended outside the uterus
III		Carcinoma has extended outside the uterus, but not outside the true pelvis
IV		Carcinoma has extended outside the true pelvis or has obviously involved the mucosa of the bladder or rectum; bullous edema, as such, does not permit a case to be allotted to stage IV
	a	Spread of the growth to adjacent organs
	b	Spread to distant organs

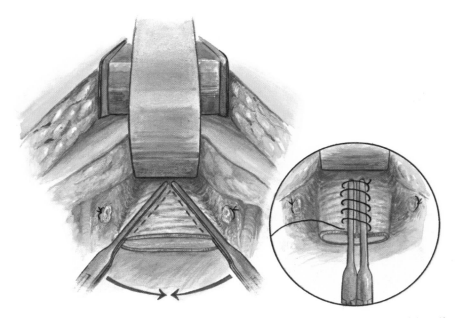

FIGURE 13.22. Transabdominal repair of cystocele is performed by dissecting the bladder further off the anterior vaginal wall in the same plane as in abdominal hysterectomy. Place two Masterson clamps downward at the apex of the dissection of the bladder and angle them toward the cardinal ligaments, forming an inverted "V". This is continued from the same plane in which the bladder was dissected off for abdominal hysterectomy. An additional 2 cm will suffice. Excise the vagina in one layer. Bring the clamps to the midline and tie a suture of 2-0 Vicryl or chromic catgut at the apex and place the suture loosely in an over-and-over fashion. Open the clamps and remove them; pull the suture up snugly. A final pass is made through the tissues and the suture is knotted. Close the vagina in the usual transverse fashion after hysterectomy with a far-and-near type suture. The use of nontraumatic clamps greatly facilitates this operation and minimizes tissue reaction. Take care to place the distal suture beyond the tip of the V so as to occlude any small arteries that retract. Manage the patient as in any cystocele repair.

therapy. The association of radiation therapy and surgical procedures in the treatment of stage I and II endometrial cancers is summarized in Table 13.3. In endometrial cancer as well as cervical cancer careful planning and coordination of radiation therapy and associated surgical procedures will produce a result far superior to that achieved by an ill-conceived excision preceding proper planning.

If an incidental appendectomy is planned, use the simple purse-string suture technique with 3-0 braided nylon atraumatic suture and cross-clamping of the appendix as described in Chapter 20.

Following the appendectomy, remove the pack from the pelvis; ligate small bleeding points or use the cautery. If the procedure is performed for malignant disease, hemostatic clips are most helpful in outlining any residual disease.

Wound Healing

Wound healing studies indicate that the peritoneum regenerates relatively quickly. Approximate the peritoneal margins with 3-0 suture of Vicryl or 2-0 chromic catgut. Take note of the precise position of the ureters on the

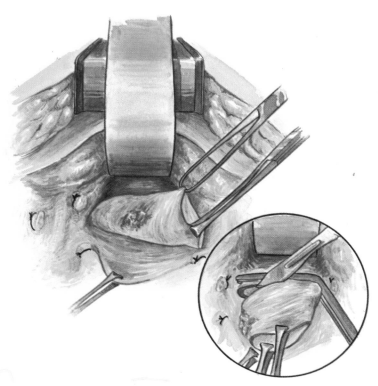

FIGURE 13.23. Vaginectomy may be needed when carcinoma in situ extends into the vagina. Mark the margins of the lesion with a colposcope prior to surgery. Mark the distal end with Allis clamps fixed to the vagina that can be easily felt, thereby obtaining an accurate excisional margin. Once the hysterectomy is carried downward to the stage of the cardinal ligaments, with strong upper traction and using straight Masterson clamps, take small bites of tissue, remaining close along the vagina with the bladder and ureters retracted laterally with narrow Deaver retractors. Once the desired length of the vagina to be resected is obtained and the margin is verified by feeling the Allis clamps through the vagina, make a sharp incision into the vagina and excise the specimen. Secure the margins of the vagina and close the vagina in the usual fashion. It may not be possible to approximate the cardinal ligaments when significant vagina is excised, but little difficulty usually arises. Should the patient wish vaginal function and a significant portion of the vagina is excised, use a skin graft. Place it immediately if the area is well vascularized or pull the peritoneum down to bridge the upper defect.

proximal peritoneal surface. Do not place sutures proximal to the doubly ligated ovarian vessels as hematoma will result, with large extraperitoneal collections of blood in some patients. If, at this time, any hematoma is noted in the ovarian vessels, carefully isolate the vessels, dissect upward, and doubly ligate in the technique described and excise the distal hematoma.

If the hysterectomy was performed for endometriosis or pelvic inflammatory disease where the peritoneal surface has already been greatly compromised, little normal pelvic peritoneum may remain. If both ovaries have been removed, the sigmoid may be allowed to fall into the pelvis and the omentum may be pulled downward. If the left ovary is left in place, however, a retrosigmoid tumor may form, which appears grossly like a simple serous cystadenoma. Serosal surface forms about the ovary and, if continued ovulation occurs, a retrosigmoid mass of some proportion may result, requiring later laparotomy. If the ovaries are to be left in, they should be

TABLE 13.3. Therapy for Endometrial Cancer[a]

Stage	Surgery[b]	Irradiation
I	TAH, BSO 1 to 5 days following radium removal	Preoperatively: 7,000 rads to vaginal surface and 2,000 mg–hr uterine fundus, Fletcher-Suit tandem and ovoids (Underwood technique) Postoperatively: Add 2,000 rads parametrial and 2,000 rads whole pelvis if more than 50% myometrium involved
	Alternate Plan	
G1	TAH, BSO	Postoperatively: 4,000 rads total more than ⅓ myometrial invaded
G2	TAH, BSO	Postoperatively: 4,000 rads total pelvis if any myometrial invasion
G3	TAH, BSO, nodal sampling pelvis and para-aortic nodes	Postoperatively: 4,000 to 5,000 rads total pelvis; add 4,000 rads surface dose vaginal ovoids if more than 50% myometrium involved; add 4,000 to 4,500 rads to para-aortic portals if nodes positive
II	TAH, BSO 1 to 5 days following radium removal	Preoperatively: 4,000 rads total pelvis, 1,000 rads parametria, 4,000 rads surface vagina; and 2,000 mg–hr uterus
III	Explore, do TAH if possible	Preoperatively: 4,000 rads total pelvis, 1,000 rads parametria, 4,000 rads surface vagina, and 2,000 mg–hr uterus or 5,000 rads total pelvis
IV		Individualize irradiation and perform surgery for fistula

[a] This table outlines combined therapy programs. The best results will be obtained when therapy is individualized.

[b] TAH, total abdominal hysterectomy; BSO, bilateral salpingo-oophorectomy.

pulled well up out of the pelvis and, if on a long ovarian vascular pedicle, they should be sutured to the lateral pelvic wall peritoneum. The sigmoid may be used, freely sutured directly to the bladder flap as needed, as bowel obstruction from adhesions to the sigmoid colon is remarkably rare.

Should drainage be necessary, the author prefers suction drainage of the Hemovac type. Place the catheters retroperitoneally by inserting the trocar through the abdominal wall, taking care to palpate the inferior epigastric vessels, and inserting the trocar into the retroperitoneal space behind the round ligaments. This is led downward into the side of the abdominal hysterectomy out the opposite abdominal wall with the catheters left in until the drainage does not exceed 30 ml/24 hr. There is little rationale for the use of Penrose drains through the vagina or through stab wounds throughout the lower abdomen as they produce very little drainage and increase the access of bacteria.[11] Suction catheters are inert; they are associated with very few complications in themselves and produce adequate suction to extract serum, blood, or any other materials that accumulate. The author does not favor the use of a T-tube type drain after abdominal hysterectomy as the drain is in the area of the pelvic–vaginal cuff, an area that is subjected to the most trauma during abdominal hysterectomy; the drain provides a site of access to traumatized tissues containing abundant amounts of suture material, which, experimentally, greatly increases the incidence of wound infections.[11]

Postoperative Management

Meticulous care in the recovery area and during the subsequent postoperative period is important. The patient may require intravenous fluids for the first 24 hr; lactated Ringer's solution in D5W is suitable, and the dosage should rarely exceed 3000 ml/day. If the patient should have gastric suction for some other reason, then $\frac{1}{2}$ normal saline might be substituted for lactated Ringer's to provide an adequate amount of chloride and avoid any tendency toward alkalosis. Patients are encouraged to ambulate as soon as possible and the Foley catheter should be removed as soon as the patient is capable of voiding. Encouraging the patient to cough is the most effective postoperative procedure to avoid atelectasis; the author does not routinely use positive pressure breathing. A small disposable plastic respirator may be used to encourage increased respiratory volume. Obtain routine blood gases during surgery, and in patients with compromised cardiopulmonary symptoms obtain blood gases in the recovery room. Give the patient a Fleets enema on the second postoperative day and order a diet as tolerated when the patient passes flatus. Check the hemoglobin and hematocrit on the second postoperative day. They should not differ greatly from the preoperative levels in the average patient.

Remove skin sutures on the sixth or seventh postoperative day. Monofilament nylon suture properly placed will produce minimal skin reaction. In a transverse incision with absorbable subcuticular skin closure, the ends of the suture may be cut the evening before discharge.

One day prior to discharge prescribe estrogen replacements for those patients in whom the uterus was removed for benign disease. In patients having significant bleeding, prescribe an iron preparation. Although the patient's hemoglobin level may be within the normal range, iron stores may have been depleted.

The author recommends that a surgical associate, who may be a nurse clinician, have a prolonged uninterrupted visit with the patient prior to discharge to instruct her in postoperative care, diet, and level of activity. In addition, the patient is provided with printed instructions and a return appointment in 2 weeks. The author also provides the patient with a copy of the pathology report for her retention.

Postoperative Complications

White et al. have reviewed in detail the complications of hysterectomy occurring in a composite series of clinic, university, and private patients.[15] This study is summarized in Table 13.4. While the private patients had fewer complications, the composite picture is useful for the house officer and practicing surgeon alike reviewing possible complications that may occur.

The Professional Activity Study of 12,026 hysterectomies from multiple hospitals showed a morbidity rate of 31%.[12] This high morbidity rate, however, is not inherent in the procedure of abdominal hysterectomy. Richardson studied various techniques employed in abdominal hysterectomy over a period of years on his service in the Crawford W. Long Hospital. His initial series of patients were operated on with Heaney clamps, self-retaining retractors, and 1 chromic suture. Richardson noted a febrile morbidity of 22% in these patients and a transfusion rate of 48%. When Richardson and co-workers altered their technique to a much less traumatic one with fine suture and nontraumatic handling of tissues, the febrile

147

TABLE 13.4. Complications after Abdominal Hysterectomy in 300 Patients

Complication	No. of Patients
Urinary tract infection	132
Febrile postoperatively (temperature greater than 100.4°F for 2 days)	108
Abdominal wound infection	17
Intestinal obstruction	17
Pneumonia or atelectasis	15
Urinary retention	9
Vaginal cuff hematoma or infection	7
Postoperative shock	3
Bladder injury	1
Ureteral injury	1
Associated other complication	9
Death	3

morbidity rate fell to 2.4% and the incidence of transfusions fell to 3.5%.[13]

The author has observed a similar variability in morbidity, transfusion, and complication rates in gynecologic surgery based primarily on the handling of tissues and techniques and suture material used. There is little justification today for the occasional operator or the untrained surgeon performing with great difficulty, excessive blood loss, and complication-ridden postoperative course a procedure that may be performed simply, in a brief period of time, with a short hospital stay by a more experienced and skillful surgeon using more modern suture materials, instruments, and techniques. Careful review of complications in pelvic surgery will define those parameters useful in minimizing the complications of this abdominal procedure.

The mortality rate for abdominal hysterectomy is 0.2%; while modern techniques permit performance of hysterectomy without great consideration for mortality, note that 20 women die for every 10,000 hysterectomies performed.[9] Both the patient and the surgeon should consider the benefits to be derived from surgery worth the risk, though slight, of the patient's dying.

References

1. Andrews, W.C., and Larsen, D.C.: Endometriosis: Treatment with hormonal pseudopregnancy and/or operation. *Am. J. Obstet. Gynecol.* **118**:643–651, 1974.
2. Blaustein, A.: *Pathology of the Female Genital Tract.* New York, Springer-Verlag, 1977.
3. Carter, B.: Treatment of endometriosis. *J. Obstet. Gynaecol. Br. Commonw.* **69**:783–789, 1962.
4. Christopherson, W.M., Gray, L.A., and Parker, J.E.: Microinvasive carcinoma of the uterine cervix: Long term follow up study of 80 cases. *Cancer* **38**:629–632, 1976.
5. Dmowski, W.P., and Cohen, M.R.: Antigonadotropin (Danazol) in the treatment of endometriosis: Evaluation of post-treatment fertility and three-year follow-up data. *Am. J. Obstet. Gynecol.* **130**:41–48, 1978.
6. Gray, L.A.: Endometriosis of the bowel: Role of bowel resection, superficial excision and oophorectomy in treatment. *Ann. Surg.* **177**:580–587, 1973.
7. Green, T.H.: Urinary stress incontinence: Differential diagnosis, pathophysiology, and management. *Am. J. Obstet. Gynecol.* **122**:368–400, 1975.

8. Hammond, C.B., Rock, J.A., and Parker, R.T.: Conservative treatment of endometriosis: The effects of limited surgery and hormonal pseudopregnancy. *Fertil. Steril.* **27:**756–766, 1976.

9. Ledger, W.J., and Child, M.A.: The hospital care of patients undergoing hysterectomy: An analysis of 12,026 patients from the Professional Study Activity. *Am. J. Obstet. Gynecol.* **117:**423–433, 1973.

10. Long, R.T., Sala, J.M., and Spratt, J.S.: Endometrial carcinoma recurring after hysterectomy: A study of 64 cases, with observations on effective treatment modalities and implications for alteration of primary therapy. *Am. J. Obstet. Gynecol.* **29:**318–321, 1978.

11. Peacock, E.E., and Van Winkle, W.: *Wound Repair.* Philadelphia, Saunders, 1976.

12. QRB Editorial: Controversy or perversity? Quality Rev. Bull. Vol. 3, No. 3, p. 11, March 1977.

13. Richardson, A.C., Lyon, J.B., and Graham, E.E.: Abdominal hysterectomy: Relationship between morbidity and surgical technique. *Am. J. Obstet. Gynecol.* **115:**953–961, 1973.

14. Rubio, C.A., and Thomassen, P.: A critical evaluation of the Schiller test in patients before conization. *Am. J. Obstet. Gynecol.* **125:**96–99, 1976.

15. White, S.C., Wartel, L.J., and Wade, M.E.: Comparison of abdominal and vaginal hysterectomies: A review of 600 operations. *Obstet. Gynecol.* **37:**530–537, 1971.

16. Williams, T.J.: The role of surgery in the management of endometriosis. *Mayo Clin. Proc.* **50:**198–203, 1975.

14 Radical Hysterectomy

James W. Daly

The anatomic theory of the radical hysterectomy was described by the German surgeon Ries in 1895, but it was performed for the first time by an American, John Clark, at Johns Hopkins Hospital.[7] In 1898 Wertheim began to do this operation for carcinoma of the cervix, and in 1912 he published a monograph that included 500 cases.[9] This procedure, together with the Schauta vaginal hysterectomy, became the mainstay of the surgical attack on cervical cancer in Europe and Great Britain. However, in the United States, radium and then radium and external radiation therapy were the most commonly practiced methods of treatment for cervical cancer until Meigs reintroduced radical hysterectomy and bilateral pelvic node dissection to American surgeons in 1944.[3] Meigs, in contrast to the European surgeons, advocated complete and routine removal of the pelvic lymph nodes in every case. Interestingly enough, the radical abdominal hysterectomy is often called the Wertheim operation in the United States, while many European surgeons refer to it as the Meigs operation. The procedure described in this chapter is based largely on the technique first described by Okabayashi in 1921[5] and expanded by Yagi in 1955.[10]

Radical hysterectomy and pelvic node dissection is a proven and time-honored method of cure for the smaller Ib and IIa carcinomas of the cervix. The procedure allows an immediate and detailed evaluation of the extent of the tumor, and in younger women it is possible to preserve ovarian function. In the smaller cervical cancers it is unusual for metastasis to occur in the adnexae; therefore, their removal is not necessarily part of the operation. Of great advantage is the avoidance of late radiation damage to the pelvic tissues and organs such as the small bowel, bladder, and rectum.

The operation is not suitable for patients with large cervical tumors and those that extend beyond the medial third or half of the paracervical and paracolpal tissue. It is probably best to treat patients with parametrial disease with radiotherapy since it is often difficult to get beyond the tumor with a surgical approach. Elderly patients (those over 65 or perhaps 70) and those with a compromised pulmonary or cardiovascular system may do better with radiotherapy. Patients who are extremely obese are technically difficult to operate upon; bleeding in these patients may be extremely troublesome.

A significant disadvantage to the operation described in this chapter is postoperative bowel and bladder denervation and dysfunction.[6,7] If one is not prepared to handle this problem postoperatively and teach the patient how to use her bladder and to take care of her bowels, then one should not use this particular technique.

All patients operated upon with this technique will have some degree of bowel and rectal denervation and subsequent dysfunction. The magnitude of the problem will vary from patient to patient, but they all have some injury and the situation is usually permanent. However, with proper care and teaching the patient can overcome these difficulties and lead a normal life without any significant degree of renal damage.[6,7] The incidence of ureteral and bladder fistulas has significantly decreased over the years from 15% to 1% to 5% at the present time.[2] A larger number of patients will ultimately develop ureteral strictures, perhaps 6% overall. A few patients will have incision into the rectum during the operation, and in that case it is usually best to perform a colostomy; however, if these rectal injuries are properly repaired, the colostomy can later be taken down and closed. The blood loss will vary from 1,000 to 4,000 ml, and on occasion may be even higher, but the average is probably somewhere between 2,000 and 2,500 ml. Occasionally a patient develops a postoperative lymphocyst, but it is generally asymptomatic and causes no significant problems. It can, however, obstruct the ureter or become infected, or both, and in that instance further surgery is necessary.

Preoperative Evaluation

The diagnostic evaluation of the patient with carcinoma of the cervix begins with a detailed history and physical; for it is only after this examination that one can determine whether a patient is truly a technical or medical candidate for the surgical approach. The patient should have a chest x-ray and an intravenous pyelogram and, if she is 40 years of age or older, an electrocardiogram. Lymphangiography is useful, although a negative test can be highly inaccurate. If indeed one or more of the pelvic nodes is positive, this finding may dictate that the node dissection should include the para-aortic as well as the pelvic nodes. Cystoscopy should be done in the larger cervical lesions, but in those where the lesion is small and obviously confined to the cervix, cystoscopy is not necessary.

The patient should have a complete blood count and a urinalysis with a urine culture. It is also wise to culture the cervix for gonococcus; if the patient develops a postoperative gonococcal infection the complications can be severe. Blood urea nitrogen, serum creatinine, and electrolytes should be obtained. It is also wise to do a liver profile. Prior to surgery, colposcopy should be performed so that a mucosal lesion in the vagina is not overlooked.

Operative Technique

The surgical anatomy involved in this procedure is discussed in Chapter 13. The operation is designed to remove the primary tumor and the regional tissue into which contiguous spread of the cancer occurs as well as the primary (pelvic) and, less often, secondary nodes (aortic). The technique is illustrated in Figures 14.1 through 14.18.

The tissues that may contain contiguous spread are the paracervical and paravaginal tissues and the upper third of the vagina. These paracervical and paravaginal tissues are in essence the cardinal and the uterosacral

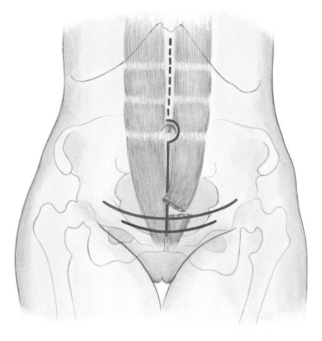

FIGURE 14.1. Open the abdomen through a midline incision from the xyphoid to the pubis, passing to the left of the umbilicus. While a muscle-cutting, lower abdominal transverse incision produces good exposure of the pelvis, para-aortic lymph node dissections or biopsies are compromised through this incision. Carefully explore the abdomen, including the liver and para-aortic and pelvic nodal areas. Biopsy any suspicious areas on the peritoneal surface and obtain any free fluid in the abdomen for cell washings. Make certain the stomach is empty and was not distended during the induction of anesthesia. A Levine tube is used to keep the stomach decompressed and in the postoperative period for the management of ileus, which frequently occurs with para-aortic nodal dissection. Pull the transverse colon anterior to the wound and cover it with moist laparotomy tape.

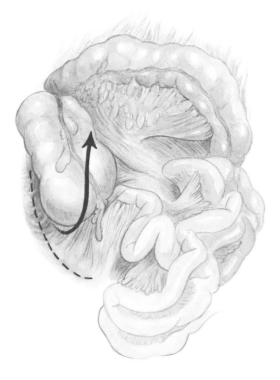

FIGURE 14.2. Grasp the uterus at the cornual areas with Masterson clamps and pull sharply to the left, putting the right round ligament on tension. Ligate and divide the round ligament close to the right pelvic wall. Open the peritoneum inferiorly to where the external iliac artery exits the abdomen; place a medium Deaver retractor at this lower margin. Incise the peritoneum in a cephalad fashion up the right peritoneal gutter lateral to the cecum for 10 cm. Lift the cecum and put tension on the medial peritoneum. If no retroperitoneal dissection is planned, proceed to Figure 14.8.

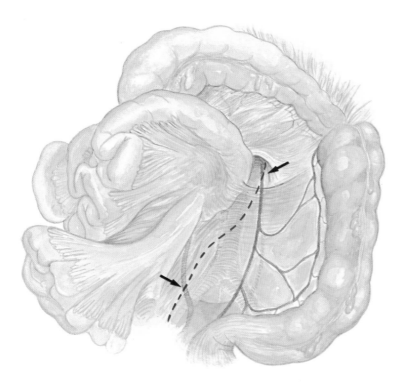

FIGURE 14.3.   Transfer the small bowel to the patient's right side, maintain the tension on the peritoneum, and incise with a scissor diagonally across the abdomen, following the route of the small bowel mesentery up to the ligament of Treitz. Use a fiberoptic light to transilluminate, avoiding the right ovarian vessels, ureter, and inferior mesenteric vein. Carefully identify the structures in the left retroperitoneum as the overlying colon and superior rectal artery obscure their identification. Identify both ureters, as they are the margins of this dissection. Secure any small bleeders with clips or cauterization and avoid staining the retroperitoneal fat as this makes dissection more difficult. Exteriorize the small bowel and cover it with warm laparotomy tapes. Place a wide Deaver at the margins of the duodenum to produce exposure to the upper margins of the wound. Use care with the upper abdominal retractors to avoid injury to the liver and spleen and pressure necrosis of the underlying colon. Frequently check the retractors to make certain no injuries are being produced.

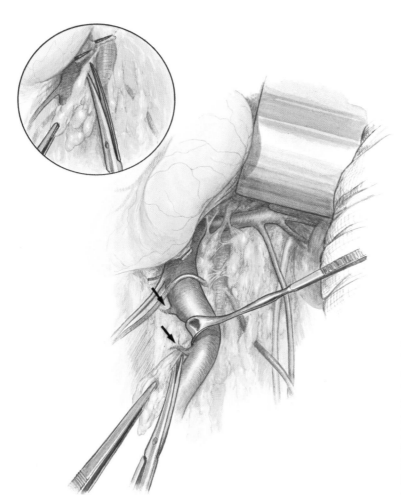

FIGURE 14.4.   Begin the dissection in the area of the right common iliac vein by grasping the fibroareolar tissue with Adson-Brown thumb forceps and pull up sharply. Dissect upward over the vena cava in this plane to the duodenum as it crosses the aorta and vena cava. Inset: Carefully expose the left renal vein with the large Deaver retractor and remove the nodes about and inferior to it using small clips, long delicate Nelson scissors, and long Adson-Brown thumb forceps. Avoid damage to the lumbar veins, which enter the vena cava in this area.

153

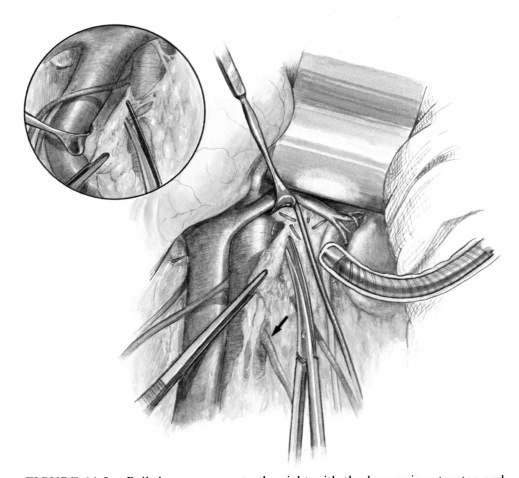

FIGURE 14.5. Pull the vena cava to the right with the long vein retractor and remove the nodes lying between the vena cava and aorta (inset). Secure these lymphatics with small clips. Enter the adventitial sheath over the aorta and identify the inferior mesenteric artery, which exits the aorta superior and lateral to the bifurcation. While shown preserved in these drawings, the inferior mesenteric may be sacrificed without undue risk if this will facilitate exposure or dissection. Clamp the inferior mesenteric artery loosely with a Gemini clamp and observe any vascular changes in the lower colon. If no evidence of vascular insufficiency is noted in the colon, ligate the inferior mesenteric with 2-0 nylon and secure with an additional suture ligature. Continue the dissection anterior to the aorta up to the duodenum to the level of the left renal vein. Lift this vein with a vein retractor and secure the lymphatics at this level with multiple clips. Remove the node chain and dissect lateral and inferior to the aorta to remove the additional group of nodes in that location. Be certain to secure the upper margin of this chain of nodes as they go under the renal vein to avoid lymph accumulations in the retroperitoneum.

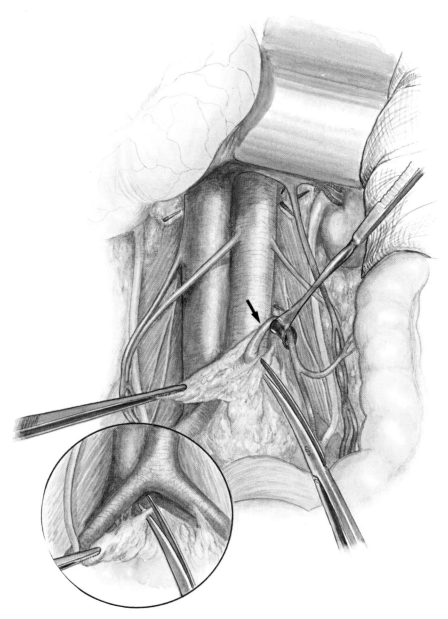

FIGURE 14.6.   Bring the nodal mass downward toward the pelvis and dissect it free of the inferior mesenteric artery. Again, pay attention to the lumbar vessels as they exit the aorta in this area. Dissect the nodal chain downward anteriorly and superior to the common iliac artery to the point where the ureter crosses this vessel. Perform a similar dissection on the right side and remove the fat pad overlying the bifurcation of the vena cava which often contains nodal tissue. Inset: Remove the remaining common iliac nodes from around the common iliac artery and vein to the point where the ureter and ovarian vessels cross the bifurcation of the common iliac artery. Avoid injury to the ureter by constant visualization. Continuously monitor retraction on the upper abdominal viscera as the deep retractors may produce the injuries previously noted. Remember that vascular anomalies are common, particularly in the venous system, and be alert to isolate and clip such unsuspected vessels. Save time by placing a dry pack against a small vessel that is difficult to visualize and dissect in other areas. Often the bleeding will have stopped after a period of pressure application. Avoid mass ligation of lymphoid tissue in the upper reaches of the incision as damage to branches of the celiac axis or other abdominal vessels may occur if the area is not well exposed.

155

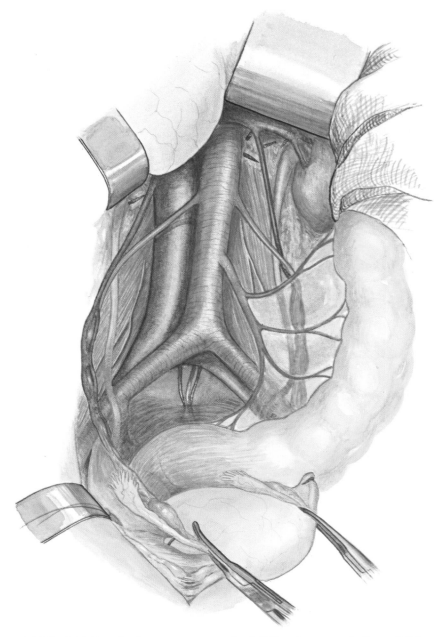

FIGURE 14.7.   Drains are not required following completion of this procedure. Close the peritoneal incision with continuous 2-0 or 3-0 absorbable suture. Carefully inspect the upper abdominal viscera, colon, and small bowel; replace them in the abdomen with warm packs; replace the large Deaver retractors above and proceed with distal lymph node dissection.

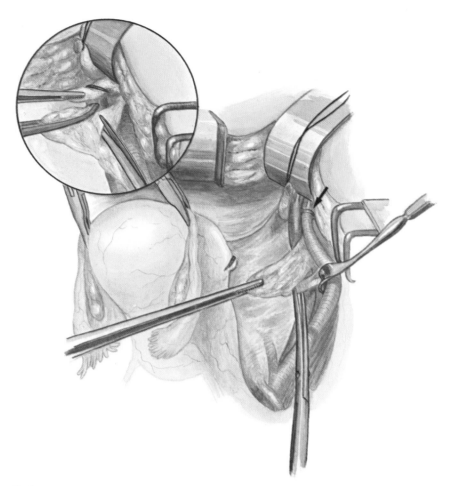

FIGURE 14.8.   Identify the ovarian vessels and separate them from the
ureter. Doubly ligate the ovarian vessels with 2-0 Nurolon, employing a
distal suture ligature, and clip the specimen side vessels; divide them between the uterus and ovary if they are to be retained. Continue the lymphadenectomy by extending the dissection plane in the adventitia of the
great vessels along the anterior surface of the external iliac artery to the
point where the vessel leaves the abdomen. Avoid or clip the circumflex
iliac vein at the arrow as it crosses anterior to the external iliac artery.
Dissect the fibrofatty tissue and lymph nodes along the psoas muscle and
genitofemoral nerve and direct these medially. Avoid severing the genitofemoral nerve. Pull the nodal tissues medially near the inguinal ligament,
exposing the external iliac artery and vein. Medial to the external iliac
vein, lymphatic tissue and numerous lymphatic channels from the groin
should be pulled upward and clipped. Inset: Dissect downward toward
the pelvic floor into the paravesical space and enter the adventitial sheath
covering the external iliac vein. Dissect these tissues free using Adson-
Brown thumb forceps, long delicate Nelson chest scissors, and sponge
sticks to produce planar tension on the tissues.

157

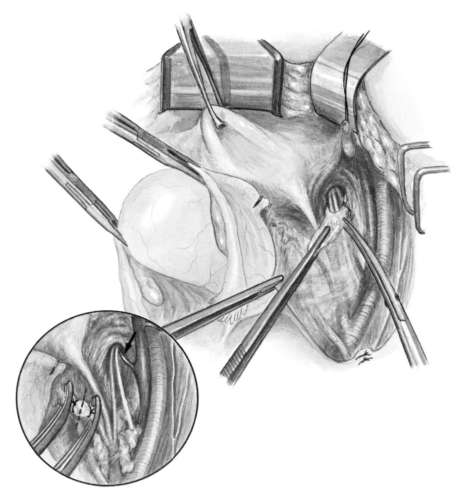

FIGURE 14.9. Continue the dissection cephalad between the external iliac artery and vein and reflect these tissues medially. Clip the rather constant bleeder at the junction of the external and internal iliac artery and vein securely. Expose the obturator nerve, artery, and vein. The nerve is easily palpated. Secure the vein if necessary with a small clip and dissect this node group upward and medially. With initial entrance into the pelvic floor through the paravesical space, the great vessels along the pelvic wall and ureteral entrance into the pelvis are now clearly seen. Isolate and preserve the superior vesical artery and the artery to the ureter from the internal iliac arising 2 to 3 cm from the bifurcation. Inset: Irrigate the pelvis and secure any bleeders. Follow the ureter downward and identify the uterine artery. It is usually serpiginous and most commonly arises from the internal iliac or superior vesical artery. Elevate it with a Gemini clamp and doubly ligate with 2-0 or 3-0 nonabsorbable suture. Leave the specimen side long for ease in identification when dissecting the ureteral tunnel. Note the anomalous obturator vein at the arrow; a variety of vascular patterns are found in the pelvis. Perform a similar dissection on the opposite side by pulling the uterus sharply to the right; enter the retroperitoneum by dividing the round ligaments as before, and initiate the dissection of the plane anterior to the external iliac artery. Strong traction with Masterson clamps upward toward the patient's right shoulder will produce the best initial exposure.

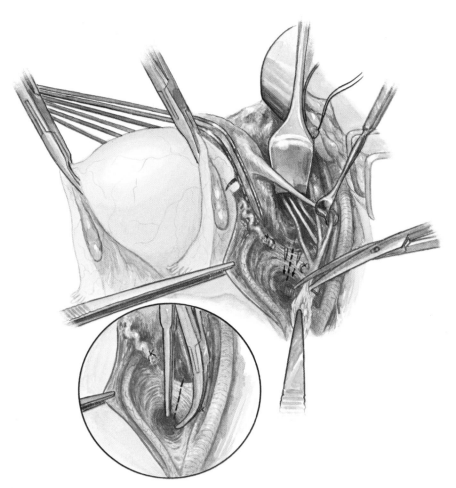

FIGURE 14.10. Complete nodal removal of any tissues lying in the perirectal space and bluntly dissect both the pararectal and paravesical spaces to the floor at the levator muscles. Pull the superior vesical artery from the area with a vein retractor and visualize the cardinal ligament (web) separating the paravesical and pararectal spaces. If slender, secure with a row of clips and divide sharply. Remember that once employed it is difficult to apply a clamp across clips if they do not work. Inset: The web may be clamped by a long curved Masterson clamp to the pelvic wall and may be secured with a swaged 0 chromic catgut or heavy silk figure-of-eight sutures. A straight Masterson clamp may be applied medially on the specimen or the vessels may be clipped. When clips are applied, remember that strong traction may avulse them from the vessels and the area should be inspected to avoid unsuspected blood loss. When pelvic wall bleeding occurs, figure-of-eight sutures or clips may be needed. Do not suture too deeply as the sciatic nerve lies close by.

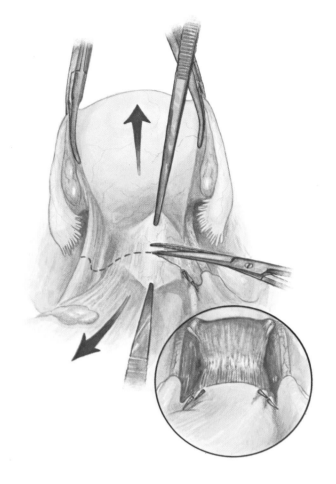

FIGURE 14.11. Pull the uterus sharply and firmly toward the pubis, putting the rectum in tension. Open the peritoneum across the cul-de-sac, being careful of the ureters on each side. Sharply dissect the rectum down 3 to 4 cm from its attachment to the vagina. Identify the uterosacral ligaments on each side; they are best identified by palpation between the surgeon's fingers. Divide and clip them with large clips close to their origin on the sacrum. Inset: Carry this dissection down parallel to the sacrum and toward the vagina. It is necessary to clip the uterosacrals on both sides due to the hemorrhoidal vessels in these ligaments. The uterus will rise out of the pelvis as these ligaments are severed. Continue the dissection until all palpable uterosacral ligaments have been divided.

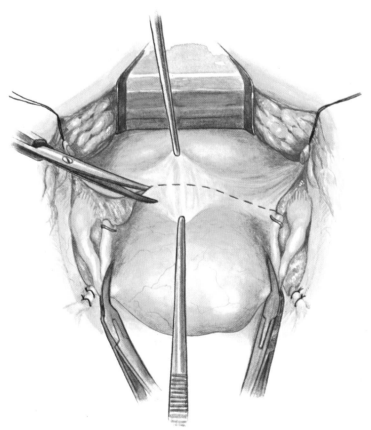

FIGURE 14.12. Pull the uterus up cephalad and open the vesicouterine fold. The anterior bladder pillars are clamped with Gemini clamps and suture ligated with fine absorbable suture.

160

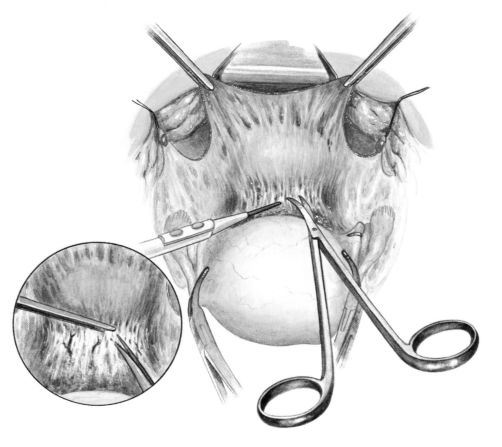

FIGURE 14.13. Grasp the bladder with Adson-Brown thumb forceps and sharply dissect the bladder off the anterior vagina for 5 to 6 cm. This utilizes the same plane as simple hysterectomy; however, the dissection is more extensive and the vaginal muscularis should be left intact using the vesical margin of this plane.

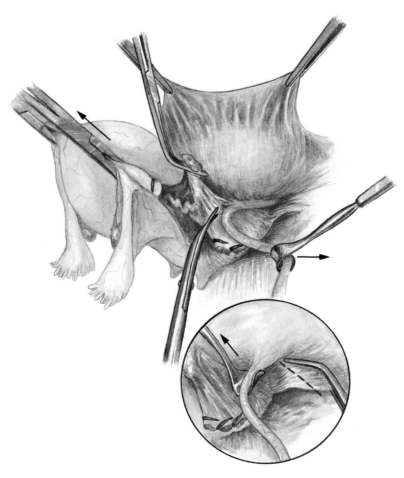

FIGURE 14.14. Free the ureters from the medial peritoneum just cephalad to the uterus and hold the ureters laterally, defining the ureteral tunnel. Pull the uterus strongly to the opposite side and cut the ureters from their tunnel with fine sharp Metzenbaum scissors. Ligate any bleeders. This dissection is facilitated by pulling sharply upward with Gemini forceps on the stump of the uterine artery, freeing the ureter all around with sharp dissection. Dissect holding the ureter downward as the lower vagina is approached and sever the ureteral vaginal attachment with scissors. The ureteral tunnel is comprised of numerous venous sinusoids attached to both bladder and vagina and is variable in size. Inset: If thin, only sharp incision is required along the dotted line. If more substantial, individual clamping with Gemini clamps and 3-0 or 4-0 absorbable suture may be required. Do not employ clips this near the vaginal margin, on the bladder, or in the bladder muscle.

161

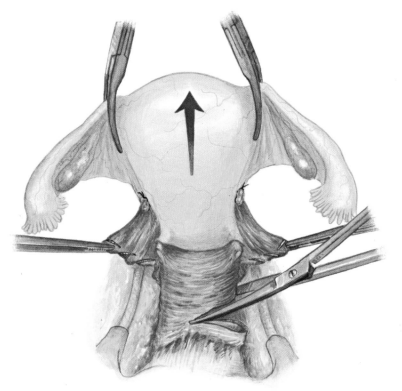

FIGURE 14.15. Hold the uterus upward anteriorly and sever any remaining uterosacral or other ligamentous structures. Hold the stumps of the cardinal ligaments away from the uterus and any remaining lateral bladder pillars will become apparent. These structures contain nerve tissue and may contain several large veins. Clamp and suture ligate any remaining vessels. Dissect any remaining bladder off the anterior surface of the vagina to the chosen margin of excision. Clamp the tissue lateral to the vagina with Masterson clamps, transect, and suture ligate these remaining tissues. Cut across the vagina above the bladder and rectal reflection. Secure the remaining vagina anteriorly, laterally, and posteriorly with Allis clamps.

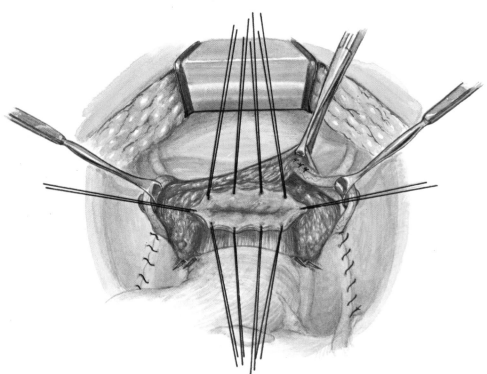

FIGURE 14.16. Ligate the edges of the open vagina with a figure-of-eight suture. Do not use a running lock as this narrows the vaginal opening. Tie the sutures but leave them long. Irrigate the pelvis copiously with saline and seek any remaining bleeders. Catch the edge of the bladder where the superior vesical artery joins the dome and hold it on tension. Support the ureter with the superior vesical artery for 3 to 4 cm cephalad to the bladder, taking care not to obstruct either structure. Place sump drains through separate stab wounds beneath the tied round ligaments and place them medial to the pelvic vessels but lateral to the ureter. Place the tip of the sump in the obturator fossa.

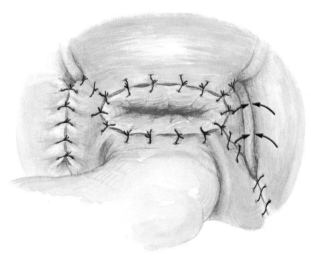

FIGURE 14.17. Sew the bladder flap anterior to the anterior vaginal wall using long chromic sutures previously placed in the vagina; sew the posterior vaginal flap to the rectal peritoneum in a similar fashion. Reperitonealize the area lateral to the vagina for several centimeters in a similar fashion. Sew the peritoneum covering the bladder to the peritoneum covering the rectum such that a pouch of open vagina is created. The ureters are now in the peritoneal cavity. Prepare a hammock for them by oversewing the peritoneum over the distal ureter, making certain that no stricture exists where the ureter enters the peritoneal tunnel. Sew the peritoneum over the ureters and complete any peritoneal closure if necessary near the aorta. If the peritoneum is of poor quality due to heavy irradiation or adhesions, the ureters may be placed extraperitoneally and the remaining peritoneum may simply be closed after the vaginal vault is closed with interrupted Smead Jones sutures of 3-0 absorbable suture. This produces a closed vagina and places the ureters in an extraperitoneal fashion. If no peritoneum remains be certain to close the vagina and prepare an omental carpet to cover the pelvis and distal ureters.

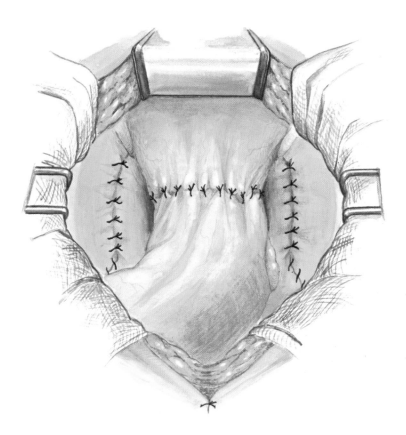

FIGURE 14.18. Following complete reperitonealization, place the drains extraperitoneally and attach them to suction. The lengthened vagina lies in the midline. The aortic peritoneum incision should meet the lower pelvic closure. Obtain careful needle and instrument counts, remove all laparotomy packs from the abdomen, and close the wound in layers of 0 braided nylon or wire in a Smead Jones fashion. No subcutaneous stitches are used and the skin is closed with 3-0 nylon.

163

ligaments. In stage I and IIa disease up to 25% of patients may have nodal metastasis. These patients have a 5% to 10% chance of also having para-aortic disease. About 25% of the patients who have pelvic nodal metastasis also have para-aortic spread, so when there is definite evidence of nodal disease in the pelvis it is probably wise to perform a para-aortic node dissection. Therefore, in the complete operation the nodes along the aorta and vena cava from the renal vessels down are removed along with the lymph nodes in the pelvis. The uterus and upper third of the vagina are also removed, along with almost the entire uterosacral and cardinal ligaments. The operation is useful for cancers confined to the cervix, i.e., the smaller stage Ib and IIa cancers, carcinoma of the upper vagina, and stage II carcinoma of the endometrium.

In most patients with recurrent cervical cancer after radiation this type of operation will not be suitable because of the size of the tumor, the involvement of adjacent organs, or prior radiation therapy. However, in very selected patients, radical hysterectomy may be suitable, although one must be willing to accept a higher complication rate due to the devascularization of the pelvis following radiation therapy.

Postoperative Management

On the morning of operation the patient is given 5,000 units of heparin subcutaneously, and this dose is administered every 12 hr until the patient is fully ambulatory. The author has noted that heparinization with a very low dose of heparin has increased the operative bleeding slightly, but no associated postoperative hemorrhages or wound hematomas have been noted. With the use of chemical prophylaxis the number and severity of pulmonary emboli have decreased and the author has noted no postoperative deaths due to pulmonary embolization.

Pelvic node dissection will predispose the patient to a large postoperative and intraoperative loss of serum and serum albumin. If left uncorrected this can lead to a deficit in intravascular volume, tachycardia, and postoperative edema. Therefore, the patient is given 25 g salt-poor albumin during the operation and an additional 50 to 75 g on the day of operation. For the next several days, 50 to 75 g of albumin is given and the serum protein concentration is closely monitored. A simple and inexpensive way to monitor the serum proteins is to measure the serum solids, since this is equivalent to total protein. The serum solids should be kept between 6 and 7 g/dl.

Another problem that occurs with retroperitoneal dissection is an accumulation of lymph and serum along the pelvic sidewalls that may become infected or ultimately lead to a lymphocyst. Therefore, both sides of the pelvis and the deep pelvic cavity should be drained. The author prefers the use of sump drains, finding them more efficient than the closed Hemovac system. The sumps are left in until each side drains less than 30 ml/day; this usually occurs on the fourth or fifth postoperative day. Under no circumstances should the sump tubes be irrigated, since this can lead to a serious pelvic infection.

The third problem associated with retroperitoneal dissection is ileus. It is therefore wise to insert a nasogastric tube during the operation and maintain the patient on nasogastric suction for several days. Once the patient's bowel activity has returned and she is passing flatus the tube can be withdrawn.

The operation described in this chapter will almost completely remove all the autonomic nerves to and from the bladder and, to a lesser extent, the rectum. The usual postoperative hospital stay is 7 to 10 days. Postoperatively the patient will have little, if any, bladder sensation, and alarming amounts of urine may accumulate in the bladder. It is necessary to leave a Foley catheter or, if one chooses, a suprapubic cystotomy catheter in the bladder for 4 to 6 weeks postoperatively. Then the catheter is withdrawn and the urine cultured. The patient is then taught to use the Credé maneuver (suprapubic pressure) and is told to void every 2 or 3 hr during the day, by the clock, using the abdominal musculature and the mechanical pressure of the hands to completely evacuate the bladder. She is also told to use a mild laxative such as milk of magnesia and to keep her bowel working and as empty as possible. The patient returns after 1 week and the residual urine is checked. If it is less than 150 ml the catheter can be left out. It is necessary to check the patient again for residual in 1 month and in 3 months, and to continue to reinforce timed voiding with the suprapubic maneuver. The patients will, over a period of time, recover some of their bladder sensation but it is usually not normal.

While the catheter is in place the author gives pharmacologic prophylaxis against infection and maintains this for several weeks after the catheter is withdrawn. Then, when the residual is checked, the urine is again cultured. Approximately 3 months after surgery an intravenous pyelogram is performed to see if there has been ureteral damage or stricture.

Results

Hoskins et al. surveyed the recent literature for results of radical hysterectomy and pelvic lymphadenectomy. They analyzed a total of 1,874 cases reported by 9 authors and summarized the results as follows[1]:

Survival for stage Ib	81.9%
Survival for stages Ib and IIa	74.2%
Ureterovaginal fistula rate	4.8%
Operative mortality	1.3%

In Symmond's series of 64 patients, included in the 1,874 cases, no urinary tract fistulas were noted.

When the primary cervical cancer is larger than 1 cm, approximately 10% of radical hysterectomy specimens have one or more nodes showing microscopic cancer. When microscopic nodal disease is found, the patient should receive 5,000 rads in 5 weeks to the whole pelvis postoperatively. In their own series of 224 patients, Hoskins et al. report that 75% survived 3 years.[1]

References

1. Hoskins, W.J., Ford, J.H., Lutz, M.H., et al.: Radical hysterectomy and pelvic lymphadenectomy for the management of early invasive cancer of the cervix. *Gynecol. Oncol.* **4:**278–290, 1976.
2. Macaset, M.A., Lu, T., and Nelson, J.H., Jr.: Ureterovaginal fistula as a complication of radical hysterectomy. *Am. J. Obstet. Gynecol.* **124:**757–760, 1976.

3. Meigs, J.V.: Carcinoma of the cervix—The Wertheim operation. *Surg. Gynecol. Obstet.* **78:**195–199, 1944.

4. Nelson, J.H., Jr.: *Atlas of Radical Pelvic Surgery,* 2nd ed. New York, Appleton-Century-Crofts, 1977.

5. Okabayashi, J.: Radical abdominal hysterectomy for cancer of the cervix uteri. *Surg. Gynecol. Obstet.* **33:**335–341, 1921.

6. Roman-Lopez, J.J., and Barclay, D.C.: Bladder dysfunction following Schauta hysterectomy. *Am. J. Obstet. Gynecol.* **115:**81–90, 1973.

7. Seski, J.C., and Diokno, A.C.: Bladder dysfunction after radical abdominal hysterectomy. *Am. J. Obstet. Gynecol.* **128:**643–651, 1977.

8. Speert, H.: *Obstetric and Gynecologic Milestones: Essays in Eponymy.* New York, Macmillan, 1958.

9. Wertheim, E.: The extended abdominal operation for carcinoma uteri: Based on 500 operated cases (Gradd, H. transl.). *Am. J. Obstet. Gynecol. Dis. Women Child.* **66:**169–232, 1912.

10. Yagi, J.: Extended abdominal hysterectomy with pelvic lymphadenectomy for carcinoma of the cervix. *Am. J. Obstet. Gynecol.* **69:**33–47, 1955.

Myomectomy

15

Leiomyomas of the uterus occur in approximately 20% of women over 30 years of age in this country.[8] Of the women who have leiomyomas of significant size, approximately 40% demonstrate infertility[10]; 50% of the patients in whom no other cause of infertility is demonstrated become pregnant on removal of the myoma.[11] It is apparent that, in well-selected patients, myomectomy does increase fertility and it is an alternative for uterine preservation in those patients desiring childbearing capabilities.

The mechanism of myomas in infertility is not known.[11] It is generally agreed that small myomas have little effect on fertility; however, as the size approaches 2 cm, particularly if they are multiple, the incidence of infertility may increase. If the leiomyomas are submucosal in location, they may interfere with proper nidation by distending the endometrium over the leiomyoma, producing a relatively less vascular endometrium. A large leiomyoma may disturb the normal uterine artery and it may also distort the intramural portion of the fallopian tube. Obviously, the larger the tumor the more difficulty one might anticipate. Additionally, submucosal leiomyomas are commonly associated with menorrhagia and may require treatment prior to or in an interval between pregnancies. Where continued fertility is desired, myomectomy is performed in these patients.

Pathology

The cut surface of leiomyomas will project above the surrounding myometrium and may often compress it. This compression produces a capsule of use in myomectomy. The blood vessels to the leiomyomas enter through this capsule.[2] The arteries are derived from the adjacent uterine vessels and enter the leiomyomas from different poles. They then branch and penetrate toward the center. The blood supply is decreased toward the center of the tumor and degenerative changes usually start there. The veins are usually beneath the capsule. Thus, in myomectomy, the capsule is used as a surgical plane but sutures are placed through it to provide hemostasis.

Leiomyomas may undergo various degenerative changes. Persaud noted that 65% showed one or more alterations. Hyaline degeneration was most common, but myxomatous, mucoid, cystic, fatty, and red changes

167

were also seen; 8% of leiomyomas calcify and there is little or no correlation with the clinical picture and the type of degeneration observed.

Preoperative Evaluation

Myomectomy is indicated in those patients in whom a symptomatic lesion exists and in the patient who wishes uterine preservation. If the patient is infertile for 1 year or more and no other cause of infertility is present, myomectomy is suggested. The procedure is reserved for the patient with a leiomyoma larger than 2 cm.

Myomectomy in pregnancy is rarely necessary. Gainey and Keeler noted that only 0.05% of 355,550 pregnancies were complicated by leiomyoma.[3] Stevenson found excellent results in 17 cases of myomectomy during pregnancy with 83% of the pregnancies progressing to term.[11] In 14 of these patients, subserosal tumors were found. Although undergoing torsion with necrosis, these tumors would not be expected to have significant influence on the uterine cavity. Three of his patients did have intramural leiomyomas and these were removed without subsequent complication of the pregnancy.

Pelvic examination will generally disclose the presence of a leiomyoma. A uterine sound is used to detect the presence of a submucosal leiomyoma. The patient should have a hysterosalpingogram to document the presence of such a tumor prior to surgery. A dilatation and curettage is performed in all myomectomy patients to rule out the presence of a coexistent malignancy. Hysteroscopy has recently been reported by Neuwirth to be an alternative to abdominal myomectomy, although he indicates this option is still under clinical investigation.[7]

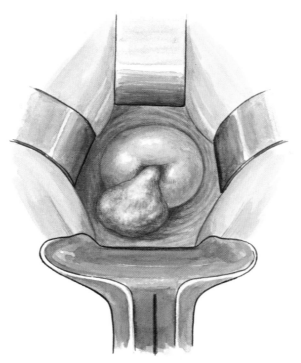

FIGURE 15.1. A leiomyoma presenting through the cervix that is amenable to vaginal excision.

Operative Technique

If the leiomyoma presents vaginally and the patient desires continued fertility, a tonsil snare is passed over the leiomyoma and it is excised (Figures 15.1 and 15.2). The patient is placed on antibiotics prior to excision as these patients usually have associated parametritis due to the inflammatory reaction surrounding the leiomyoma. If the leiomyoma is submucosal or intramural in location, direct incision through an abdominal approach with excision is performed (Figures 15.3 and 15.4). Subserous myomas do not usually interfere with fertility or produce bleeding problems and they would not be treated unless large in size. When multiple myomectomies are considered, complete one excision at a time to minimize blood loss.

Cervical leiomyomas are discussed in Chapter 13.

When the surgeon proceeds without delay, no tourniquet or clamps are placed across the uterine blood supply; instead the author recommends the use of a hemostatic solution. While Pituitrin produces a superior vasospastic reaction in the pelvis, its use is associated with cardiac abnormalities and the author does not recommend it for general use. Six drops of Neo-Synephrine in 30 ml of saline is quite satisfactory and is injected into the uterine wall surrounding the mass with a 22-gauge needle. The use of well-placed sutures followed by a brief period of pressure is usually adequate for hemostasis.

Postoperative Management and Results

In the vaginal approach the postoperative orders are the same as for a patient who undergoes a dilatation and curettage. For the abdominal ap-

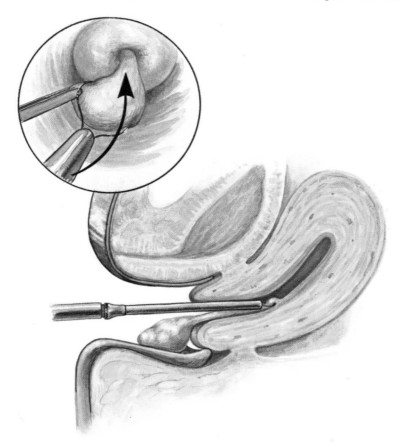

FIGURE 15.2. If the leiomyoma has a relatively narrow stalk, it is removed vaginally with a tonsil snare. Inset: Pass the extended wire of the tonsil snare around the leiomyoma and grasp it with thumb forceps. Slide the tonsil snare to the base of the leiomyoma and close it, cutting the pedunculated leiomyoma free. Curette the uterine cavity to make certain that no malignancy has been obscured by the symptoms of bleeding and discharge that usually accompany prolapsed leiomyoma.

169

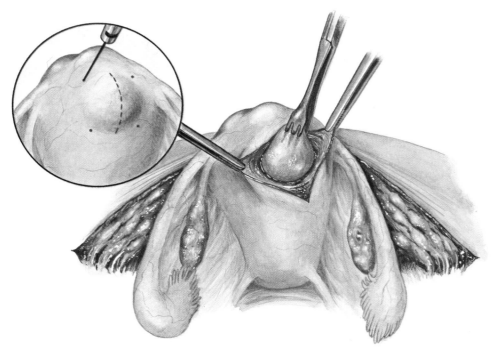

FIGURE 15.3.   Inject the leiomyoma with a dilute solution of Neo-Synephrine in its periphery in the substance of the capsule where the blood supply originates; make the incision in the capsule overlying the tumor taking care not to incise the tubal lumen (inset). Grasp the leiomyoma firmly with the thyroid clamp and pull upward. The plane of dissection lies in the capsule surrounding the substance of the leiomyoma and it may be enucleated from this capsule.

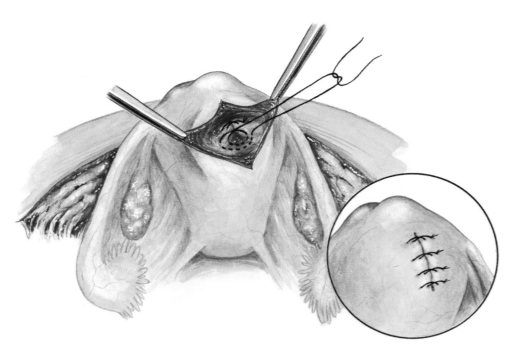

FIGURE 15.4.   Close the uterus in two layers. Using 0 chromic catgut on a general closure swaged needle, place the first layer deep in the substance of the capsule and uterine muscle in a Smead Jones or pulley-type fashion. When the uterine cavity is entered, invert the mucosa but do not close the mucosa as a separate layer. Inset: Use the same type of suture in the outer layer to close the uterine defect.

proach, laparotomy postoperative orders are employed. Regardless of the approach, place the patient on antibiotics for 3 days.

The absence of uterine involution, inflammatory changes of pregnancy, and problems with hemostasis promote better uterine healing in myomectomy than in cesarean section. Uterine rupture after myomectomy is rare in subsequent pregnancies. Brown et al. reported the delivery of 120 term infants without uterine rupture; 96 were delivered vaginally and 24 by cesarean section.[1] Many obstetricians today, however, will deliver all patients after myomectomy by cesarean section except if the myoma was subserous. If the uterine cavity has been entered or multiple myomectomies performed, cesarean section is considered obligatory.[5] Where careful preoperative evaluation has excluded other causes of infertility, a pregnancy rate of 36.8%[1] to 50%[11] has been observed following myomectomy for infertility.

Myomectomy should be regarded as a temporizing procedure to gain time for reproductive efforts. Loeffler and Noble noted a 60% recurrence rate for menorrhagia and 75% recurrence of irregular bleeding in the 5-year period following myomectomy performed for these reasons.[6] The occurrence of additional leiomyomas can be expected. Brown et al. found that 28% of myomectomy patients had recurrent leiomyomas in a 2-year period of follow-up, and 15% of these patients required hysterectomy. Ingersoll and Malone followed a group of 125 myomectomy patients.[4] Leiomyomas recurred in 47%. When the myomectomy was performed for multiple and large tumors, the recurrence rate was 58.8%. Twenty percent of the 125 patients had subsequent hysterectomies for leiomyomas that had recurred.[4]

References

1. Brown, A.B., Chamberlain, R., and TeLinde, R.W.: Myomectomy. *Am. J. Obstet. Gynecol.* **71**:759–763, 1956.
2. Faulkner, R.L.: The blood vessels of the myomatous uterus. *Am. J. Obstet. Gynecol.* **47**:185–197, 1944.
3. Gainey, H.L., and Keeler, J.E.: Submucous myoma in term pregnancy. *Am. J. Obstet. Gynecol.* **58**:727–737, 1949.
4. Ingersoll, F.M., and Malone, L.J.: Myomectomy: An alternative to hysterectomy. *Arch. Surg.* **100**:557–561, 1970.
5. Krantz, K.E.: Personal communication.
6. Loeffler, F.E., and Noble, A.D.: Myomectomy at the Chelsea Hospital for Women. *J. Obstet. Gynaecol. Br. Commonw.* **77**:167–170, 1970.
7. Neuwirth, R.S.: A new technique for and additional experience with hysteroscopic resection of submucous fibroids. *Am. J. Obstet. Gynecol.* **131**:91–94, 1978.
8. Novak, E.: *Gynecological and Obstetrical Pathology,* 2nd ed. Philadelphia, Saunders, 1947.
9. Persaud, V. and Arjoon, P.D.: Uterine leiomyoma. *Obstet. Gynecol.* **35**: 432–436, 1970.
10. Rubin, I.C.: Myomectomy in the interest of fertility. *Trans. N.J. Obstet. Gynecol. Soc.* **2**:7, 1957.
11. Stevenson, C.S.: Myomectomy for improvement of fertility. *Fertil. Steril.* **15**:367–384, 1964.

16 Infertility Surgery of the Fallopian Tube

Jamil A. Fayez

One-half of the women who desire to bear a child but who are unable to have tubal abnormalities. In most cases the tubes are either occluded or surrounded by peritoneal adhesions.[5] Gynecologists have long been interested in surgical correction of these defects, but initial results were quite poor. Greenhill surveyed 107 gynecologists in 1936 who were members of The American Association of Obstetricians and Gynecologists or The American Gynecologic Society. Eighty-two percent had never performed a tubal implantation and the entire group had performed 818 tuboplastic operations. Thirty-six live births resulted from these procedures for an incidence of 1 live baby per 22 operations. The majority of gynecologists surveyed were definitely opposed to tubal infertility surgery.[7]

The gynecologist who trained using Heaney clamps, 1 chromic suture and whose primary surgical experience was in extirpative surgery was ill-suited to delicate reconstructive procedures. Therefore there were generally poor results and such patients were frequently referred to university hospitals. Physicians with a special interest in infertility surgery gradually developed.

Refinements in technique and new technological advances in eye and reconstructive surgery were gradually applied to tubal repair. Hellman reported use of polyethylene splints in 1951[8] and Rock and Mulligan suggested hoods to protect the fimbria of the tube from agglutinizing during the postoperative period.[11]

Greenhill resurveyed the literature in 1956 and collected reports from surgeons specifically interested in infertility surgery who had extensive experience in tubal reconstructive surgery. Twenty-one hundred and thirteen plastic tubal operations were collected for a total of 313 live births or 1 baby per 6 tubal operations.

Swolin, using meticulous surgical technique made possible by the application of the operating microscope to surgery, noted improved results.[13] Splinting devices were discarded and indications continued to be refined.

Continuing developments in optics, microsuture material, adhesion retardants, and micro instruments allowed greater delicacy in operative manipulation, anastomosis, and hemostasis. Improved rates of tubal patency, resumption of physiological tubal function, and diminished tubal adhesions are being observed. The ultimate reward will hopefully be a high postoperative pregnancy rate with the absolute minimum number of tubal pregnancies. Remember that it has been repeatedly shown that the percentage of tubal patency far exceeds the percentage of pregnancies.[13]

Anatomy and Physiology

The oviducts vary from 8 to 14 cm in length and are covered by peritoneum throughout their entire length. The lumen of the oviduct is lined by a simple layer of columnar cells, of both ciliated and secretory types. The ciliated cells are more easily damaged by pelvic infection. The epithelium rests directly on the muscularis as there is no tubal submucosa. Tubal surgery works best if at least 65% of the cells are ciliated; if the percentage is lower, the results of reconstructive surgery are not good.

Each tube is divided into an interstitial portion, isthmus, ampulla, and infundibulum. The fimbria ovarica is the longest strand of the fimbriae. It contains muscle and forms a shallow gutter that is attached to the ovary. When surgeons approach damaged fimbriae they must remember that there is in fact a normal attachment to the ovary.

The primary physiological consideration in this surgery stems from the differential anatomy of the oviduct. The heavier musculature and the acute angulation of the interstitial portion suggest that the cornu may serve as a sphincter controlling access to the ampulla.[14] The isthmic and ampullary portions show different anatomy, suggesting different physiological functions. In the more lightly muscled ampullary portion, ciliary and peristaltic action appears to be the primary function.[2] The major physiological functions of the oviduct are the process of ovum pick-up, ovum transport, sperm transport, sperm capacitation, fertilization, embryo transport, and early embryo nourishment.[10]

Preoperative Evaluation

Select only those patients who have no other identifiable cause for infertility. These patients then must have adequate tubal diagnostic tests to determine if they might benefit from tuboplasty. Preoperative hysterosalpingography will demonstrate the absence of intrauterine lesions, the site of tubal obstruction, and the presence or absence of ampullary rugae. Women whose tubal lumina have maintained rugae are said to have a better prognosis.[15] Laparoscopy accompanied by intrauterine injection of dye and gentle tubal manipulation is the most reliable test as it reveals the condition of the fimbriae and the degree of tubal fixation; it permits assessment of the pathology at the site of occlusion and hence permits a better selection of patients. After laparoscopy, all patients must be counseled in the presence of their husbands and advised precisely of what can be accomplished by the contemplated surgery, particularly with regard to the chances of a term pregnancy.

The following factors are considered contraindications of tuboplasty:

1. Age over 38 years old: after this age there is a marked decrease in the fertility rate.

2. A recent history of active inflammatory disease: 6 months should elapse after successful treatment before tuboplasty is attempted.
3. A history of pelvic tuberculosis: these patients may develop generalized peritonitis and the results are exceedingly poor.
4. Obesity: The procedure is extremely difficult if the tubes cannot be elevated almost to the level of the abdominal wall; however, obesity is only a relative contraindication.
5. Less than 5 cm of tube remaining on both sides of the cauterized area as revealed by laparoscopy.
6. Previous sterilization by fimbriectomy with resection of the infundibular–fimbrial mechanism.
7. Contraindications to pregnancy.

Operative Strategy

Adherence to the general principles as outlined by Gomel can improve the results of reconstructive tubal surgery and help prevent postoperative pelvic adhesions.[6]

Perform all procedures during the proliferative phase of the menstrual cycle as diminished operative bleeding, improved tubal healing, and convenient hydrotubation timing are present during this phase.

The damage due to surgical handling causes the formation of peritubal adhesions, fibrosis, poor revascularization, and a disturbance of patency. Talc and starch, the two materials used to dust sterile gloves, have been shown to cause intraperitoneal granuloma formation. Therefore, gloves must be rinsed prior to opening the peritoneal cavity. Minimum handling of tissues with atraumatic surgical instruments is also imperative. Threads from gauze sponges have also been found in association with granulomas. The mesothelium of reproductive organs is easily scraped off, predisposing the tissue to adhesion formation. Irrigation with normal saline and suction should be used throughout the entire procedure to clear the operative field, avoid tissue desiccation and minimize tissue trauma.

Instrumentation

In tuboplasty the use of light instruments that can be held by the fingertips is mandatory. The author uses fine opthalmic microsurgical instruments such as Castro viejo needle holders and scissors and opthalmic straight or curved scissors delicate enough for fine fingertip control. Straight bayonet-type forceps with fine tips are employed for tying fine sutures. Use 7-0 Prolene or 7-0 Vicryl; the former is nonabsorbable and has minimal associated tissue reaction due to the fact that biodegradation takes place long after the healing process is completed. Ideally, the needle should be tapered, about 5 mm in length, and have a curvature of about 135 degrees. If smaller suture is chosen, use a small needle as much of the tissue damage is produced by the needle. 8-0 suture, for example, should be armed with a 130-μ needle.[4]

Meticulous hemostasis can best be achieved with a bipolar forceps providing coagulation at low voltage. Grasp tissues to be coagulated so that the tips do not contact each other as the current will be short circuited and no coagulation will occur. Use an intermittent stream of saline solution to avoid burning adjacent tissues.

Hoods and stents result in fibrosis of the tubal wall and in unnecessary destruction of the delicate ciliated mucosa of the endosalpinx; the present consensus is to avoid the use of artificial devices to maintain tubal patency.

Exposure

Carefully divide any pelvic adhesions. Pack the cul-de-sac with laparotomy tapes soaked in normal saline containing 4 mg dexamethasone per liter. Elevate the uterus and adnexae anteriorly to allow positioning of the operating microscope so that the surgeon may sit and rest his forearms comfortably.

Intraoperative Tubal Patency Test

Probes should never be used to test tubal patency because the technique has proved to be excessively traumatic; histopathological studies often disclosed the presence of translocated mucosal cells within the muscular layer.

Patency of the tube or the site of tubal occlusion can be visualized during the procedure through intrauterine dye instillation: Occlude the lower uterine segment with an atraumatic clamp and inject a solution of indigo carmine diluted in normal saline utilizing a 30-ml syringe with an 18-gauge needle transfundal into the uterine cavity. Patency is confirmed when spillage from the tube occurs. This procedure also facilitates location of the mucosal lining of the tubal lumen, since the endosalpinx is stained dark blue. Patency of the distal portion of the tube in cases of midsegment reanastomosis is established by perfusion with the same dye solution using a bulb syringe inserted through the fimbria.

Pelvic Lavage

When the procedure is completed, the patient is put in the reversed Trendelenburg position and the pelvis is washed several times with warm normal saline solution, removing all blood clots and debris that may be left after surgery. Before closure of the abdomen, 200 ml low molecular weight dextran solution mixed with 8 mg dexamethasone is introduced intraperitoneally. Dextran is reported to have an antithrombotic effect and a silicon-like function that hinder adhesion formation.[9]

Medication

Antihistamines and pharmacologic doses of glucocorticoids preoperatively, intraoperatively, and postoperatively probably reduce the physiological response to surgical trauma. The use of these agents suppresses the initial inflammatory exudate associated with surgery and also inhibits fibroplasia within the fibrinous exudate. In view of the fact that large doses of corticoids may diminish the body's resistance to infection, a broad-spectrum antibiotic must be administered concurrently. In the author's institution, all patients are given 8 mg Decadron and 25 mg Phenergan in separate syringes intramuscularly 2 hr before operation. Beginning 4 hr postsurgery, the same intramuscular dose is repeated at 6-hr intervals and continued through the third postoperative day. As noted, the medications must be separated to eliminate the formation of a precipitate.

Ampicillin, 1 g every 6 hr, is administered intravenously beginning 2 hr prior to surgery and is continued for 72 hr postoperatively; then it is given in a dose of 250 mg every 6 hr orally for 10 days.

Hydrotubation

The value of postoperative hydrotubation has been demonstrated by Grant, who reported significant improvement in his results through frequent treatments.[6] For a number of years, the author has been utilizing hydrotubation in all patients who had tuboplasty. The author is convinced from his unpublished data that hydrotubation plays a major therapeutic role in maintaining tubal patency. The purpose is to remove tubal agglutinations and to flush out mucus and blood. Neomycin, 0.5%, and 4 mg dexamethasone are added to normal saline to a total volume of 50 ml. By means of a hysterosalpingogram cannula, the solution is injected through the cervix gently and slowly. It is advised that the patient be given 50 mg Demerol intravenously 15 min prior to the procedure.

Postoperative Management

All patients should have hysterosalpingography with aqueous contrast medium 10 weeks postoperatively to assess the results; this should be done during the proliferative phase of the cycle. Swolin advocated a second-look laparoscopy, particularly in fimbrioplasty and in salpingoneostomy cases.[13] The author agrees and performs laparoscopy 12 weeks postoperatively.

Intercourse should be avoided for 6 weeks and contraceptive measures be practiced for 3 months postoperatively.

It is imperative to watch closely all patients subjected to reconstructive tubal surgery. The incidence of ectopic in those patients who subsequently become pregnant is approximately 10%.[12] The patients must be made aware of this fact and of its signs and symptoms.

Patients who are unable to achieve a successful term pregnancy within the first 18 months after surgery should be encouraged to adopt. Nearly 75% of those who became pregnant did so within the first year after surgery and 82% conceived within 18 months.[1]

Macroscopic versus Microscopic Tuboplasty

Gynecologic microsurgery is a comparatively new field and is expanding rapidly. The introduction of microsurgical techniques to gynecology has greatly raised the expectations of those who are interested in infertility surgery. The brief experience with the operative microscope has shown that the use of microsurgery yields an impressive improvement in patency and pregnancy rate over the results obtained with gross surgery.[2]

Most infertility surgeons believe that magnification is essential in tubal surgery. Some surgeons use the operating microscope; others are satisfied with magnifying loupes that offer a 4 power magnification. In general the operating microscope is mandatory for all types of tubal reanastomosis; usual magnifications used are between 6 and 16 times. For other infertility operations for tubal reconstruction, loupes that magnify 4 times are often sufficient. The use of the microscope requires special training prior to any attempt by the gynecologist to employ it for tuboplasty. For those wishing to apply microsurgery to the fallopian tube, the New Zealand white rabbit is a useful surrogate patient.[3]

Operative Technique

For the sake of simplicity, and to enable a comparison of his results with others using similar techniques, the author has adopted the following classification since 1974:

1. Salpingolysis: Lysis of peritubal and/or periovarian adhesions to facilitate the tubo-ovarian pick-up mechanism.

2. Fimbrioplasty: Dilatation and/or deagglutination of fimbrial phimosis leaving almost normal fimbria.
3. Salpingoneostomy: Technique for opening the distal tubal obstruction in which no identifiable fimbriae are seen.
4. Anastomosis, either end to end or tubouterine.
5. Cornual implantation: Implantation of the isthmic or ampullary segment into the uterine cavity through an artificially made cornual opening.

Salpingolysis

The term *salpingolysis* refers only to excision of peritubal and periovarian adhesions producing an abnormal tubo-ovarian relationship. These adhesions are usually due to previous pelvic inflammatory disease, previous surgery, or endometriosis. The tubes are patent and infertility is due to impaired ovum pick-up.

Separation of these adhesions is often feasible via laparoscopy and this should be considered as the primary approach. To prevent the recurrence of adhesions, the pelvis should be washed thoroughly with normal saline, and then dextran mixed with dexamethasone is instilled and left in the pelvic cavity. Corticosteroids and antihistamines are administered parenterally as described before.

If separation of the adhesions by laparoscopy is impractical, then laparotomy is performed using extra care in handling the tissues. Blunt digital manipulation should be avoided as lysis should be performed under visual control using microsurgical instruments. The adhesions are stretched with fine-toothed forceps and excised; care must be exercised not to cut the serosal surface (Figure 16.1). A magnifying loupe, though not mandatory, facilitates better dissection in the fimbrial–ovarian region. Bleeding is controlled by constant irrigation; rarely, a microsurgical electrode is necessary; tissue forceps, sutures, and sponges should never be used. Full tubal and ovarian motility should be restored, with the fimbria ovarica kept intact. Large defects and denuded areas should be reperitonealized with 7-0 poly(glycolic acid) suture; minor ones should be left to reperitonize spontaneously.

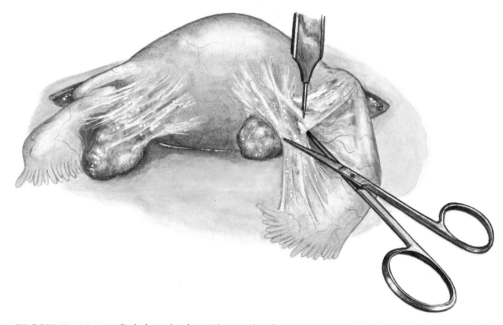

FIGURE 16.1. Salpingolysis. The adhesions are stretched with fine-toothed forceps and excised with eye scissors.

After completion of salpingolysis perform transuterine lavage with indigo carmine to verify tubal patency. Wash the pelvis with normal saline and instill dextran mixed with dexamethasone prior to closure. Glucocorticoids, antihistamines, and antibiotics are used as usual. No hydrotubation is recommended.

Fimbrioplasty

Fimbrioplasty is the correction of partial fimbrial closure by gently teasing apart fimbrial strands and agglutination. Fimbrial phimosis is usually due to bacterial salpingitis or endometriosis, a ruptured appendix, or less often an ectopic pregnancy or generalized peritonitis. This condition is almost always associated with periadnexal obstructive bands. During the diagnostic laparoscopy, some fimbriae are noted with infundibular filling and minimal spillage of dye. Such pathology is surgically corrected during laparoscopy by lysing the adhesions first, and then dilating the fimbrial end by carefully inserting probes and forceps into the small terminal orifice.

If laparotomy is to be performed, the peritoneal adhesions are excised first, then dye is injected transfundally to distend the fimbrial ends. Gently tease apart the fimbria with a microforcep or delicate hemostat (Figure 16.2). This procedure should be repeated a few times in several directions to free the fimbriae and establish a normal opening. A magnifying loupe, though not mandatory, aids the surgeon in performing an accurate and delicate separation of the fimbrial strands. Bleeding is usually minimal. No sutures are used to hold back the fimbria unless it is clear that obstruc-

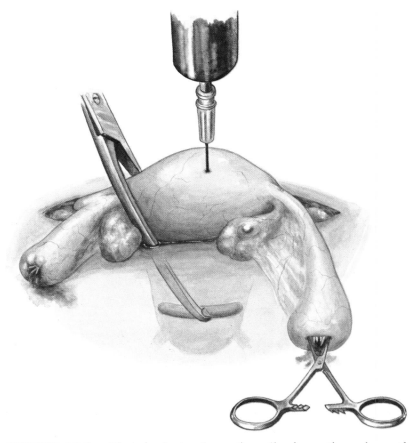

FIGURE 16.2. Fimbrioplasty. Lyse the adhesions; then clamp the cervix and inject transfundal dye to distend the fimbrial ends. To separate the fimbrial agglutinations insert a small closed hemostat into the fimbrial opening and gently spread within the lumen.

tion would surely recur without their use. If necessary, evert the fimbria with a minimum of 7-0 Vicryl suture.

An intraoperative tubal patency test, pelvic lavage, and medications (including antibiotics) are used as previously described. Hydrotubation is started on the first postoperative day when the patient is discharged from the hospital. Hydrotubation is tedious but the author has found that it improves the pregnancy rate.

Salpingoneostomy

This operation involves the establishment of a new stoma in the fimbriated end of a blocked tube such as in a hydrosalpinx. The subtle anatomy of the fimbriae and the importance of their role in ovum pick-up make successful repair difficult. The main problem is not so much the making of a stoma but that of keeping an opened functioning tube. Patients whose hysterosalpingograms show small terminal dilatations and linear mucosal markings have better results than those who have large terminal dilatations without luminal markings.

After the tubes are freed of any adhesions by careful, sharp dissection, a Buxton-type uterine clamp is applied to the cervix and indigo carmine solution is injected transfundal into the uterine cavity. On close observation by the naked eye, or preferably by using a magnifying loupe, one sees a dimple at the distended distal end of the tube. The whitish dimple is stretched with fine-toothed forceps and the infolded fimbria is teased out after the blocked end is opened with a pointed eye forceps (Figure 16.3). Intraoperative procedures and postoperative follow-up are similar to those of fimbrioplasty.

Anastomosis

An anastomosis may be a midsegment reconstruction—which includes

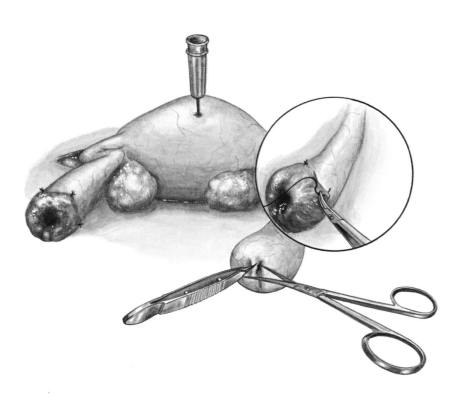

FIGURE 16.3. Salpingoneostomy. The initial procedure is to tease out the infolded fimbria by progressively dilating the lumen after opening it with a pointed eye scissors at the dimple. By adhering to this technique, one encounters minimal bleeding that can easily be controlled by constant irrigation. If this fails, make an X-shaped incision at the bulbous extremity of the tube, thus forming four mucosal flaps. The redundant portion is trimmed back to healthy fimbriated mucosa; in large hydrosalpinges a large amount of thinned out tube must be excised. The mucosa is turned inside out so as to form a pouting mucosal stoma. The mucosal edges of this everted cuff are folded back for about 8 mm and secured to the serosa by four interrupted 7-0 Vicryl sutures. Bleeding points are coagulated individually with the microelectrode under an intermittent stream of saline solution.

ampullary to ampullary, ampullary to isthmic, and isthmic to isthmic—or a tubouterine anastomosis—which involves ampullary to cornual or isthmic to cornual. Each of these five varieties has its own special technical problems and a different prognosis.

End-to-End Anastomosis Most end-to-end anastomoses of the midportion of the tube are usually performed to restore tubal patency following a previous tubal ligation, and less commonly for tubal pregnancy or endometriosis. Favorable results can be expected if the damaged segment is not too extensive as the length of the remaining tube is critical. The site of sterilization is important; ligation in the isthmus region is easier to reverse than that in the ampulla because there is better approximation and more muscle around the site. The Irving and Pomeroy methods offer the best hope of successful reversals, while laparoscopic diathermy offers the least hope. The new methods of sterilization such as the silastic band or the Hulka clip may produce less damage to the tube and thereby offer a greater chance of successful restoration of fertility.

All candidates for tubal reconstruction should undergo diagnostic laparoscopy. If this reveals that there is less than 5 cm of tube remaining on both sides, tubal reconstruction should not be attempted. It has been estimated that more than 50% of applicants with previous tubal sterilization have been denied the benefit of reconstructive surgery due to the fact that only a small portion of the tube remained intact.[2]

Microsurgical techniques are mandatory in this type of tubal repair as they undoubtedly enhance the degree of accuracy. Anastomosis under the operative microscope has resulted in a significant improvement in pregnancy rate and a great decrease in tubal gestations. The improvement is credited to the minimal tissue trauma and the precision made possible by higher magnification and finer suture material.[2]

The obstructed ends are resected with fine scissors while hemostasis is obtained with constant irrigation (Figure 16.4). The muscularis of the mesentric edges of both cut ends of the left tube are approximated with 7-0 Prolene. Anastomosis is completed by serosal approximation of the right tube (Figure 16.5).

When there is parity in the caliber of the two lumina to be approximated, the technique of oblique resection is highly recommended.[5] The occluded segments are resected at an oblique angle, with the mesenteric edge longer in the isthmic portion and shorter in the ampullary segment.

Patency may be tested by transfundal perfusion of indigo carmine solution prior to abdominal closure. Intraoperative and postoperative management are similar to those for the salpingoneostomy procedure with the exception of the frequency hydrotubation. For end-to-end anastomosis hydrotubation is performed only on the fourth and seventh postoperative days.

Tubouterine Anastomosis The most common cause of cornual occlusion is destruction of the isthmic portion of the tube following laparoscopic sterilization via electrocautery. Other causes of cornual occlusion are salpingitis isthmica nodosa and inflammatory luminal fibrosis at the uterotubal junction. Several authors have demonstrated that in such cases the intramural portion of the tube is usually patent.[6] Therefore, tubouterine implantation, which has been the traditional approach to cornual occlusion for a long time, has recently been replaced by tubouterine anastomosis using the operating microscope. Anastomosis has a major advantage over

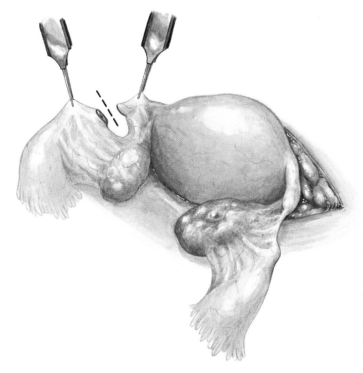

FIGURE 16.4. Midsegment anastomosis. This technique requires the identification of the proximal obstructed end by intrauterine injection of indigo carmine dye after the cervix has been occluded with a Buxton-type uterine clamp. Patency of the distal segment is established by retrograde fimbrial perfusion. The obstructed ends are resected with fine scissors while hemostasis is obtained by constant irrigation and, when necessary, microelectrode coagulation. Do not use any splints with this particular type of end-to-end anastomosis.

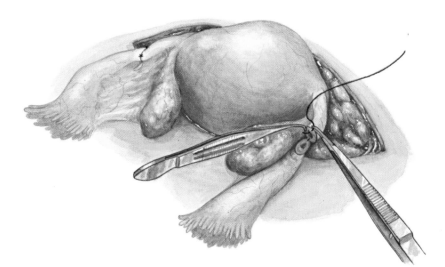

FIGURE 16.5. Midsegment anastomosis. End-to-end anastomosis is performed in two layers. The first stitch individually picks the muscularis of the mesentric edges of both ends of the tube (6 o'clock) and the 7-0 Prolene suture is tied with three knots. The second stitch approximates the muscularis of the two segments at 3 o'clock. In a similar pattern, the third stitch is taken at 9 o'clock, while the fourth approximates the antimesenteric edges at 12 o'clock. Two sutures are placed to close the gap in the mesosalpinx. Finally, the serosa is approximated with four interrupted stitches of the same suture material.

implantation because it leaves the intramural portion intact, which thus retains its anatomical and physiological significance. The convoluted anatomical features of the intramural portion are impossible to reconstruct surgically and the chances of restoring physiological function to this portion of the tube after implantation are poor.[2] Another advantage of anastomosis over implantation is that the myometrium is not weakened and, therefore, vaginal delivery rather than cesarean section is the more likely outcome.

Indigo carmine solution is injected into the uterine cavity with a cervical clamp. Both cornua are inspected by a magnifying device, preferably the operating microscope. Repeated thin slices about 1 mm thick are taken from the cornua until the patent area is reached. The patency of the distal segment of tube is ascertained by injecting the dye through the fimbrial

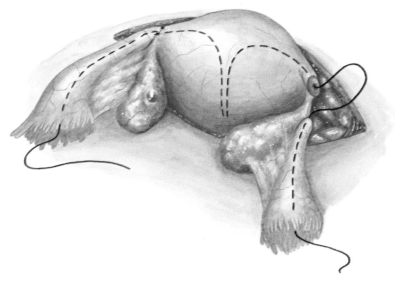

FIGURE 16.6. Tubouterine anastomosis. A splint consisting of 1-0 or 2-0 mono-filament nylon is introduced into the intramural portion of the tube and passed into the uterine cavity. The other end of the splint is introduced into the cut end of the distal segment and brought out through the fimbria. End-to-end anastomosis is performed in two layers using 7-0 Prolene. Four anastomatic sutures are placed in the muscularis of both segments at 6, 3, 9, and 12 o'clock and tied without tension. Adequate epithelial opposition is enhanced by the use of the microscope. The gap in the mesosalpinx is closed, then the serosal layer is approximated with the same suture material.

end. Hemostasis is accomplished by coagulation with a microelectrode under intermittent irrigation with normal saline solution (Figure 16.6).

The splint is removed from the uterine cavity via the vagina on the fourth postoperative day. The intraoperative and postoperative management, including hydrotubation, are the same as for the midsegment anastomosis procedure.

Cornual Implantation

This procedure consists of the implantation of either the isthmic or ampullary segment into the uterine cavity. It is used only when an anastomosis at the cornua is not possible due to the occlusion of the intramural segment of the tube (Figure 16.7). The intraoperative and postoperative management, including hydrotubation, are similar to those for the anastomosis procedure.

Results

The outcome of tuboplasty depends mostly upon the extent of the tubal disease and the type of procedure performed. The age of the patient at the time of the operation, whether surgery was done for one or both tubes, and the duration of follow-up are other factors that should be considered when comparisons of results are made. In general the best results are obtained after the salpingolysis procedure followed by the anastomosis procedure. Salpingoneostomy gives the worst results as it is rarely followed by term pregnancies. The preliminary reports regarding microsurgical techniques have shown a significant increase in pregnancy rates and a sharp decline in the incidence of tubal gestations. The most recent data show that the over-

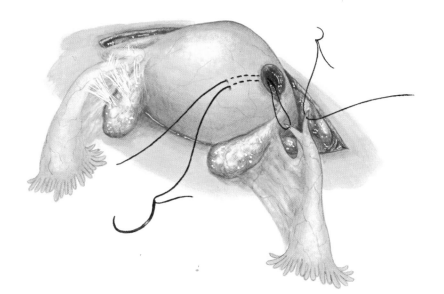

FIGURE 16.7. Cornual implantation. The endometrial cavity is identified by the blue staining, and the bivalved cut end of the tube is approximated to be implanted into the uterine cavity with a 6-0 Vicryl suture for each flap. Notice the larger needle used to traverse the thick uterine wall.

all term pregnancy rate by gross surgical procedure is about 30% versus 60% for microsurgical procedures; the ectopic pregnancy rate has dropped from about 20% to less than 10%.[5] For a more comprehensive review of the results following different types of tuboplasty, the reader is referred to the detailed review by Siegler.[12]

Immediate postoperative complications should be extremely rare. Pelvic infection, including bilateral pyosalpinx, intestinal obstruction, and wound disruption, have been reported but have never been encountered by the author.

Delayed complications are usually due to prolonged handling of the tissues causing the formation of peritubal adhesions, gross fibrosis, poor revascularization and, most catastrophic of all, recurrent tubal occlusion. These complications interfere with ovum pick-up and transport, resulting in tubal pregnancy. Therefore, minimum handling of tissues with microsurgical instruments is imperative.

Surgery for Fertility Control

Tubal ligation is one of the many methods being practiced by gynecologists for sterilization of women. There have been a great number of surgical techniques employed for tubal sterilization, such as abdominal or vaginal tubal ligation, partial or complete tubal resection, and the different types of laparoscopic procedures. Although there are many methods available for tubal ligation, this discussion will be limited to the techniques commonly practiced at the author's institution. Laparoscopic procedures are discussed in detail in Chapter 2.

Prior to performing any type of tubal sterilization, the patient and her husband should have a complete explanation of all alternative methods of family planning. They should be fully aware that this sterilization is permanent. All possible complications, including failure rates, should be discussed in detail.

Patients who are 24 years old or younger should be advised against surgery, because it is usually women in this age group who come back requesting the reversal of their tubal ligation. Once decided, these patients should have only the Pomeroy technique performed because its reversal is

183

easier and its corrective results are better. Patients whose ages range between 24 and 34 years should have only Pomeroy tubal sterilization for the same reasons mentioned above. Patients who are 35 years of age or older should have fimbriectomy or the Irving technique performed. Fimbriectomy in which the distal third of the tube is amputated is the most effective surgical technique for sterilization and it is irreversible. The Irving technique and vaginal tubal sterilization are rarely practiced at the author's institution. The most common indication for their use is as experience for residents in training, so that they may become familiar with the pros and cons of these techniques. In patients with high parity, especially when there is a need for extensive vaginal plastic surgery, the treatment of choice is vaginal hysterectomy and vaginal repair.

Timing

Sterilization accompanying cesarean section is conveniently timed, and it is practiced commonly at the author's institution. The ideal time for puerperal tubal ligation is during the first 48 hr after delivery. The advantages of this early sterilization include easy access to the uterus by a small subumbilical incision and the convenience of combining postpartum and postoperative convalescence with no additional hospitalization. Patients who are at risk during the immediate postpartum period may have their surgery done 6 weeks after delivery or at any later period.

Incisions

A patient who is not obese and whose uterus is mobile on bimanual examination so that the fundus can be manipulated to a point directly beneath the anterior abdominal wall is a good candidate for the minilaparotomy approach. A transverse or longitudinal skin incision approximately 2 to 5 cm in length is made just above the pubic bone. After the uterus is steadied with a tenaculum and a cannula, the patient is placed in the frog position to permit manipulation of the uterus, which is brought up to the incision during the operation. Fixation of the pelvic organs due to previous infection or any other cause is a contraindication, as is excessive obesity, which would require a larger incision to obtain adequate surgical exposure.

Postpartum tubal ligation is done through a transverse or longitudinal subumbilical incision about 2 to 5 cm in length. The surgeon manually pushes the uterus to the left side to get hold of the right tube and then to the right side to bring the left tube up through the incision.

Operative Technique

The Pomeroy technique is perhaps the simplest and the most common. If appropriately done, the failure rate should not exceed the other methods of sterilization. The advantage is that the tube is not extensively damaged and therefore re-establishment of patency when desired is possible (Figure 16.8).

Fimbriectomy or amputation of the distal third of the tube is simple and perhaps the most effective technique for sterilization. The tube is identified, elevated with forceps, crushed about 2 cm from the fimbrial end, and tied with 0 chromic surgical gut. The only disadvantage of this technique is its irreversibility. In all tubal sterilizations, positively identify the tubes by visualizing the fimbria and follow the tube back to the chosen operative site. Division of the round ligaments has little effect on fertility.

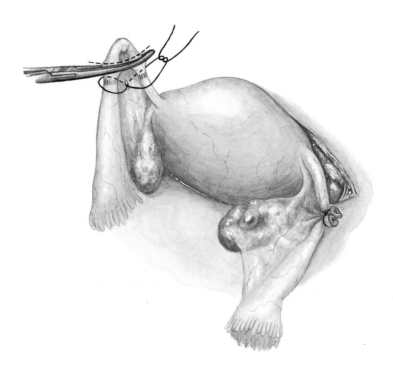

FIGURE 16.8. Pomeroy technique for tubal ligation. Elevate the tube near the middle, crush it about 1 cm from the apex of the loop, and apply a figure-of-eight chromic catgut suture around the crushed areas. Excise the knuckle above the ligature.

The Irving and vaginal sterilization techniques are rarely justified in the laparoscope and minilaparotomy era. They are time consuming and have more postoperative complications.

Results
Complications should be rare. Occasionally, the uterus is perforated by the elevating cannula and requires a hemostatic stitch. Bleeding from a torn mesosalpinx should be easily controlled by a ligature. Wound complications such as hematomas or infections should be extremely rare because the incision is so small.

Recovery from minilaparotomy is rapid. Ordinary physical and social activities can be resumed in 1 week. The postpartum course should not be affected by the puerperal tubal ligation.

References

1. Bronson, R.A., and Wallach, E.E.: Lysis of periadnexal adhesions for correction of infertility. *Fertil. Steril.* **28**:613–619, 1977.
2. Diamond, E.: Microsurgical reconstruction of the uterine tube in sterilized patients. *Fertil. Steril.* **28**:1203–1210, 1977.
3. Editorial comment on reversibility of tubal ring sterilization. *Obstet. Gynecol. Surv.* **33**:138–139, 1978.
4. Garcia C.: Symposium. Probing the causes of infertility–clinicians in the laboratory. *Contemporary Ob/Gyn* **13**:58–98, 1979.
5. Gomel, V.: Reconstructive surgery of the oviduct. *J. Reprod. Med.* **18**:181–190, 1977.
6. Grant, A.: Infertility surgery of the oviduct. *Fertil. Steril.* **22**:496–503, 1971.
7. Greenhill, J.P.: Evaluation of salpingostomy and tubal implantation for treatment of sterility. *Am. J. Obstet. Gynecol.* **33**:39–51, 1937.
8. Hellman, L.M.: The use of polyethylene in human tubal plastic operations. *Fertil. Steril.* **2**:498–504, 1951.

9. Neuwirth, R.S., and Khalaf, S.M.: Effect of thirty-two percent dextran 70 on peritoneal adhesion formation. *Am. J. Obstet. Gynecol.* **121**:420–426, 1975.
10. Pauerstein, C.J.: Overview. In: *The Fallopian Tube: A Reappraisal.* Philadelphia, Lea & Febiger, 1974, p. 1.
11. Rock J., Mulligan W.J., and Easterday, C.L.: Polyethylene in tuboplasty. *Obstet. Gynecol.* **3**:21–29, 1954.
12. Siegler, A.M.: Surgical treatments for tuboperitoneal causes of infertility since 1967. *Fertil. Steril.* **28**:1019–1032, 1977.
13. Swolin, K.: Fifty fertility operations. Literature and methods. *Obstet. Gynecol. Surv.* **23**:382–384, 1968.
14. Thibault, C.: Physiology and pathophysiology of the fallopian tube. *Int. J. Fert.* **17**:1–13, 1972.
15. Young, P.E., Egan, J.E., Barlow, J.J. et al.: Reconstructive surgery for infertility at the Boston Hospital for Women. *Am. J. Obstet. Gynecol.* **108**: 1092–1097, 1970.

Selected Bibliography

Behrman, S.J. and Kistner, R.W. eds.: *Progress in Infertility.* Boston, Little, Brown and Company, 1968.

Kistner, R.W. and Patton G.W.: *Atlas of Infertility Surgery.* Boston, Little, Brown and Company, 1975.

Ectopic Pregnancy

17

The incidence of ectopic pregnancy in the United States is 1 in 100 live births, and Schneider calculates from this figure that there are 30,000 ectopic gestations per year.[9] From 5.9%[2] to 10%[9] of maternal deaths in the United States are due to ectopic pregnancy, occurring predominantly in females 26 to 30 years of age.[2] In Breen's series of 654 ectopic pregnancies, 89% of patients had previously been pregnant demonstrating a high fertility index in this group of patients[2]; 10% to 20% of ectopic pregnancies resulted from tubal surgery for infertility.[3] Of the 654 ectopic pregnancies, 97.7% were located in the tube; the others were located in the abdomen or ovary. Of the 639 tubal gestations, 41% occurred in the distal third of the tube, 38% in the middle third, and the remaining 21% in the proximal third interstitial portion or in the fimbria[2] (Figure 17.1). The common denominator in this group of patients is delay in transport of the ovum fertilized in the ampulla of the tube to the normal implantation site in the uterus.

One of the more common predisposing factors to ectopic pregnancy is pelvic inflammatory disease with salpingitis and resultant fibrosis, peritubal adhesions, and diverticula. An increase in pelvic inflammatory disease is seen in the younger population associated with earlier sexual relations and the use of intrauterine devices.[8] Additionally, intrauterine devices seem to increase the rate of ectopic pregnancies as they inhibit intrauterine implantation.[4]

At laparotomy, gross evidence of pelvic inflammatory disease may be found in patients with ectopic pregnancies; however, 50% of patients have grossly normal adnexae. Remember that the normal external appearance of a fallopian tube may not be a true reflection of the condition of the tubal mucosa. Additional predisposing factors include the presence of ectopic endometrium in the tube, transperitoneal migration of the ovum (implicated in 20% to 50% of cases by the finding of a corpus luteum in the contralateral ovary), and inflammatory changes of a prior ectopic pregnancy. Over 50% of the patients who have an ectopic pregnancy become infertile.[3] The data for the incidence of recurrent tubal gestational implantations with the different kinds of tubal reconstructive surgery vary in the literature. An average figure would be 20% for tubal reimplantation, midsegment tubal anastomosis, and salpingostomy.

187

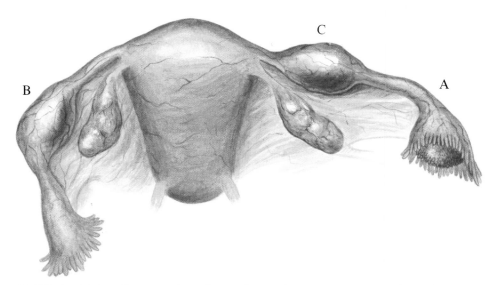

FIGURE 17.1. Common locations of ectopic pregnancy. **A** Distal third of the tube. **B** Middle third of the tube. **C** Proximal third of the interstitial portion of the tube. The distal third is the most common site.

Preoperative Evaluation

The most common symptom in ectopic pregnancy is abdominal pain, usually in the lower abdomen, which occurs approximately 3 to 5 weeks after the missed menses. When shoulder pain occurs, it is safe to assume the ectopic pregnancy has ruptured. If the lesion is in the fimbria or distal ampulla, distention in the peritoneal surfaces occurs later and symptoms are not noticed as soon. Vaginal bleeding occurs in 80% of patients, usually in scanty amounts.[2]

Physical findings are quite variable. The most common are a fullness in the cul-de-sac and tenderness on motion of the cervix in approximately 87% of patients, localized tenderness in 60%, and rebound tenderness in 52%. Approximately 50% of patients have a mass on examination and, depending on the progress of the disease, as many as 50% are admitted in shock, usually on a hemorrhagic basis.[2]

A number of women present with vague abdominal symptoms consisting primarily of pain without specific findings; one should be highly suspicious of ectopic pregnancy in these patients. Diagnostic laparoscopy is indicated and often reveals blood in the peritoneal cavity, tubal distention, and bleeding from the tube.

Laboratory test findings are variable. The most reliable procedure is culdocentesis, which documents bleeding of the pregnancy into the abdomen. Breen reported nonclotting blood in 90% of patients who had a culdocentesis.[2]

A routine pregnancy test is positive in 50% of the patients,[3] but the beta-subunit human chorionic gonadotropin radioimmunoassay is much more sensitive and will detect pregnancy after trophoblastic cells have begun to actively grow, as early as 2 weeks following implantation.[6]

Ultrasound is useful as a diagnostic tool in the evaluation of a gestational sac in the uterus or fallopian tube. Levi and Delval report that diagnostic ultrasound has an overall 80% accuracy rate when used to confirm a clinical finding in the female pelvis; however, it is only 37% accurate in the diagnosis of an ectopic pregnancy. Of the 27 cases they examined, there were 6 mistaken diagnoses, 2 false negatives, and 9 doubtful diagnoses.[5]

Operative Strategy

The patient who desires no further children presents a relatively simple surgical problem after diagnosis is made. Salpingectomy is the standard treatment for ectopic pregnancy (Figure 17.2). If the patient chooses, tubal ligation may be performed in the opposite tube as well.

The difficulty in the management of ectopic pregnancy occurs in those patients who desire continued fertility, and a great deal of controversy surrounds the most effective means of treating these patients. The difficulty of evaluating the noninvolved tube by gross inspection has been noted. It is also difficult to estimate the damage to the tubal epithelium in the nonin-

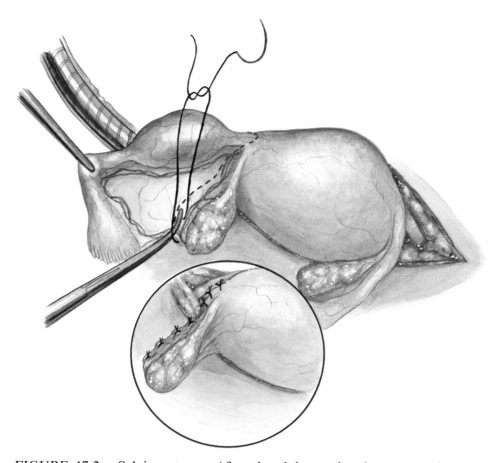

FIGURE 17.2. Salpingectomy. After the abdomen has been opened and the pregnancy site identified, place a fiberoptic light source behind the broad ligaments, transilluminating the blood vessels as they course through the meso-ovarium. Place Gemini artery forceps and divide the mesentery between clamps. Secure each bite on the ovarian side with suture ligatures of 3-0 or 4-0 braided nylon. Incise the junction of the tube and uterine cornua; close these incisions as well. Carefully inspect the excision site for any additional bleeding and always identify the ureter prior to placing the first clamp along the ovary. If bleeding occurs in the ovary, the ovary is excised at this time. Irrigate any blood from the peritoneal cavity, and close the abdomen and wound in layers, using 2-0 absorbable suture in the peritoneal cavity. Approximate the rectus muscles with interrupted sutures of 2-0 absorbable suture material and use continuous absorbable sutures of 2-0 chromic catgut in the anterior rectus fascia. The skin is approximated with 4-0 absorbable subcuticular sutures or 3-0 nylon subcuticular closure with 5-0 nylon interrupted sutures to even any ridges produced.

volved tube caused by the inflammatory changes resulting from the current ectopic pregnancy. If the diagnosis is unruptured ectopic pregnancy, conservative surgery is recommended if the patient has a fertile husband, is 35 years of age or less, has no other contraindications to future pregnancy, is in satisfactory condition at the time of laparotomy, and is appraised of the increased risk in surgery to maintain her fertility. Bronson disscusses in detail the strategy to maximize fertility.[3]

The tube must be excised when the rupture of the tubal implantation has led to hemorrhage and extensive tubal damage. When hemorrhage extends into the mesosalpinx and meso-ovarian, oophorectomy is also indicated.

Experience is accumulating which shows that conservation of the involved tube increases the likelihood of future fertility without greatly increasing subsequent risk of recurrent ectopic pregnancy. As most implantations occur within the ampulla or are attached to the fimbria, the pregnancy may be expressed and separated from the tube without difficulty.[3] Timonen and Nieminen have evidence that the incidence of recurrent ectopic pregnancies may be higher with expression of the tubal gestation as compared to salpingostomy. This may be due to retained trophoblastic tissue.[10] Tompkins suggests surgical removal of the ectopic pregnancy under direct vision by incising the antimesenteric aspect of the tube, securing hemostasis, and leaving the tubal incision open.[11]

When the pregnancy is farther from the end of the tube, a linear incision over the ectopic pregnancy and removal of the gestational sac and trophoblastic tissue is recommended (Figure 17.3). If the pregnancy is of the less common isthmic variety, excision of that portion will probably be required. Cornual reimplantation may be done at a later date by a surgeon who has a particular interest in infertility surgery.[3] In Timonen and Nieminen's series of 92 patients with linear salpingostomy, 76 had bilateral tubal patency. Recurrent ectopic pregnancy following linear salpingostomy occurred in 12% of patients and 30% had normal term pregnancies.[10] While oophorectomy has been advocated when salpingectomy is necessary to decrease the incidence of tubal pregnancies due to transmigration, Bender's data indicate that the incidence of recurrent ectopic pregnancy is approximately the same with salpingo-oophorectomy as with salpingectomy.[1]

Postoperative Management

Apprise the patient of the increased incidence of repeat ectopic pregnancies. If sterilization results from the procedure, the patient needs to fully understand the thinking behind the decision. Finally, if additional surgical procedures are necessary to improve the patient's fertility, refer the patient to a surgeon experienced in microsurgery.

Routine appendectomy may be performed with surgery for tubal pregnancy if the patient is in good condition and the appendix is easily exposed. Onuigbo noted a 25% febrile morbidity rate in a series of 264 laparotomies for ectopic pregnancy irrespective of incidental appendectomy.[7] Routine appendectomy is not done if any reconstructive procedure has been performed in an attempt to maintain fertility.

Schneider et al. reviewed maternal mortality due to ectopic pregnancy and found an impressive delay between the onset of symptoms and definitive therapy as well as an average delay of 3 days between consultation and

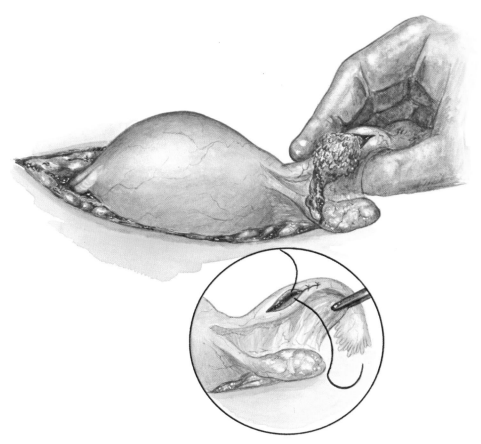

FIGURE 17.3.   Surgery of ectopic pregnancy farther from the end of the tube. Make an incision over the tubal pregnancy, applying pressure with the finger and thumb beneath the ectopic gestation. Using a No. 15 blade, incise each layer in entering the tubal lumen. Express the products of conception and irrigate the tubal lumen. Secure hemostasis with a very fine tipped cautery or 4-0 or 5-0 absorbable suture. Gently irrigate any adherent blood clots remaining from the tubal lumen. Inset: Close the tube by suturing small portions of the muscularis, avoiding the mucosa. If the tube cannot be approximated due to edema or hemorrhage, secure hemostasis with ties and delicate cautery and leave the tube open.

hospital admission.[9] All facets of delay were generally higher in patients treated in university hospitals. They postulate that laparoscopic investigation, aggressive surgical management, and adequate blood replacement would save up to 75% of the patients who die of ectopic pregnancy.

References

1. Bender, S.: Fertility after tubal pregnancy. *J. Obstet. Gynaecol. Br. Emp.* **63:**400–403, 1956.
2. Breen, J.L.: A 21 year survey of 654 ectopic pregnancies. *Am. J. Obstet. Gynecol.* **106:**1004–1019, 1970.
3. Bronson, R.A.: Tubal pregnancy and inferility. *Fertil. Steril.* **28:**221–228, 1977.
4. Landesman, R., Coutinho, E.M., and Saxina, B.B.: Detection of human chorionic gonadotropin in blood of regularly bleeding women using copper intrauterine contraceptive devices. *Fertil. Steril.* **27:**1062–1066, 1976.
5. Levi, S., and Delval, R.: Value of ultrasonic diagnosis of gynecological tumors in 370 surgical cases. *Acta Obstet. Gynecol. Scand.* **55:**261–266, 1976.

6. Milwidsky, A., Adoni, A., Miodovnik, M. et al.: Human chorionic gondao-tropin (β-subunit) in the early diagnosis of ectopic pregnancy. *Obstet. Gynecol.* **51**:725–726, 1978.
7. Onuigbo, W.T.B.: Elective appendectomy at salpingectomy for ectopic pregnancy. *Obstet. Gynecol.* **49**:435–437, 1977.
8. Ory, H.W.: A review of the association between intrauterine devices and acute pelvic inflammatory disease. *J. Reprod. Med.* **20**:200–204, 1978.
9. Schneider, J., Berger, C.J., and Cattell, C.: Maternal mortality due to ectopic pregnancy. *Obstet. Gynecol.* **49**:557–561, 1977.
10. Timonen, S., and Nieminen, U.: Tubal pregnancy, choice of operative method of treatment. *Acta Obstet. Gynecol. Scand.* **46**:327–339, 1967.
11. Tompkins, P.L.: Preservation of fertility by conservative surgery for ectopic pregnancy. *Fertil. Steril.* **7**:448–455, 1956.

Surgery of the Ovary

18

To care for a patient with ovarian disease, the surgeon must have appropriate training in gynecologic pathology. He must be able to recognize the gross ovarian pathological changes in situ to make proper surgical decisions. Close interaction between pathologist and gynecologist, careful consideration of the patient's reproductive wishes, and skillful application of modern techniques in surgery, chemotherapy, and irradiation therapy are required for optimal results. The basic concepts and surgical techniques for the care of ovarian surgical disease will be outlined in this chapter.

Surgical Anatomy

The ovarian arteries are two of the three vessels providing significant blood supply to pelvic viscera that do not arise as branches of the internal iliac artery. The arteries to the ovary arise from the aorta, course downward, and divide into branches that enter the hilus of the ovary. The remaining portion of the ovarian artery continues to anastomose with the uterine arteries alongside the uterus.

The ovarian veins exit from the hilum of the ovary to form a pampiniform plexus that unites near the brim of the pelvis into two or three veins that subsequently join as they course upward. The veins from the right ovary enter the inferior vena cava and the left ovary drains into the left renal vein. The lymph vessels of the ovary are joined by those situated in the periaortic area at the level of the renal artery.

The proximal ovary is attached to the uterus by the ovarian ligament. Its distal end is surrounded by the fallopian tube and the ovary itself lies between two folds of peritoneum called the meso-ovarium. The endocrine and reproductive activities of the ovary, its rich blood supply, and its exposed position in the abdominal cavity make it host to a myriad of pathological conditions of inflammatory, metabolic, or neoplastic etiology. Detailed discussion of these numerous pathological abnormalities and their gross and microscopic characteristics is beyond the scope of this text. The reader is referred to the Selected Bibliography for readings on this topic.

Preoperative Evaluation

The patient's history is of particular importance when the lesion is a functional cyst. Note the patient's last menstrual period, use of oral contraceptives, history of pelvic pain, previous pelvic inflammatory disease, use of an intrauterine contraceptive device, and other symptoms of the genitourinary and gastrointestinal systems. Likewise, historical data and symptoms suggesting the possibility of pregnancy, ascites, or abdominal distention are important.

In patients with ovarian cancer, Piver et al. observed abdominal distention as the initial symptom in 44% of patients and pelvic or abdominal pain in 33%; 15% of patients had no symptoms and the mass was detected on routine pelvic examination.[36]

On pelvic examination note the size of the lesion, its mobility, the presence of tenderness or nodularity, and the condition of the opposite ovary. Do a Papanicolaou smear with a sampling of the uterine cavity to determine the possible presence of coexistent uterine malignancy.

Sonography is useful in the evaluation of suspected ovarian masses. Lawson and Albaretti reported observations in 251 cases of suspected pelvic masses studied by gray scale ultrasonography. The presence or absence of a mass, its consistency, and its location were identified correctly in 91% of patients. Most inaccuracies were associated with a misreading of the distended loops of bowel and errors in technique. Diagnostic errors were also more common at the lower limits of the resolution of the technique.[27]

Review of the usefulness of liver and spleen scans on the author's service has shown them to be unreliable in the evaluation of ovarian malignancy.

A lymphangiogram is particularly useful in suspected cases of dysgerminoma, and computerized tomography is sometimes useful in the evaluation of periaortic nodal disease.

Chest x-ray, intravenous pyelogram, barium enema, and protocscopy are recommended in the evaluation of all ovarian masses except those associated with pregnancy and those mobile cystic masses in which irradiation of the young patient's ovaries would be unlikely to provide data valuable enough to merit the irradiation.

The surgeon must be constantly aware of the high incidence of metastatic cancer of the ovary presenting as a primary lesion in the older patient. A thorough preoperative evaluation of other sites for possible malignancies is recommended where metastasis is suspected. An upper gastrointestinal series, mammography, and cystoscopy are indicated.

Two groups of laboratory studies are currently prominent in the literature. The first is a chemical profile consisting of urinary nonesterified cholesterol, plasma placental lactogen, and chorionic gonadotropin. These levels are often elevated in ovarian cancer: 72% of patients have high plasma placental lactogen levels and 45% have high human chorionic gonadotropin levels. There is little correlation between blood levels and the disease course, and the current clinical usefulness of these studies is limited.

The second group of studies consists of tests of tumor-associated antigens. These have been investigated since 1930, and three are currently of interest. Carcinoembryonic antigen, α-fetoprotein, and ovarian cystadenocarcinoma antigen have recently been studied by several investigators; however, the reproducibility of such studies, particularly with ovarian cystadenocarcinoma antigen, limit their current usefulness. The development of a reliable tumor marker for ovarian cancer would revolutionize the current management of such cancers.

Laparoscopy is most helpful in the evaluation of adnexal masses, particularly in young patients; but if a clear-cut indication for laparotomy is present, laparoscopy is an unnecessary prolongation of the preoperative evaluation.

Following the preoperative clinical evaluation, laparotomy is performed if any one of the following conditions exists[22]:

1. Any solid ovarian neoplasm.
2. Any premenarchal or postmenopausal ovarian cyst.
3. Any ovarian cyst over 5 cm in size followed through at least one menstrual cycle but not responding to suppressive therapy.
4. Any ovarian cyst less than 5 cm in diameter that has persisted through three menstrual cycles.
5. Signs and symptoms that suggest torsion or rupture of an ovarian cyst producing an acute abdomen.
6. Any ovarian cyst that causes pain severe enough to interfere with normal activities.
7. Unexplained ascites.

The most important diagnostic test in an ovarian mass meeting the criteria for laparotomy is the laparotomy itself. Laparotomy must not be compromised by an inadequate incision. The surgeon should carefully observe any fixation or adhesions of the mass, note the presence or absence of ascites, and obtain peritoneal fluid for cytological study; if no peritoneal fluid is present, peritoneal washings are performed. The omentum is biopsied and excised if ovarian malignancy is present in the ovaries. A careful exploration is made of the liver and peritoneal gutters as well as the pelvic and aortic lymph nodes, kidneys, large and small bowel, pancreas, stomach, and diaphragm. If malignancy is present, a total abdominal hysterectomy and bilateral salpingo-oophorectomy with removal of the omentum and all gross cancer is indicated.

A histologic classification of ovarian tumors is presented in Table 18.1; a system of surgical staging carcinoma of the ovary is given in Table 18.2.

Operative Technique

Choice of Incision

In the young patient with a freely movable cystic mass and a high probability of this mass being benign on tissue examination, a Pfannenstiel-type transverse incision is adequate. Mobile cystic masses can be easily elevated into the wound and adequately exposed without difficulty. In all other patients with adnexal masses, make a midline incision capable of being extended to the xyphoid.

The operative permit must allow for a wide latitude of procedures such as bowel resection, temporary or permanent colostomy, and pelvic or periaortic node biopsy. Thorough bowel preparation, including mechanical cleansing, antibiotics, and vitamin K is indicated with large or fixed masses (Chapter 19).

One must be aware of the upper abdominal pathology in ovarian cancer. Piver found 83% of ovarian cancer patients referred to him postoperatively had an incision inadequate for upper abdominal exploration.[36] Piver

195

TABLE 18.1. Histologic Classification of Ovarian Tumors
(World Health Organization)

I. Common "epithelial" tumors
   A. Serous tumors
      1. Benign
         a. Cystadenoma and papillary cystadenoma
         b. Surface papilloma
         c. Adenofibroma and cystadenofibroma
      2. Of borderline malignancy (carcinomas of low malignant potential)
         a. Cystadenoma and papillary cystadenoma
         b. Surface papilloma
         c. Adenofibroma and cystadenofibroma
      3. Malignant
         a. Adenocarcinoma, papillary adenocarcinoma, and papillary cystadeno-
           carcinoma
         b. Surface papillary carcinoma
         c. Malignant adenofibroma and cystadenofibroma

   B. Mucinous tumors
      1. Benign
         a. Cystadenoma
         b. Adenofibroma and cystadenofibroma
      2. Of borderline malignancy (carcinomas of low malignant potential)
         a. Cystadenoma
         b. Adenofibroma and cystadenofibroma
      3. Malignant
         a. Adenocarcinoma and cystadenocarcinoma
         b. Malignant adenofibroma and cystadenofibroma

   C. Endometrioid tumors
      1. Benign
         a. Adenoma and cystadenoma
         b. Adenofibroma and cystadenofibroma
      2. Of borderline malignancy (carcinomas of low malignant potential)
         a. Adenoma and cystadenoma
         b. Adenofibroma and cystadenofibroma
      3. Malignant
         a. Carcinoma
            i. Adenocarcinoma
           ii. Adenoacanthoma
          iii. Malignant adenofibroma and cystadenofibroma
         b. Endometrioid stromal sarcomas
         c. Mesodermal (müllerian) mixed tumors, homologous and heterologous

   D. Clear cell (mesonephroid) tumors
      1. Benign: adenofibroma
      2. Of borderline malignancy (carcinomas of low malignant potential)
      3. Malignant: carcinoma and adenocarcinoma

   E. Brenner tumors
      1. Benign
      2. Of borderline malignancy (proliferating)
      3. Malignant

   F. Mixed epithelial tumors
      1. Benign
      2. Of borderline malignancy
      3. Malignant

   G. Undifferentiated carcinoma

   H. Unclassified epithelial tumors

II. Sex cord stromal tumors
   A. Granulosa–stromal cell tumors
      1. Granulosa cell tumor

TABLE 18.1 *(Continued)*

      2. Tumors in the thecoma–fibroma group
        a. Thecoma
        b. Fibroma
        c. Unclassified
   B. Androblastomas; Sertoli–Leydig cell tumors
      1. Well differentiated
        a. Tubular androblastoma; Sertoli cell tumor (tubular adenoma of Pick)
        b. Tubular androblastoma with lipid storage; Sertoli cell tumor with lipid storage (folliculome lipidique of Lecene)
        c. Sertoli–Leydig cell tumor (tubular adenoma with Leydig cells)
        d. Leydig cell tumor; hilus cell tumor
      2. Of intermediate differentiation
      3. Poorly differentiated (sarcomatoid)
      4. With heterologous elements
   C. Gynandroblastoma
   D. Unclassified

III. Lipoid (lipoid) cell tumors

IV. Germ cell tumors
   A. Dysgerminoma
   B. Endodermal sinus tumor
   C. Embryonal carcinoma
   D. Polyembryoma
   E. Choriocarcinoma
   F. Teratomas
      1. Immature
      2. Mature
        a. Solid
        b. Cystic
           i. Dermoid cyst (mature cystic teratoma)
           ii. Dermoid cyst with malignant transformation
      3. Monodermal and highly specialized
        a. Struma ovarii
        b. Carcinoid
        c. Struma ovarii and carcinoid
        d. Others
   G. Mixed forms

V. Gonadoblastoma
   A. Pure
   B. Mixed with dysgerminoma or other form of germ cell tumor

VI. Soft tissue tumors not specific to ovary

VII. Unclassified tumors

VIII. Secondary (metastatic) tumors

IX. Tumor-like conditions
   A. Pregnancy luteoma
   B. Hyperplasia of ovarian stroma and hyperthecosis
   C. Massive edema
   D. Solitary follicle cyst and corpus luteum cyst
   E. Multiple follicle cysts (polycystic ovaries)
   F. Multiple luteinized follicle cysts and/or corpora lutea
   G. Endometriosis
   H. Surface-epithelial inclusion cysts (germinal inclusion cysts)
   I. Simple cysts
   J. Inflammatory lesions
   K. Parovarian cysts

TABLE 18.2.   Staging of Primary Carcinoma of the Ovary[a] (International Federation of Gynecologists and Obstetricians)

Stage	Characteristic
I	Growth limited to the ovaries
a	Growth limited to one ovary; no ascites
i	No tumor on the external surface; capsule intact
ii	Tumor present on the external surface and/or capsule ruptured
b	Growth limited to both ovaries; no ascites
i	No tumor on the external surface; capsules intact
ii	Tumor present on the external surface and/or capsule(s) ruptured
c	Tumor either stage Ia or stage Ib, but with ascites[b] present or positive peritoneal washings
II	Growth involving one or both ovaries with pelvic extension
a	Extension and/or metastases to the uterus and/or tubes
b	Extension to other pelvic tissues
c	Tumor either stage IIa or stage IIb, but with ascites[b] present or positive peritoneal washings
III	Growth involving one or both ovaries with intraperitoneal metastases outside the pelvis and/or positive retroperitoneal nodes
	Tumor limited to the true pelvis with histologically proven malignant extension to small bowel or omentum
IV	Growth involving one or both ovaries with distant metastases
	If pleural effusion is present there must be positive cytology to allot a case to stage IV
	Parenchymal liver metastases equals stage IV
Special category	Unexplored cases that are thought to be ovarian carcinoma

[a] Based on findings at clinical examination and surgical exploration. The final histology after surgery is to be considered in the staging, as well as cytology as far as effusions are concerned.
[b] Ascites is peritoneal effusion which in the opinion of the surgeon is pathological and/or clearly exceeds normal amounts.

et al. reviewed laparoscopic findings in previously treated patients with stage I ovarian cancers: 11% had diaphragmatic metastasis, 13% aortic lymph node metastasis, 8% pelvic lymph node metastasis, 3% omental metastasis, and 32% positive peritoneal washings.[35]

An adequate incision is an absolute prerequisite for operating on the pelvic mass that may be an ovarian cancer. Not only is the incision important for surgical excision, but in addition subsequent follow-up treatment programs will be based on the findings of the original laparotomy. Careful, thorough abdominal surgery and detailed, precise recording of the intraoperative findings are vital for the care of the patient with this devastating disease.

Unilateral Benign Ovarian Tumors

The gross characteristics of benign ovarian tumor are a smooth capsule, cystic mass, unilateral location, mobility, lack of adhesions, no excrescences or solid areas palpable through the cyst, the absence of ascites, and a negative abdominal exploration. When such gross characteristics are present and the patient wishes to maintain fertility, cystectomy (Figure 18.1), oophorectomy (Figure 18.2), or salpingo-oophorectomy (Figures 18.3 through 18.6) is performed, depending on the size of the tumor. Excise the specimen intact and give it to the pathologist. If the diagnosis suggests the possibility of bilateral disease such as serous cystadenoma, the opposite ovary is biopsied. If the diagnosis is dermoid, the biopsy can be omitted

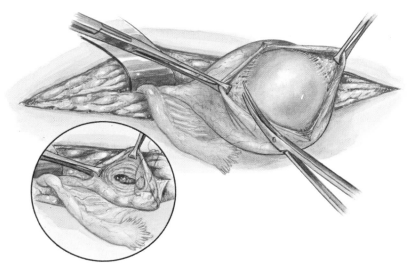

FIGURE 18.1. Cystectomy. In the patient with a simple ovarian cyst, grasp the ovary between the thumb and index finger. Using a No. 15 blade, make an incision through the fibrous ovarian capsule overlying the cyst. Grasp the fibrous wall with intestinal Allis clamps and pull laterally. With fine Metzenbaum scissors, dissect the areolar tissue that lies between the cyst wall and the ovarian capsule. Attempt to excise this structure intact and give it to the pathologist. If there is any evidence that malignancy exists, do not attempt this type of excision. Inset: Close the ovarian defect with one or two layers of far-and-near stitches going through the ovary and grasping the edges to approximate the ovary. Use swaged intestinal needles and 3-0 or 4-0 absorbable suture.

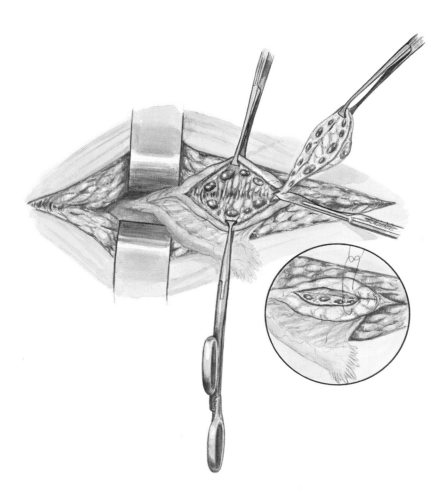

FIGURE 18.2. Oophorectomy. Expose the ovary and grasp the meso-ovarium with the left hand. Using a No. 15 blade, incise a wedge of tissue which extends well into the hilum of the ovary. This procedure is useful in Stein-Leventhal syndrome and to rule out the presence of malignancy in the opposite ovary. Inset: Make a parallel incision and excise the wedge of ovarian tissue. Place intestinal Allis clamps on the edge and close the defect with modified far-and-near sutures of 3-0 or 4-0 absorbable suture.

199

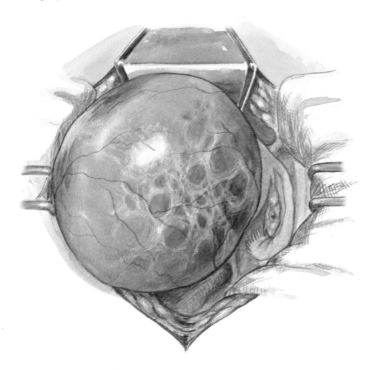

FIGURE 18.3.   Salpingo-oophorectomy. Mobilize the large ovarian mass into the wound, freeing any adhesions to adjacent viscera. Unless the pedicle is very long, the retroperitoneal approach is the best and produces fewer problems with bleeding.

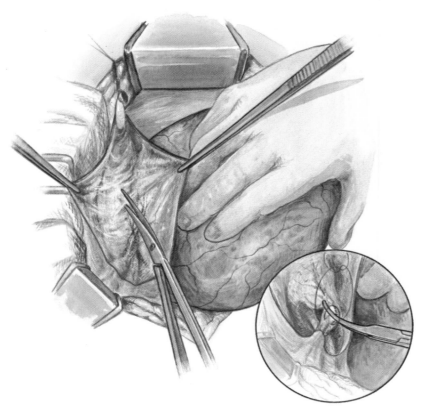

FIGURE 18.4.   Cut the round ligament and secure it with a 3-0 Nurolon suture. Incise sharply back over the psoas muscle using fine Metzenbaum scissors. Grasp the cut edges with Adson-Brown thumb forceps and pull laterally. Identify the ureter as it lays on the medial fold of the peritoneum coursing up toward the ovary as well as the ovarian vessels. Inset: Pass a 3-0 Nurolon suture around the ovarian vessels and ligate them. Place a curved Masterson clamp proximally toward the ovary and place a transfixation suture of 3-0 Nurolon through the ovarian vessels between the clamp and the free tie. Cut the ovarian vessels.

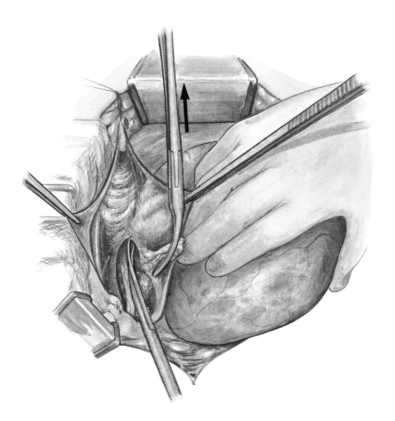

FIGURE 18.5. Using the ovarian vessels for traction, cut the peritoneum parallel to the ureter while applying traction to the ovarian mass and elevating it out of the pelvis. Avoid placing large clamps where the ureter cannot be clearly visualized. Small bleeders are secured with 3-0 Nurolon ties or small clips.

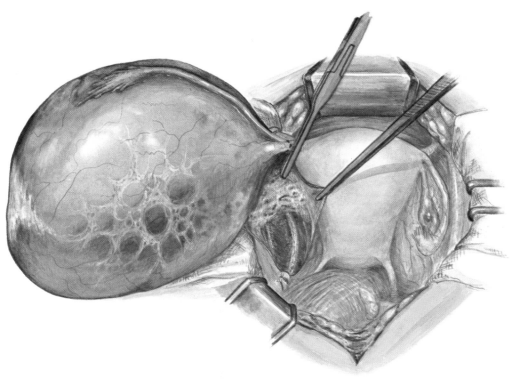

FIGURE 18.6. Once the mass is mobilized out of the pelvis, place Masterson clamps across the utero-ovarian vessels and the tube and excise the mass from the pelvis. Secure hemostasis of the ovarian vessels with a 2-0 Nurolon suture. Close the peritoneal defect with a continuous 3-0 absorbable suture taking care to avoid the ureter. Avoid placing any sutures above the ligated ovarian vessels as this is a pampiniform plexus of veins and any puncture will produce hematoma above the ligature.

201

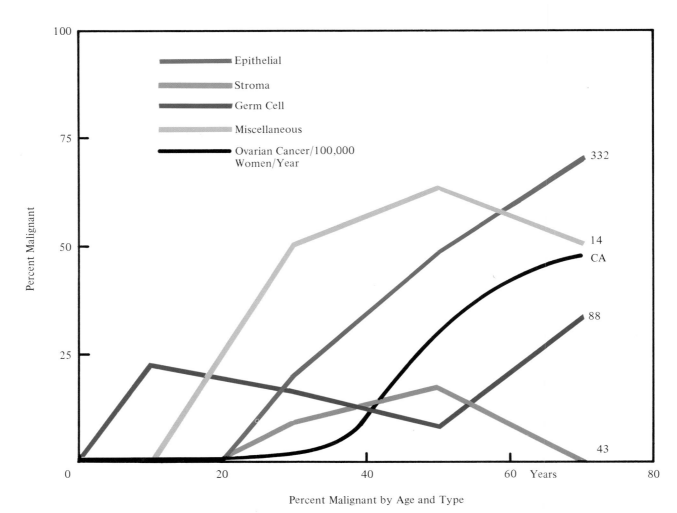

Percent Malignant by Age and Type

FIGURE 18.7.   Types of ovarian neoplasms seen in a 10-year period at the University of Kansas Medical Center plotted according to age and percentage malignant. The total number of each type is noted at the right. The extreme rarity of ovarian tumors under the age of 20 is evident, as is the absence of epithelial neoplasm in this group. The increase in ovarian cancer incidence per 100,000 women is also plotted and parallels the increase in epithelial neoplasms, which comprise 80% of such cancers. Adapted from Masterson, B.J., and Smith, S., Review of 447 ovarian tumors (unpublished data) and Cramer, D.W., and Cutler, S.J., *Am. J. Obstet. Gynecol.* **118**:443–460, 1974.

in the contralateral ovary if it appears grossly normal.[37] If the biposy is negative, no further surgery is necessary. Every effort is made during the ovarian biopsy to avoid unnecessary trauma to the remaining ovary and to minimize ovarian and peritubal adhesions.

One must maintain perspective in evaluating adnexal masses. There are no physiological adnexal masses in children and postmenopausal women. In women in the reproductive years 95% of palpable adnexal masses are physiological ovarian cysts. These cystic masses require no specific treatment and will resolve during observation for a span of two menses.[37]

In a study of young women with palpable adnexal masses that did not resolve, Ranney and Chastain found 66 endometriomas, 43 tubal pregnancies, 30 paramesonephric cysts, 22 polycystic ovaries, 12 pyo- and hydrosalpinx, and 11 physiological cysts; there were 24 dermoid tumors, 19 serous cystadenomas, 7 mucinous cystadenomas, and 7 fibroids.[37] Malignant ovarian neoplasms rarely occur in the early reproductive years; therefore, one must blend a healthy conservatism in this group with agressive investigation and therapy in the older patients (Figure 18.7).

Residual Ovarian Syndrome

An occasional patient will be seen who has had hysterectomy with one or both ovaries still present and a pelvic mass. Many have pelvic pain, but some are asymptomatic. Operative findings include extensive adhesions between the ovary and adjacent viscera.[15] The ureter and sometimes the iliac vessels may be pushed medially by this cystic retroperitoneal mass. Take care in the dissection and be sure to visualize the ureter as it will be hard to palpate in the scar tissue. Most ovaries will contain follicle cysts or corpus luteum and the malignancy rate is only 3% to 10%.[15] To avoid this situation, remove the ovaries in the patient over 35 or suspend them well out of the pelvis if they are left in the younger patient.

Bilateral Benign Tumors

The same pathological characteristics may be present bilaterally. If the patient wishes to maintain fertility, remove the most involved ovary for frozen section study. If the tumor is histologically benign, resect the benign disease from the less involved ovary. Blum and Meidan followed this plan of management in 18 patients.[10] Menstrual function was present in 17 patients; 9 conceived and delivered within 3 years of surgery. Most of the tumors in the series were bilateral dermoid cysts.

Pelvic Inflammatory Disease and Tuboovarian Abscess

Ninety percent of patients with acute pelvic inflammatory disease (PID) respond to antibiotic therapy. In the study by Cunningham et al. 92% became asymptomatic 4 days after either tetracycline or penicillin treatment for acute PID.[16] In addition, some patients will require drugs active against anaerobic bacteria or gram-negative aerobes, intravenous fluids, and bed rest.

Approximately 5% of patients with acute PID develop abscess formation. This abscess may lie outside the tube, be of tubovarian location, or consist of a pyosalpinx. Conservative therapy consisting of inpatient management, antibiotics, and fluids is recommended. Where the diagnosis is uncertain, laparoscopy is indicated.

Approximately 30% of pelvic abscesses merit colpotomy drainage. The requirements for colpotomy drainage are midline location of the abscess with fluctuation of the contents, surgical accessibility via the cul-de-sac, and obliteration of adjacent peritoneum to avoid drainage of the abscess contents into the peritoneal cavity (which produces generalized peritonitis).[21] Uhrich and Sanders discussed the sonographic characteristics of pelvic masses. The predominantly unilocular abscess is effectively drained vaginally by dissecting the rectovaginal septum, whereas the multilocular abscess, usually at a distance from the midline of the pelvis, is difficult to drain.[43] In patients in whom colpotomy drainage cannot be established, abdominal exploration is indicated if increasing rebound tenderness, increasing abscess size, a failure to defervesce, and abdominal rigidity occur.

Immediate exploration is indicated in those patients in whom rupture of the abscess is suspected. Symptoms of rupture include severe pain, often in the left lower abdomen, increasing signs and symptoms in the upper abdomen, and pain on examination. Diarrhea, chills, a rapid pulse, and ileus are the signs of a ruptured tuboovarian abscess. An elevated temperature is usually not observed.[17]

Daly and Monif note that 70% of patients survive if brought to surgery within 12 hr of the time of rupture, whereas 80% die if surgery is not promptly performed. If no surgical intervention is undertaken, 100% of patients die.[17]

Ten percent of patients with pelvic abscess need early surgical intervention, and in general that procedure should consist of total abdominal hysterectomy and bilateral salpingo-oophorectomy. Examine the pelvic veins for separative pelvic thrombophlebitis and, if present, ligate them very high and administer anticoagulants.

Unilateral salpingo-oophorectomy is acceptable in the patient who has a strong desire for children and whose contralateral adnexa appears normal on gross examination. A surprising 10% to 30% of patients managed conservatively may eventually become pregnant. The patient must understand that as many as 20% of patients with pelvic abscess are subject to more extensive surgery due to persistent pelvic inflammatory disease or associated symptoms.

Stein-Leventhal Syndrome

Oligomenorrhea or amenorrhea, ovulatory failure, hirsuitism, and sometimes obesity associated with bilateral polycystic ovaries with a fibrous capsule comprise the Stein-Leventhal syndrome.[41] Endocrine studies usually show elevated plasma testosterone, androstenedione, and sometimes 17-ketosteroid levels. Plasma luteinizing hormone is elevated, whereas follicle-stimulating hormone is consistently low.[28] Laparoscopy will confirm the diagnosis and sonography can demonstrate the ovarian changes as well.

Clomiphene citrate produces ovulation in the majority of patients.[19] Should clomiphene not produce a prompt response, wedge resection is suggested, as it produces a return of ovulatory function in 95% of patients and most who desire to can become pregnant.[41] Babaknia et al. reported 28 ovarian tumors and 36 other pelvic lesions in 181 cases of Stein-Leventhal syndrome, calling attention to the need for exploration and microscopic study of palpable pelvic masses in this condition if the laparoscopic appearance is at all atypical.[6] The surgeon is reminded that pelvic adhesions occur following a surgical procedure in the lower abdomen and pelvis; therefore, special attention to surgical technique is recommended to minimize pelvic adhesions following wedge resection as the adhesions may lead to infertility. Weinstein and Polishuk studied 57 patients who had an ovarian wedge resection and observed that 14% developed pelvic adhesions that resulted in infertility.[44]

Malignant Tumors Amenable to Unilateral Salpingo-oophorectomy

Epithelial Lesion   The borderline epithelial lesion that is unilateral and encapsulated may be managed with unilateral salpingo-oophorectomy when reproductive capabilities are an overriding concern.[18] The difficulty in treating this lesion lies in obtaining a final diagnosis of borderline status at the time of surgery. Likewise, one may manage stage Ia well-differentiated grade 1 epithelial tumors that are unilateral and encapsulated the same way. Williams and Dockerty reported 65 patients with low-grade epithelial malignancies of the ovary: 26 patients had mucinous cystadenocarcinoma, 25 serous cystadenocarcinoma, and 14 endometroid carcinoma.[48] No deaths from malignancy of the ovary resulted in the entire group of patients with unilateral intracystic, grade 1 cancer. In the contralateral ovary, 31% of patients had serous ovarian tumors and 14% had malignant tumors. Frozen section must, therefore, confirm a normal contralateral ovary, even one grossly normal in appearance.

The criteria for conservative management of epithelial ovarian tumors are as follows: occurrence in a patient under 35 years of age, intercystic location, unruptured, nonadherent, of low grade, and opposite ovary uninvolved by the tumor process on microscopic examination. As only 8% of epithelial tumors occur in women under 40,[9] these criteria are rarely met; however, approximately 50% of patients will achieve pregnancy if some ovarian tissue can be left behind.

Germ Cell Tumors   Germ cell tumors are amenable to unilateral salpingo-oophorectomy in two specific types of tumors: dysgerminoma and mature teratoma. The dysgerminoma must be under 10 cm in size, unilateral, well encapsulated, and without metastasis or mixed elements. When the lesion does not meet these criteria, total abdominal hysterectomy, bilateral salpingo-oophorectomy, and irradiation therapy are indicated.[1] Unilateral salpingo-oophorectomy as the initial surgical treatment does not significantly change the 10-year postoperative survival rate.[4]

Although cystic mature teratomas have a 2% malignancy rate,[42] if the teratoma is well encapsulated, unilateral salpingo-oophorectomy is acceptable. Most cases of cystic mature teratomas are unilateral and occur during the reproductive years.

All reported cases of solid mature teratomas have been unilateral, hence well-encapsulated lesions may be treated with unilateral salpingo-oophorectomy.[42]

Stromal Tumors, Granulosa Cell Carcinoma, and Sertoli–Leydig Tumors These tumors, which are unilateral and encapsulated, permit the preservation of the opposite ovary as they are rarely bilateral.[45] Remember that as many as 20% of granulosa cell tumors have associated endometrial cancer; therefore, uterine curettage is essential for an accurate diagnosis.

Bilateral Salpingo-oophorectomy and Hysterectomy

Bilateral salpingo-oophorectomy and total abdominal hysterectomy are indicated in those patients with benign ovarian tumors who do not wish to preserve their fertility. When malignant tumor is present, a thorough abdominal exploration, total abdominal hysterectomy, bilateral salpingo-oophorectomy, omentectomy, and removal of all gross cancer consistent with good surgical judgment is standard therapy.

Parker et al. observed statistically different long-term survival rates in patients with epithelial carcinoma of the ovary in whom the omentum was removed[33] (Figures 18.8 and 18.9). Biopsy the omentum in all patients with possible malignant lesions of the ovary and remove the omentum in all patients who receive definitive therapy for ovarian cancer. The details of omental vascular anatomy are reviewed by Alday and Goldsmith.[2]

Place catheters for radioactive chromic phosphate (^{32}P) administration in patients with stage I epithelial malignancy of the ovary and give it in the immediate postoperative period (Figures 18.10 and 18.11). Chromic phosphate has been shown to achieve approximately a 90% 5-year survival rate in stage I ovarian cancer. Chromic phosphate, which emits pure beta irradiation, is adequate to destroy small clusters of malignant cells. It has a

205

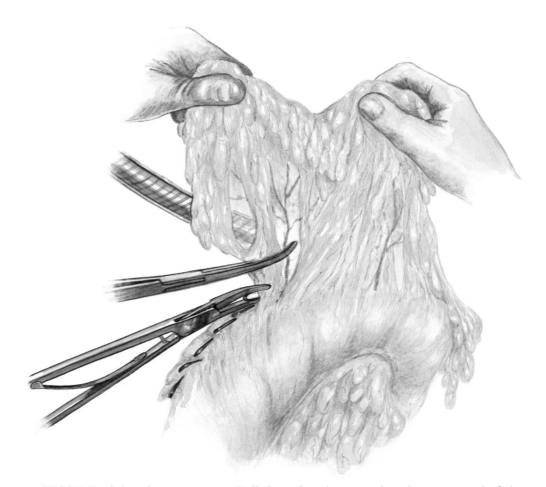

FIGURE 18.8.   Omentectomy. Pull the colon downward at the upper end of the laparotomy wound into the field. Place a fiberoptic light source behind the omentum, transilluminating it. Identify the vessels seen, beginning from left to right; pull the omentum upward and divide it using hemoclips on the side proximal to the colon and a series of hemostats above the clips.

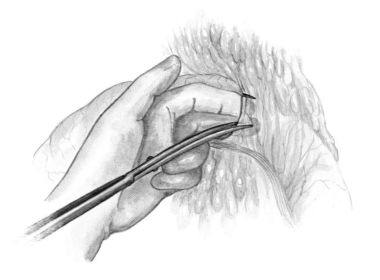

FIGURE 18.9.   When the omentum is to be excised from the margins of the stomach, divide the filmy adhesions that attach the omentum to the colon by inserting the fingers in this cleavage plane. Using sharp dissection, completely free the omentum from the colon. Use hemoclips if any bleeding vessels are encountered. Pull the omentum down from the stomach; identify the gastroepiploic vessels and ligate them using hemoclips and a series of hemostats opposite the clipped vessels. Excise the rest of the omentum between the clips and hemostats. Avoid the underlying colonic vessels during this excision.

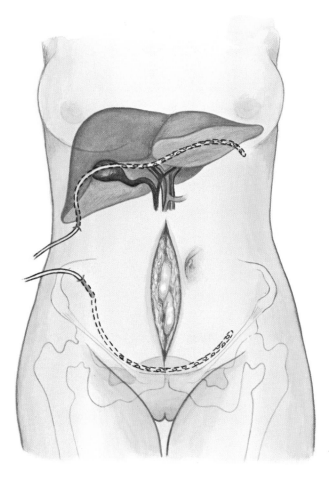

FIGURE 18.10. When administration of chromic phosphate is anticipated in the postoperative period, always insert radioisotope administration tubes. If the histologic diagnosis is in doubt, insert the tubes. If clinical indications are not present, their use causes little morbidity and they can be removed. Small or medium Hemovac tubes are adaptable by cutting two to three extra holes with sharp scissors, taking care not to weaken the structural integrity of the tube. Use a Hemovac needle and place the needles in a diagonal fashion through the abdominal wall to allow partial closure on removal of the tubes so that spill will be minimized. Take care to avoid the anastomosis between the superior and inferior epigastric vessels which can be palpated through the abdominal wall. Secure the tubes with braided nylon suture placed in a circular fashion 3 to 4 mm from the tube edge; leave the sutures untied and rolled in a gauze edge taped to the abdomen. The tubes will be ready for closure on removal of the administration tubes. Lay the tubing into the abdomen.

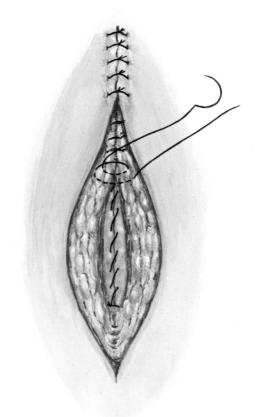

FIGURE 18.11. Chromic phosphate is important and differs from the usual wound closure. No drains can be used when chromic phosphate is to be administered; the peritoneal closure should be separate and differs from the usual far-and-near wound closure. Close the peritoneum with a continuous 2-0 chromic suture, everting the edges and making the closure as watertight as possible. Place a separate far-and-near layer of 0 nylon sutures. Make certain the longer limb does not enter the peritoneum. Close the skin with interrupted 3-0 monofilament vertical mattress sutures.

maximum penetration of approximately 4 mm and the isotope has a half-life of 14 to 15 days.[35] Administration is usually 10 μCi in 200 ml volume.

Hilaris and Clark reported survival rates of 92% in patients with stage I ovarian cancer who received ^{32}P and 77% in a similar group who did not.[24] Patients with ruptured tumors are also candidates for radiocoloid administration. If the diagnosis is in doubt, place catheters. Remove them if the pathological diagnosis is benign.

External radiation of the pelvis is used in patients with stage II ovarian cancer in whom little tumor remains after surgery in combination with intraperitoneal ^{32}P or chemotherapy. Mansfield notes a 47% 5-year survival rate as opposed to 33% when no irradiation was given.[29] Shielding of the liver and kidney prevents therapeutic doses from going to the common sites of spread in advanced ovarian cancer. Most treatment protocols emphasize surgery and chemotherapy for stage III ovarian disease.[18]

If the lesion is of the serous type, the administration of alkylating agents such as oral phenylalanine mustard 1 mg/kg in divided doses over a 5-day period once a month is appropriate. If the patient has a poorly differentiated lesion, more aggressive therapy such as Adriamycin and Cytoxan with the addition of progestational agents is advised. Buchler et al. reported on 62 patients with stage III ovarian carcinoma treated with irradiation, five-drug chemotherapy, or single chemotherapeutic agents.[11] Of the 62 patients, 27 had a favorable response when treated with surgery and chemotherapy or surgery and irradiation. The difference in survival time between the two groups was not significant: the median survival was 24.6 months after surgery and chemotherapy and 21.6 months after surgery and irradiation. Significant side effects were seen following multidrug therapy. If gross tumor remains following surgery, use chemotherapy alone.

Patients with minimal residual disease have a better prognosis, and the surgeon must make every effort consistent with good surgical judgment to remove all resectable epithelial ovarian cancer.[12,33] It is difficult for a surgeon trained in the anatomic surgical technique of Halstead to debulk a patient with ovarian cancer and not feel it is meddlesome at best or destructive at worst.

Fisher has reviewed modern laboratory data suggesting that tumor cells are released into the bloodstream very early in the natural development of a tumor, but are destroyed by the host's immunologic system until it is overcome.[20] Furthermore, although lymph nodes are effective at screening particulate matter, most tumor cells entering a lymph node do not stay localized. Thus one has to consider the host as the unit involved, not the various components such as lymph or blood.[20]

Immunologic benefits from the removal of tumor bulk include the removal of serum blocking factor,[23] increased cell-mediated immunity,[47] and increased release of lymphoblasts by regional nodes.[3] While debulking does increase the proportion of growing tumor cells due to improved blood and oxygen supply, these growing cells are more sensitive to chemotherapy and irradiation than resting cells.

Finally, when the tumor mass approaches a lethal volume, lymphocyte cytotoxicity is lost and host death follows.

These immunologic concepts are useful in the treatment of epithelial ovarian cancer as most lesions are beyond complete surgical excision. Procedures must be tailored to decrease tumor burden so that host defense mechanisms and adjunctive therapy may be effective.[26] The operations are in no way anatomical, as microscopic tumor is usually present. They are useful now and will become increasingly more effective as adjunctive measures improve.

Second-Look Procedure

The second-look operation is an exploratory laparotomy that is performed at some time following the initial therapeutic surgical procedure for ovarian cancer. The concept is not new but its precise role in the surgical management of ovarian cancer remains to be defined.

The operation is useful in approximately 1 of 10 patients with advanced epithelial cancer of the ovary. Its primary use is to obtain information as to the state of disease in a patient in whom little disease is palpable. The patient should have had the original surgery at least 1 year before, received at least 1 year of chemotherapy, and clinically responded to such therapy by a marked decrease in the size of the residual disease.

Unfortunately, the majority of patients with a postoperative response to chemotherapy have clinically detectable tumor; however, approximately 50% of patients who had all visible disease resected initially are found free of disease at second-look surgery. Patients with massive unresectable disease prior to chemotherapy rarely have negative second-look results.[38] An adequate second-look procedure includes the following: sampling of any peritoneal fluid (or washings if fluid is lacking); biopsy of both gutters; observation of the diaphragm and periaortic and pelvic wall nodes; and careful exploration of the abdomen. The majority of patients in whom these examinations are negative will be long-term survivors. Piver et al. found no advantage in the incorporation of second-look operations early in the course of chemotherapy, second-look exploratory laparotomy, and whole-abdomen irradiation.[34]

Patients with pelvic masses that do not change in size over a long period of observation or chemotherapy usually have adherent masses of the small bowel. Ovarian cancer will either respond to chemotherapy or progressively grow.

Exploration is contraindicated in heavily irradiated patients, patients treated with intraperitoneal isotopes, and patients with progressive tumor at other sites. The author opposes the indiscriminate use of computerized tomography, sonography, laparoscopy, and laparotomy in patients with obvious generalized progressive ovarian cancer as little information useful to the patient is ever obtained. It remains to be seen whether second-look surgery will add any 5-year survivors to the 7% of women who now survive after presenting with ovarian cancer spread to the abdomen.[34]

Ovarian Tumors in Children and Adolescents

Ovarian malignancies are very rare in children and produce less than 50 deaths per year in the United States.[40] Most of the neoplasms in children arise from germ cells, in contrast to adults, in whom 80% or more of the primary ovarian malignancies arise from epithelium. Barber notes that the ovary in the infant and child is an abdominal organ and pelvic examination is often negative in the presence of an abdominal mass of ovarian origin.[7]

Symptoms are abdominal pain, pressure, and those symptoms associated with the phenomena of torsion, hemorrhage, or hormone production. Torsion is common due to the smooth surface and long pedicles, and acute appendicitis is the most common misdiagnosis.[30] Preoperative evaluation includes chest x-ray, intravenous pyelogram, serum studies for gonadotropins, α-fetoprotein, and carcinoembryonic antigens, and ultrasound studies. The intravenous pyelogram is a vital study; 40% of abdominal masses in the newborn are of renal origin. The lucency of the area occupied by any large cyst is a useful diagnostic finding[13] as is the calcification noted in 60% of cystic teratomas.[30]

Treatment involves excision of the involved ovary or internal genitalia, depending on the nature of the lesion. This is best done where competence in the complex pathology of these rare neoplasms is available. Excise the cyst and await frozen section diagnosis. If the tumor is solid, excise the ovary and obtain a frozen section diagnosis. If the pathologist cannot arrive at a diagnosis at the time of frozen section, close the abdomen. After the correct diagnosis is obtained, additional surgery may be indicated. If removal of the remaining uterus and ovary is being considered, it is helpful to remember that most ovarian tumors in childhood are unilateral and benign.

Multiple retention, giant follicular, theca and corpus luteum cysts account for almost all ovarian masses in newborns and are uniformly benign.[5] The most common ovarian neoplasms in infants and children are cystic teratomas and their malignant counterparts.[7] The most frequent tumors in adolescents, in order of decreasing frequency, are cystic teratoma, mucinous cystadenoma, serous cystadenoma, corpus luteum cysts, para-ovarian cysts, and endometriomas. Less common tumors are embryonal teratomas, granulosa cell tumors, dysgerminoma, endodermal sinus tumor, and carcinoma.[7]

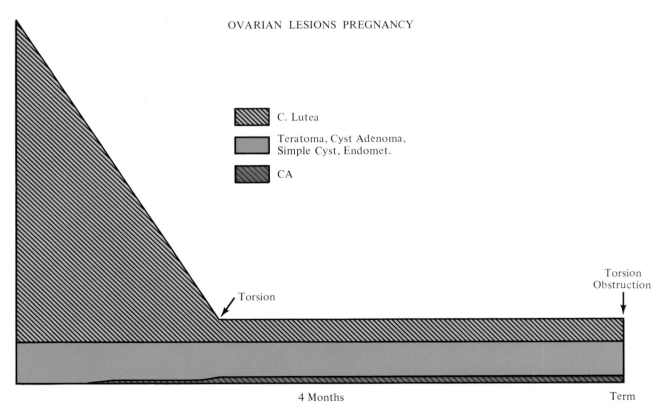

OVARIAN LESIONS PREGNANCY

C. Lutea

Teratoma, Cyst Adenoma, Simple Cyst, Endomet.

CA

Torsion

Torsion Obstruction

4 Months

Term

FIGURE 18.12. Ovarian masses in pregnancy. Note that the vast majority are corpus lutea and resolve under observation. Torsion occurs more commonly at 3 months and at term and the tumor may obstruct labor as well. Only 5% of persistent ovarian masses in pregnancy are malignant, in accord with the uncommon occurrence of epithelial malignancy in women under 40 years of age.

Ovarian Tumors in Pregnancy

Physiological enlargement of the ovary to form a corpus luteum of pregnancy is a normal event. This cystic mass rarely exceeds 6 cm in size and subsides as the placenta assumes endocrine support of the pregnancy. Ultrasound is used to document the decrease in size of this normal cystic mass. When an adnexal mass persists into the second trimester of pregnancy, exploration is indicated. Immediate exploration is necessary if the patient develops ascites, if the mass is bilateral, nodular, or solid, or if torsion or hemorrhage occur. About 1 in 1,000 pregnancies require exploration.[46] Less than 5% of the patients requiring exploration have a malignant lesion.[31] Hill et al. reported 57 ovarian masses found at exploration or seen on referral: there were 38 benign cysts such as cystic corpus luteum, 7 mature cystic teratomas, 4 endometriomas, and 5 benign and 3 malignant epithelial cystadenomas[25] (Figure 18.12).

Novak et al. reported 100 cases of ovarian tumors associated with pregnancy.[32] These cases were reference cases sent to the Emil Novak Tumor Registry over a 30-year period and are therefore the unusual and uncommon lesions, with high incidence of malignant tumors; 15 benign corpus luteum lesions were eliminated from the report. The 5-year survival rates were as follows: 75% in 45 epithelial lesions of the ovary; 76% in 33 germ cell tumors, among which dysgerminoma and dermoid were most common; and 85% in 14 gonadostromal tumors. Eight lesions included sarcomas and metastases.

In view of the coexistent pregnancy, the patient and her husband must have a clear understanding of the options available if malignant tumor, although rare, is found. Hill et al. noted little benefit in supporting the pregnancy postoperatively with progesterone to diminish abortion and found an incidence of 24% spontaneous abortions.[25]

Treatment for malignant lesions does not differ from that in the nonpregnant state, but of course the use of irradiation or chemotherapy, should the patient elect to continue the pregnancy in the face of a malignant lesion of the ovary, must be avoided.

Postoperative Management and Results

Care of the postoperative ovarian surgery patient is the same as that recommended after abdominal surgery (Chapter 13). When a malignant lesion is diagnosed by the pathologist and the surgeon does not wish to administer chemotherapy, prompt consultation regarding the initiation of chemotherapy is recommended. Likewise, when irradiation therapy is the appropriate treatment, promptly consult the radiation therapist. The intraperitoneal isotopes must be placed prior to the formation of intra-abdominal adhesions.

If the ovaries are removed, consider estrogen replacement. The author recommends combination hormone therapy to minimize breast difficulties: estrogen on days 1 to 25 of the menstrual cycle and a progestational agent on days 20 to 25 of the menstrual cycle. In contrast to endometrial cancer, malignant tumors of the ovary are not a contraindication to estrogen therapy.

The prognosis and post-treatment results for various ovarian lesions have been indicated throughout the chapter. In summary, surgery for the benign ovarian lesion is clinically successful. Pelvic inflammatory disease usually responds to conservative treatment, but ruptured tuboovarian abscess demands immediate surgical intervention.

211

Surgery remains the cornerstone of therapy in ovarian malignancies, but both chemotherapy and irradiation therapy are useful adjuncts. The 5-year survival rates for ovarian epithelial malignancy collected from various series approximate 60% to 90% in stage I, 39% to 65% in stage II, 4% to 9% in stage III, and 0% in stage IV.[8,34,39] As most patients present with stage III ovarian cancer, aggressive investigation of ovarian masses and prompt therapy of the lesion detected are vital.

References

1. Ala Alfredi, M., Vongtama, V., Tsukada, Y., et al.: Dysgerminoma of the ovary: Radiation therapy for recurrence and metastases. *Am. J. Obstet. Gynecol.* **126:**190–194, 1976.
2. Alday, E.S., and Goldsmith, H.S.: Surgical technique for omental lengthening based on arterial anatomy. *Surg. Gynecol. Obstet.* **135:**103–107, 1972.
3. Alexander, P., and Hall, J.G.: The role of immunoblasts in host resistance and immunotherapy of primary sarcoma. *Adv. Cancer Res.* **13:**1–37, 1970.
4. Asadourian, L.A., and Taylor, H.B.: Dysgerminoma: An analysis of 105 cases. *Obstet. Gynecol.,* **33:**370–379, 1969.
5. Astedt, B.: Ovarian neoplasms in newborns. *Nord. Med.* **19:**87–88, 1967.
6. Babaknia, A., Calfopoulos, P., and Jones, H.W.: The Stein-Leventhal syndrome and coincidental ovarian tumors. *Obstet. Gynecol.* **47:**223, 1976.
7. Barber, H.R.: Managing ovarian tumors of childhood and adolescence. *Female Patient* **3:**83–85, 1978.
8. Barber, H.R., and Kwon, T.H.: Current status of the treatment of gynecologic cancer by site. *Cancer* **38:** [Suppl.] 610–619, 1976.
9. Barber, H.R., Kwon, T.H., Buterman, I., et al.: Current concepts in the management of ovarian cancer. *J. Reprod. Med.* **20:**41–49, 1978.
10. Blum, M., and Meidan, A.: Late results of conservative operation for bilateral benign ovarian tumors. *Int. Surg.* **61:**561–562, 1976.
11. Buchler, D.A., Kline, J.C., Davis, H.L., et al.: Stage III ovarian carcinoma: Treatment and results. *Radiology* **122:**469–472, 1977.
12. Bush, R.S., Allt, W.E., Beale, F.A., et al.: Treatment of epithelial carcinoma of the ovary: Operation, irradiation, and chemotherapy. *Am. J. Obstet. Gynecol.* **127:**692–704, 1977.
13. Carlson, D.H., and Grimscom, N.T.: Ovarian cysts in the newborn. *Am. J. Roentgenol. Radium Ther. Nucl. Med.* **116:**664–672, 1972.
14. Carter, R.P.: Early diagnosis of ovarian cancer. In Masterson, B.J. (ed.): *Proceedings of Symposium on New Developments in Gynecologic Cancer.* Lawrence, Kans., University of Kansas Printing Service, 1978.
15. Christ, J.E., and Lotze, E.C.: The residual ovary syndrome. *Obstet. Gynecol.* **46:**551–555, 1975.
16. Cunningham, F.G., Hauth, J.C., Strong, J.D., et al: Evaluation of tetracycline or penicillin and ampicillin for the treatment of acute pelvic inflammation disease. *N. Engl. J. Med.* **296:**1380–1383, 1977.
17. Daly, J.W., and Monif, G.R.: Tuboovarian and ovarian abscesses. In Monif, G.R. (ed.): *Infectious Diseases in Obstetrics and Gynecology.* Hagerstown, Md., Harper & Row, 1974.
18. DiSaia, P.J., Townsend, D.E., and Morrow, C.P.: The rationale for less than radical treatment for gynecologic malignancy in early reproductive years. *Obstet. Gynecol. Surv.* **29:**581–593, 1974.
19. Duignan, N.M.: Polycystic ovarian disease. *Br. J. Obstet. Gynaecol.* **83:** 593–602, 1976.
20. Fisher, B.: The changing role of surgery in the treatment of cancer. In Becker, F. (ed.): *Cancer.* New York, Plenum, 1977.
21. Franklin, E.W., Hevron, J.E., and Thompson, J.D.: Management of the pelvic abscess. *Clin. Obstet. Gynecol.* **16:**66–79, 1973.

22. Gynecologic cancer. *Am. Coll. Obstet. Gynecol. Tech. Bull.* no. 24: 1–7, 1973.

23. Hellstrom, I., Hellstrom, K.E., and Sjogren, H.O.: Serum mediated inhibition of cellular immunity of methylcholanthrene-induced murine sarcomas. *Cell. Immunol.* **1:**18–30, 1970.

24. Hilaris, B.S., and Clark, D.G.C.: The value of postoperative intraperitoneal injection of radiocolloids in early cancer of the ovary. *Am. J. Roentgenol. Radium Ther. Nucl. Med.* **112:**749–754, 1971.

25. Hill, L.M., Johnson, C.E., and Lee, R.A.: Ovarian surgery in pregnancy. *Am. J. Obstet. Gynecol.* **122:**565–569, 1975.

26. Humphrey, L., Panoussopoulos, D., Volenec, F.J., et al.: The role of tumor immunity in ovarian cancer. *South. Med. J.* **70:**1186–1187, 1977.

27. Lawson, T.L., and Albaretti, J.N.: Diagnosis of gynecologic pelvic masses by gray scale ultrasonography: Analysis of specificity and accuracy. *Am. J. Roentgenol.* **128:**1003–1006, 1977.

28. Mahesh, V.B., Toledo, S.P., and Mattar E.: Hormone levels following wedge resection in polycystic ovary syndrome. *Obstet. Gynecol.* **51:**64–68, 1978.

29. Mansfield, C.: Role of radioisotope in ovarian cancer. In Masterson, B.J. (ed.): *Proceedings of Symposium on New Developments in Gynecologic Cancer.* Lawrence, Kans., University of Kansas Printing Service, 1978.

30. Moore, J.G., Schifrin, B.S., and Erez, S.: Ovarian tumors in infancy, childhood, and adolescence. *Am. J. Obstet. Gynecol.* **90:**913–922, 1967.

31. Munnell, E.W.: Primary ovarian cancer associated with pregnancy. *Clin. Obstet. Gynecol.* **6:**983–993, 1963.

32. Novak, E.R., Lambrou, C.D., and Woodruff, J.D.: Ovarian tumors in pregnancy. *Obstet. Gynecol.* **46:**401–406, 1975.

33. Parker, R.T., Parker, C.H., and Wilbanks, G.D.: Cancer of the ovary. *Am. J. Obstet. Gynecol.* **108:**878–888, 1970.

34. Piver, M.S., Barlow, J.J., Lee, F.T., et al.: Sequential therapy for advanced ovarian adenocarcinoma: Operation, chemotherapy, second-look laparotomy, and radiation therapy. *Am. J. Obstet. Gynecol.* **122:**355–358, 1975.

35. Piver, M.S., Barlow, J.J., and Lele, S.B.: Incidence of subclinical metastasis in stage I and II ovarian carcinoma. *Obstet. Gynecol.* **52:**100–104, 1978.

36. Piver, M.S., Lele, S., and Barlow, J.J.: Preoperative and intraoperative evaluation in ovarian malignancy. *Obstet. Gynecol.* **48:**312–315, 1976.

37. Ranney, B., and Chastain, D.: Ovarian function, reproduction, and later operations following adnexal surgery. *Obstet. Gynecol.* **51:**521–528, 1978.

38. Rutledge, F., Boronow, R.C., and Wharton, J.T.: Treatment of epithelial cancer of the ovary. In: *Gynecologic Oncology.* New York, Wiley, 1976.

39. Schein, P.S.: Chemotherapy in advanced ovarian cancer. *Geriatrics* **28:**89–95, 1973.

40. Silverberg, E.: Cancer statistics, 1977. *Ca—Cancer J. for Clinicians* **27:**26–41, 1977.

41. Stein, I.: Diagnosis and treatment of bilateral polycystic ovaries in the Stein-Leventhal syndrome. *Int. J. Fertil.* **3:**20–26, 1958.

42. Talerman, A.: Germ cell tumors of the ovary. In Blaustein, A. (ed.): *Pathology of the Female Genital Tract.* New York, Springer-Verlag, 1977.

43. Uhrich, P.C., and Sanders, R.C.: Ultrasonic characteristics of pelvic inflammatory masses. *J. Clin. Ultrasound* **4:**199–204, 1976.

44. Weinstein, D., and Polishuk, W.Z.: The role of wedge resection of the ovary as a cause for mechanical sterility. *Surg. Gynecol. Obstet.* **141:**417–418, 1975.

45. Wharton, L.R.: Surgery of benign adnexal disease: Endometriosis, residuals of inflammatory and granulomatous disease, and ureteral injury. In Ridley, J. (ed.): *Gynecologic Surgery: Errors, Safeguards, Salvage.* Baltimore, Williams & Wilkins, 1974.

46. White, K.C.: Ovarian tumors in pregnancy. *Am. J. Obstet. Gynecol.* **116:**544–548, 1973.

47. Whitney, R.B., Levy, J.G., and Smith, A.G.: Influence of tumor size and sur-

gical resection on cell-mediated immunity in mice. *J. Natl. Cancer Inst.* **53:** 11–116, 1974.
48. Williams, T.J., and Dockerty, M.B.: Status of the contralateral ovary in encapsulated low grade malignant tumors of the ovary. *Surg. Gynecol. Obstet.* **143:**763–766, 1976.

Selected Bibliography

Barber, H.R.K.: *Ovarian Carcinoma: Etiology, Diagnosis and Treatment.* New York, Masson, 1978.

Blaustein, A. (ed.): *Pathology of the Female Genital Tract.* New York, Springer-Verlag, 1977.

DiSaia, P., Morrow, P., and Townsend, D.: *Synopsis of Gynecologic Oncology.* New York, Wiley, 1975.

Norris, H.J.M., and Chorlton, I.: Functioning tumors of the ovary. *Clin. Obstet. Gynecol.* **17:**189–228, 1974.

Novak, E.R., Jones, G.S., and Jones, H.W.: *Novak's Textbook of Gynecology,* 9th ed. Baltimore, Williams & Wilkins, 1975.

Rutledge, F., Boronow, R.C., and Wharton, J.T.: *Gynecologic Oncology.* New York, Wiley, 1976.

Scully, R.E.: Ovarian tumors. *Am. J. Pathol.* **87:**686–720, 1977.

Management of Bowel Injuries in Gynecologic Surgery

19

This chapter deals with the operative management of the gastrointestinal tract. Lesions are discussed in two groups: first, operative injuries occurring at the operating table which require management at that time; and second, a group of procedures involving the gastrointestinal tract in association with other gynecologic conditions.

Operative Injuries

Most injuries in any surgical procedure can be traced to inadequate exposure due to poor light, unsatisfactory assistance, or poor choice of incision. Undue haste before adequate exposure is obtained is a senseless economy in surgery. There are, however, an irreducible number of operative injuries involving the gastrointestinal tract that occur in gynecologic surgery.

Small Intestine

One may injure the small bowel while opening the wound, freeing adhesions from the bowel to the anterior abdonimal wall from prior surgical procedures, or mobilizing the bowel from the pelvis in endometriosis or other conditions in which the bowel might become fixed. On noting injured small bowel, wall it off from the abdominal cavity and inspect it (Figure 19.1). If the injury is through the serosa in otherwise healthy bowel, place interrupted 4-0 Nurolon sutures transversely through the seromuscular layer covering the defect. If the muscularis is injured from a simple incision that does not devitalize the bowel and the mucosa is not injured, place a single layer of 4-0 Nurolon suture transversely in the defect. If the lumen of the small bowel is entered, one must determine the viability of the bowel surrounding the injured area. Any dead bowel wall or bowel wall that has suffered severe enough injury to make its viability questionable is then resected. If there are two injuries close to each other, resect the injured bowel and perform an end-to-end anastomosis (Figures 19.2 through 19.7).

If the injury does not involve the majority of the circumference of the small bowel, close the defect in two layers: the inner layer with interrupted 4-0 Vicryl or chromic catgut through and through the bowel wall, and the outer layer with 4-0 Nurolon suture into the submucosa, inverting the sec-

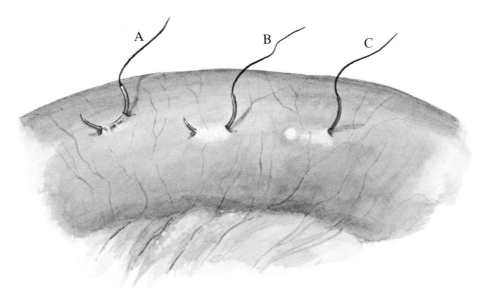

FIGURE 19.1.   Three layers of bowel used in gut surgery. Needle A is simply through the serosa; needle B enters the muscularis; and needle C enters the submucosa. The placement of sutures in the submucosa is important as this is the holding layer of the bowel. A definite resistance will be felt when the needle enters this layer, and the white circle at the needle tip is characteristic, confirming that the proper layer is being used for gut surgery.

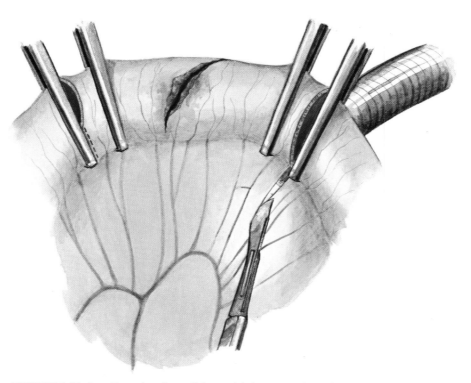

FIGURE 19.2.   Repair of small bowel injury. Isolate the bowel to be excised with Glassman nontraumatic forceps or use straight Masterson clamps, taking care not to close them fully. The fiberoptic tube light is used to transilluminate the mesentery to aid in identifying blood vessels. Ligate mesenteric vessels with 3-0 Nurolon suture ligatures or ties.

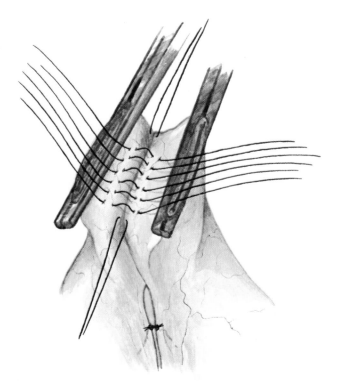

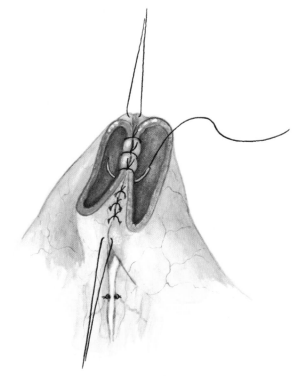

FIGURE 19.3. Trim the mesentery back from the edge of the small bowel and bring the bowel clamps together as indicated. Place lateral stay sutures of 4-0 Nurolon and attach a hemostat to each. Place an outer layer of 4-0 Nurolon interrupted sutures as shown. In end-to-end anastomosis, the posterior seromuscular layer is placed close enough to the lumen to avoid marked inversion, which produces a partial obstruction in some anastomoses.

FIGURE 19.4. Remove the Glassman clamps. Trim any devitalized tissue and secure hemostasis. Close the inner layer with interrupted 4-0 absorbable suture with the knots inside the lumen. A continuous inner layer is acceptable in unirradiated bowel. Place intestinal Allis clamps on the unsutured bowel margin to evert the edges.

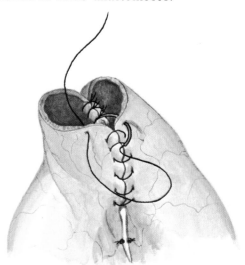

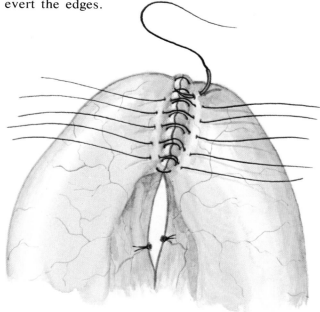

FIGURE 19.5. Continue the through-and-through inner layer around to close the circumference of the bowel. Traction on the stay suture will help invert the mucosa into the lumen. Look into the lumen to make certain that no suture has penetrated the gut and attached the opposite side, thereby obstructing the lumen.

FIGURE 19.6. Place an outer layer of 4-0 Nurolon covering the inner layer. Make certain the mesenteric border is well closed. Remove the stay suture. Palpate the lumen between the thumb and index finger and squeeze bowel contents through, further checking the security of the anastomosis.

217

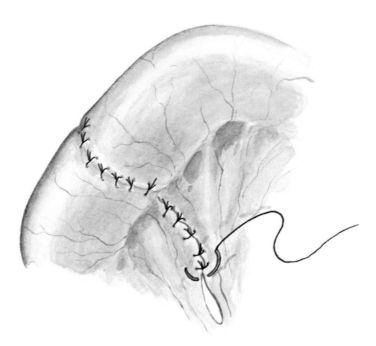

FIGURE 19.7. Close the defect in the mesentery. Avoid mesenteric vessels by transilluminating the mesentery.

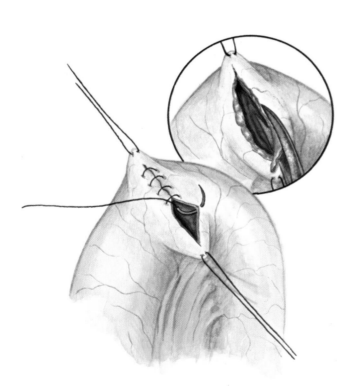

FIGURE 19.8. Two-layer repair of bowel injury. Place two stay sutures of 4-0 Nurolon. Trim any devitalized bowel wall and convert the defect to a transverse wound. Close the inner layer with 4-0 absorbable suture.

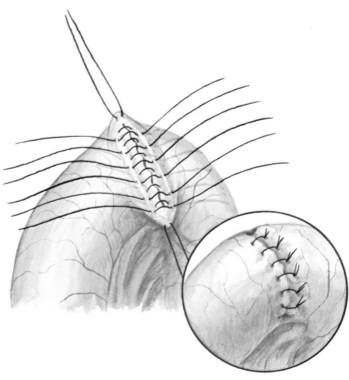

FIGURE 19.9. Place an outer layer of seromuscular suture and tie snugly but not so as to obstruct the blood supply. Remove the stay sutures.

218

ond layer (Figures 19.8 and 19.9). Note that much experimental work has shown that one-layer small bowel anastomosis is quite adequate and results in a larger lumen[12]; however, two-layer anastomosis is the most common anastomosis done and probably is safer for the surgeon occasionally operating on bowel, providing there is not too much bowel wall inversion.

After the anastomosis is complete, check the mesentery for any bleeding points and close any remaining mesenteric defect. Remove the laparotomy tapes walling off the area of repair and irrigate the abdominal cavity with warm saline. The intended procedure is then continued. Remember to inspect the bowel at the end of the procedure for continued viability.

Check the anastomosis both by palpating the lumen and by compressing bowel contents between the fingers and forcing it through the repaired lumen. The majority of anastomoses leak to some extent; therefore, the anastomosis must be in the peritoneal cavity, which has a reliable defense mechanism to prevent infection, necrosis, and ultimate dehiscence.[9] If the bowel injury is associated with a procedure for endometriosis or pelvic inflammatory disease in which a large amount of the peritoneum might be removed or with exenterative procedures in which the anastomosis would lie in an unperitonealized area, it will be at significant risk. The development of an omental pedicle to surround the anastomosis is worthwhile. Anastomoses should never lie in contact with drains or other foreign objects as this increases the failure rate.

At the time of bowel injury, begin the patient on intravenous antibiotics. These may be discontinued after 24 hr, and with small bowel injury the likelihood of abdominal infection is slight. Occasionally, a loop of small bowel may be trapped behind a retractor and not noticed until the end of the procedure. If it is still viable, the bowel should quickly resume an appearance similar to adjoining loops of bowel and the mesenteric vessels should be seen pulsating in the area immediately adjacent to the small bowel. Furthermore, elicit peristalsis by gently stimulating the injured segment of bowel. Place a warm pack over the segment in question for a few minutes. If dark blue color persists, the serosa is dull, peristalsis is absent, and the mesenteric vessels do not pulsate, the segment in question is resected, with the resection carried to an area of good blood supply. Bear in mind that successful reconstructive procedures require an unquestioned blood supply and a tension-free anastomosis.

Gastrointestinal and Other Vessels

Occasional injuries from misplaced retractors, forceful exploration, mobilization of large tumor masses, or misdiagnosis may require the gynecologist to make an immediate decision regarding vascular injuries. Gastric vessels can be ligated with impunity, as can the splenic artery and vein, the inferior mesenteric artery and vein, and the internal iliac artery and vein. Bleeding from the vena cava below the renal vein can usually be controlled with finger pressure and repaired with a running 5-0 arterial silk. The external iliac vein and the common iliac can be ligated if repair is impossible, although leg swelling may occur.

Acute loss of the superior mesenteric artery will rarely permit continued viability of the small bowel and is a life-threatening event requiring immediate consultation, careful planning, and attempted repair or grafting.[5]

Colon

In any patient in whom the possibility of entering the lower gastrointestinal tract during the course of the procedure is anticipated, meticulous preoperative preparation is essential. The patient should be advised of the possibility of a colostomy, fistula formation, or wound infection with prolonged hospitalization. Careful mechanical cleansing of the bowel is absolutely essential as it allows the surgeon to perform any necessary procedure to the colon at the time of the initial surgery and reduces the incidence of infection if the bowel is entered (Table 19.1, Figures 19.10 and 19.11). On the author's service, any patient operated on for ovarian cancer or any fixed pelvic mass goes through this protocol for bowel cleansing.

The importance of prophylactic oral antimicrobial agents in the preoperative preparation of a patient whose gastrointestinal tract may be injured has been clearly documented by Clarke et al.[3] and Goldring et al.[6] In Goldring's clinical study of 50 patients undergoing elective colon surgery, 25 were given 1 g oral kanamycin and 200 mg metronidazole every 6 hr for 3 days. Of these patients, only 2 developed wound infections, whereas 11 control patients developed postoperative infections.[6]

Irvin et al. have studied blood volume in patients with mechanical bowel preparation and found little evidence that fluid or electrolyte imbalance resulted.[8] Hypotension on induction of anesthesia is common, however, and these symptoms respond to saline or lactated Ringer's saline.

Should the surgeon accidently enter the right colon, the bacterial flora there are not significantly different from those in the small bowel, and, even in unprepared bowel, infection is much less likely than in the left colon. After it has been determined that there is no nonviable gut, two-layer closure of the injury (inner, 4-0 gut or Vicryl; outer, 4-0 Nurolon) should produce satisfactory results. The use of cecostomy as a defunctioning procedure is unnecessary. After the bowel wound has been closed, copiously irrigate the area around the wound. Intravenous antibiotics should be promptly begun at the time of injury and continued for 24 hr.

The transverse colon is rarely injured in gynecologic procedures and both hepatic and splenic flexures are well out of the operative site. The rectum and sigmoid colon, however, are intimately involved with many gynecologic tumors, pelvic masses, abscesses, and fistulas.

Serosal injury of the colon without injury to the mucosa may be oversewn with interrupted 4-0 Nurolon suture. If the unirradiated colon is perforated and the bowel has had adequate preoperative preparation with antibiotics and mechanical cleansing, simple closure in two layers will be satisfactory, particularly if the wound is clean and there has been minimal soiling of the pelvis. If in unprepared bowel the colon has been perforated or clamped with large crushing clamps that devitalized a segment of sigmoid with significant fecal contamination, resection of the devitalized tissues, two-layer closure, and proximal colostomy are necessary. The procedure of closing the injured segment and exteriorizing it to observe adequate healing, while attractive from a technical point of view, is of little benefit in gynecology because most of the injuries occur so low in the colon that it cannot

TABLE 19.1.   72-Hr Bowel Preparation

1. Liquid diet
2. Vitamin K p.o. tablet, 5 mg b.i.d.
3. Magnesium citrate, 10 oz 48 hr prior to surgery
4. Saline enema until clear 24 hr prior to surgery
5. Patient to evacuate rectum 6:30 a.m. on day of surgery
6. 48 hr prior to surgery: 1 g Kantrex p.o. every hour for 4 hr then every 6 hr until surgery and 250 mg p.o. metronidazole TID; or 1 g neomycin p.o. and 1 g erythromycin p.o. at 1 p.m., 2 p.m., and 11 p.m. on day prior to surgery

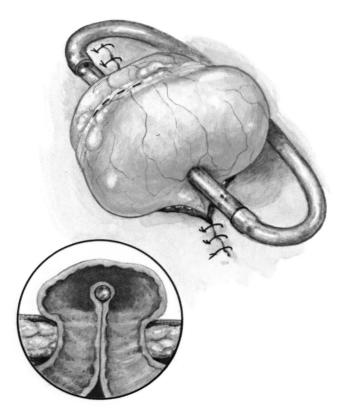

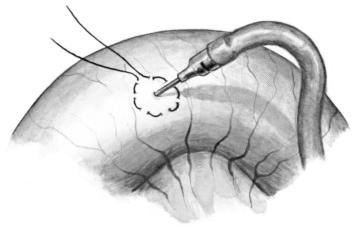

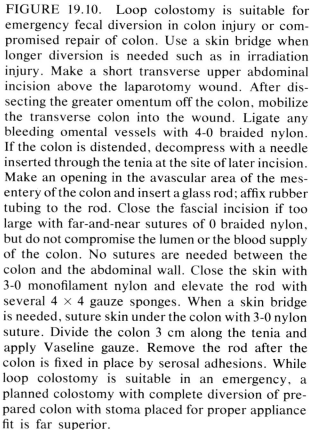

FIGURE 19.10. Loop colostomy is suitable for emergency fecal diversion in colon injury or compromised repair of colon. Use a skin bridge when longer diversion is needed such as in irradiation injury. Make a short transverse upper abdominal incision above the laparotomy wound. After dissecting the greater omentum off the colon, mobilize the transverse colon into the wound. Ligate any bleeding omental vessels with 4-0 braided nylon. If the colon is distended, decompress with a needle inserted through the tenia at the site of later incision. Make an opening in the avascular area of the mesentery of the colon and insert a glass rod; affix rubber tubing to the rod. Close the fascial incision if too large with far-and-near sutures of 0 braided nylon, but do not compromise the lumen or the blood supply of the colon. No sutures are needed between the colon and the abdominal wall. Close the skin with 3-0 monofilament nylon and elevate the rod with several 4 × 4 gauze sponges. When a skin bridge is needed, suture skin under the colon with 3-0 nylon suture. Divide the colon 3 cm along the tenia and apply Vaseline gauze. Remove the rod after the colon is fixed in place by serosal adhesions. While loop colostomy is suitable in an emergency, a planned colostomy with complete diversion of prepared colon with stoma placed for proper appliance fit is far superior.

FIGURE 19.11. Decompression of bowel. Place a purse-string suture in the segment of bowel to be decompressed. Isolate the area with laparotomy tapes. Use an 18-gauge needle and attach to wall suction. Insert the needle into the gut and aspirate. Be careful not to lacerate the opposite side of the bowel wall. Remove the needle and tubing and pull the purse-string sutures together. Discard any contaminated drapes.

be mobilized out of the pelvis. If the colon has previously been irradiated, there should be no haste in closing the colostomy protecting the repair. The surgeon should allow at least 6 to 8 weeks for the colon to heal and then perform a barium study of the distal colon before the colostomy is closed.

Surgery for Obstruction

The gynecologist is not called on to operate on patients with bowel obstruction unless he is managing a gynecologic oncology service; but he may encounter a patient who had a misdiagnosed intestinal injury or early intestinal obstruction and he needs to have some basic information in their management.

Non-neoplastic Small Bowel Obstruction

In patients with bowel obstruction, attention to preoperative details is particularly significant. Fluid and electrolyte balances should be brought within the normal range promptly. The loss of sodium chloride with 3,000 to 4,000 ml fluid into the obstructed gut is well documented. Gastrointestinal losses with high small bowel obstruction include excessive loss of chloride and potassium and resultant hypochloremic and hypokalemic alkalosis. Replacement with a sodium chloride solution with supplemental potassium is indicated. Remember that patients with high small bowel obstruction may have minimal air fluid levels on flat and upright abdominal x-ray examination.[4]

The patient with simple bowel obstruction not responding to conservative measures generally has obstruction of the distal ileum; usually it is an adhesive band or hernia, or the bowel may have been sutured into the vaginal cuff after vaginal hysterectomy or other surgical error. If exposure is difficult to obtain due to distended bowel, enter the bowel with an 18-gauge needle attached to wall suction through a small purse-string suture of 4-0 Nurolon. The contents, which consist of significant amounts of bowel gas and liquid, may be decompressed with subsequent exposure (Figure 19.11). The bowel is carefully run, beginning at the duodenum and progressing distally to the cecum. Most bowel obstructions that the gynecologist will see will be in the distal ileum. The bowel is freed and its viability is checked. Bowel contents may be pushed through the area that has been obstructed to make certain that there is no inherent obstruction in the bowel and to ascertain its viability. The serosa should glisten and the color of the bowel approximate the other small bowel; peristalsis should be present and the mesenteric vessels should be clearly pulsatile. If these conditions are met and bowel contents can be easily passed through the area of defect, nothing further need be done; however, if the obstruction has progressed to the point where the bowel has lost viability, then resection back to an area of healthy small bowel is necessary. Patients who have dead bowel would not normally be seen on the gynecology service, and in this case, as in all surgical procedures, consultation, if available, may be helpful. Remember that patients with nonstrangulating bowel obstruction have neither elevated white counts nor abdominal tenderness. Intervene early before nonviable bowel occurs as operative mortality rises dramatically when dead bowel is present.

Gastrointestinal Complications of Carcinoma of the Ovary

The gynecologist may frequently encounter gastrointestinal injuries and involvement of the bowel as a result of carcinoma of the ovary. Laparotomy of patients with carcinoma of the ovary may show the residual disease only in the distal ileum. Such patients require resection of this tumor and end-to-end anastomosis. The distal ileum may also be involved in a large pelvic mass that is resectable; in this case resection with end-to-end anastomosis may be advisable if other tumor volume is minimal. In a series of 614 cases of cancer of the ovary seen on the Gynecological Service of Memorial–James Ewing Hospital from 1947 to 1960, 8 of 94 patients (8.5%) who underwent resection of the distal ileum and right colon for invasive, advanced, and recurrent cancer of the ovary were alive after 5 years.[5] In these cases, the lesion appeared to be isolated. Forty-two patients had small bowel resection with disseminated disease and there were no 5-year survivors.

More commonly, the gynecologist may be involved with patients with ovarian cancer who have small bowel obstruction and nonresectable cancer. Burns et al.,[2] Graham and Villalba,[7] and Wheeless[13] have clearly shown that the procedure of choice in such patients is small bowel bypass. Irradiation injury is likewise best managed in this fashion. The mortality rate is greatly reduced and the surgical procedure is much less complex. Bypass may be performed in one of two ways: either an ileotransverse colostomy on a side-to-side basis (Figures 19.12–19.18) or an end-to-side ileotransverse colostomy with mucus fistula brought out to the distal end of the wound (Figure 19.19). Remember that the ileum selected must be free

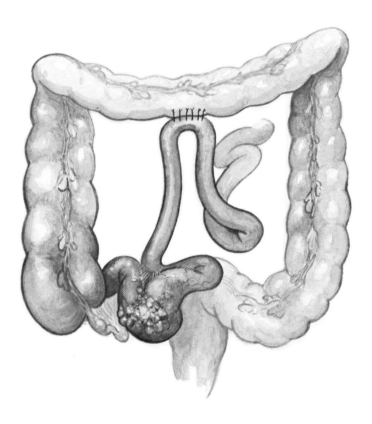

FIGURE 19.12. Side-to-side anastomosis approximating ileum and transverse colon. The anastomosis is without tension and may be buttressed with any remaining omentum.

223

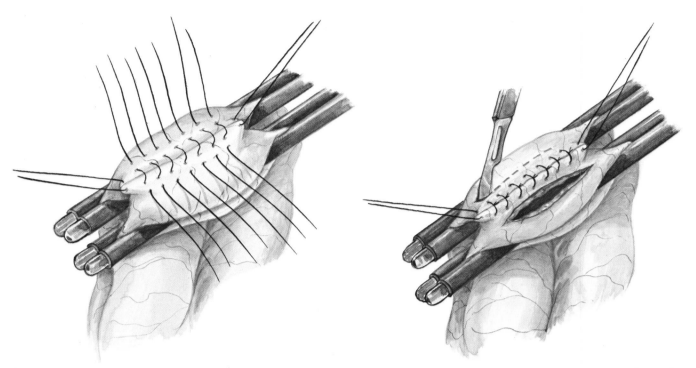

FIGURE 19.13. Select the bowel to be joined. Avoid tension or tumor at the anastomotic site. Place rubber or linen shod clamps to minimize spillage. Place a 4-0 Nurolon stay suture at each end of the bowel and an outer layer of 4-0 Nurolon joining the gut.

FIGURE 19.14. Incise sharply 8 to 10 cm from the suture line. Wall off the area with a laparotomy tape before opening the bowel. Secure hemostasis of the bowel edge.

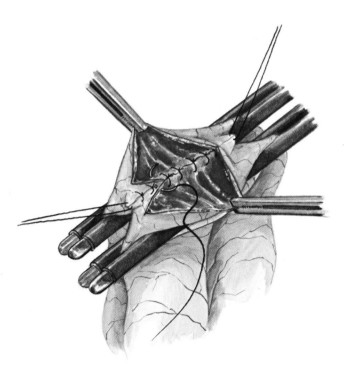

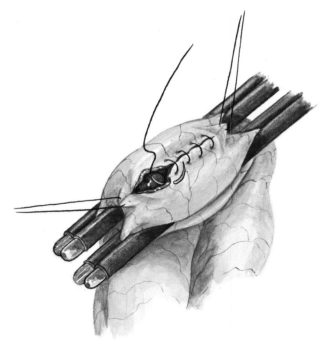

FIGURE 19.15. Place an inner layer of interrupted through-and-through 3-0 absorable suture.

FIGURE 19.16. Continue the inner layer of 3-0 absorbable suture. Use the stay suture for tension. Invert all mucosa into the lumen.

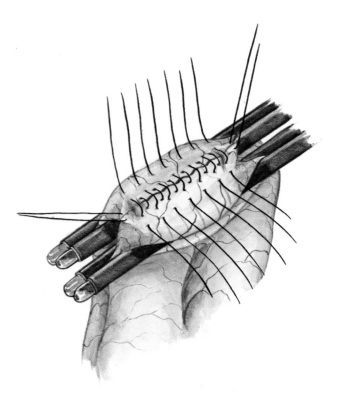

FIGURE 19.17. Place an outer layer of Nurolon covering the inner layer. As the lumen is larger in side-to-side anastomosis, use broad seromuscular bites approximating a good cuff of serosa.

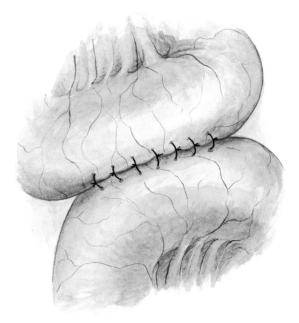

FIGURE 19.18. The stay sutures are now removed. Check the lumen between the thumb and index finger: it should be sizable. If an ileocolostomy is being performed, suture omentum about the anastomosis.

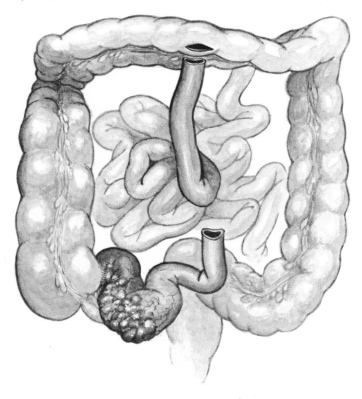

FIGURE 19.19. End-to-side anastomosis requires construction of a mucus fistula. The fistula is placed through the lower end of the midline incision and it too should be without tension. The end-to-side anastomosis is surrounded with any remaining omentum and completed with a two-layer technique similar to that outlined in side-to-side anastomosis.

225

of tumor, have an unquestionable blood supply, and reach the colon free of any tension. The omentum with good blood supply may be brought to surround this anastomosis if any remains. While the 5-year survivors are few in number, good palliation results often with an excellent quality of life.

The patient who develops colon obstruction from ovarian cancer is usually obstructed in the distal rectosigmoid and is best managed with a sigmoid colostomy and mucus fistula. When the defect is created in the anterior abdominal wall, take care to avoid injury to the anastomosis between the superior and inferior epigastric vessels. The construction of the stoma is illustrated in Figures 19.20 through 19.22. Careful selection of the colostomy site is important and is determined in part by the patient's abdominal panniculus. A preoperative visit by a stomal therapist for site selection is most helpful if colostomy is anticipated. Remember that a mucus fistula is the only exception to the dogma that one never brings a stoma through the abdominal wound. A few minutes spent carefully fashioning a stoma will avoid hours of postoperative care.

Occasionally the transverse colon becomes obstructed by ovarian cancer. The situation usually occurs when the omentum is not resected at the time of the original diagnosis and the carcinoma has produced a large cake of tumor surrounding the transverse colon. It is best to excise the transverse colon and do an anastomosis or perform a colostomy. The right colon may become obstructed and is most easily managed by ileotrans-

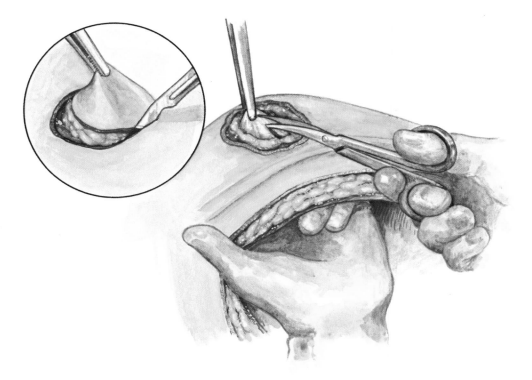

FIGURE 19.20.   Construction of the stoma in sigmoid colostomy. The defect, which goes through all layers of abdominal wall, is created by excising a cylinder of tissue approximately 1.5 inches in diameter through the skin and subcutaneous tissues, including the external oblique fascia. The inferior epigastric vessels may be palpated easily from the peritoneal surface and are to be avoided with this incision. The placement of the stoma should be determined prior to surgery, although generally it is equidistant between the anterior and superior iliac spine and umbilicus.

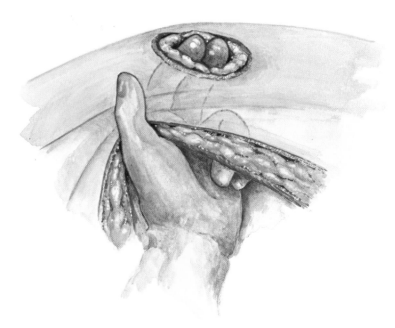

FIGURE 19.21. The middle and index fingers pass easily through the defect created.

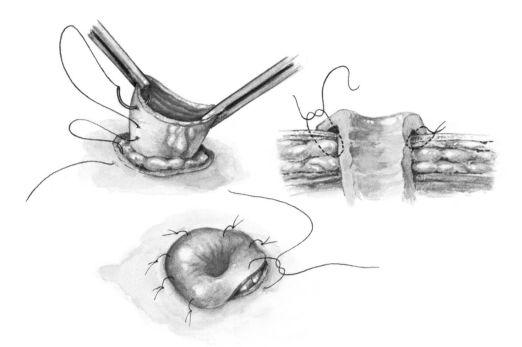

FIGURE 19.22. Whether the gut used for stoma construction is colon or small bowel, as in colostomy or ileal conduit, the skin and bowel must be joined without tension. Cut ends of the bowel should be handled with nontraumatic thumb forceps. Place a rosette stitch of 3-0 chromic catgut or 4-0 Vicryl and tie it approximating mucosa to epithelium. Handle the mucocutaneous junction gently as it is important to avoid fibrosis and later stricture.

verse colostomy, either side to side or end to side with mucus fistula; the author prefers the former. Avoid ileostomy as a diverting procedure if at all possible; the stomal problems are greater and the quality of life is poorer than with colostomy.

Surgery for Radiation Injury

Management of severe radiation injuries requires most careful consideration of numerous technical preoperative factors for satisfactory results. Patients with radiation injury to the colon and colic fistula may also have small bowel fistulas as well. The bladder may be dependent on the blood supply obtained from omental adhesions or densely adherent small bowel; mobilization of the small bowel from the bladder or pelvic floor may compromise the blood supply to these organs and adjacent bowel as well. Previously, many fistulas were due to localized injuries from radium and there was minimal damage to the remainder of the blood supply to the pelvis. Most therapeutic radiation procedures today use whole-pelvis radiation and the vascular injury encompasses the entire pelvis. The surgeon may be surprised that after mobilization of irradiated small bowel the patient often develops a postoperative fistula. This is caused by the peculiar nature of radiation injury and the destruction of small blood vessels in the structures irradiated.

The mortality rate from resection and anastomosis in these patients is high and bypass is a much safer procedure. Choose a segment of bowel for bypass anastomosis that has no evidence of intense radiation injury and meets all the requirements of viable bowel. The anastomosis is to be free of tension and the use of omentum to reinforce the blood supply is particularly important in this type of anastomosis. Photopulos has recently observed excellent healing with staple anastomosis in irradiated bowel,[10] and this method holds much promise for the future. Trimpi et al. have reviewed the laboratory and clinical experience in a large number of patients and concluded that a one-layer anastomosis excluding the mucosa and using 5-0 monofilament wire is best. One should be very alert to various malabsorption states associated with resection and bypass in irradiated small bowel, and the stagnant loop syndrome must be watched for as well. The stagnant loop syndrome or blind loop syndrome involves vitamin B_{12} malabsorption, steatorrhea, and bacterial overgrowth in the loop of the small intestine. Certain strains of bacteria, including bacteriodes, are associated with this syndrome. The definitive therapy consists of antibiotics; tetracycline has been reported to be effective, as well as clindamycin.[11]

References

1. Brunschwig, C.: Intestinal surgery for advanced cancer of the ovary. Gentil, F., and Junqueira, A.C., (eds.): In: *Ovarian Cancer*. Berlin, Springer-Verlag, 1968.
2. Burns, B.C., Rutledge, F.N., Smith, J.P., et al.: Management of ovarian carcinoma. *Am. J. Obstet. Gynecol.* **98**:374–386, 1967.
3. Clarke, J.S., Condon, R.E., Bartlett, J.G., et al.: Preoperative oral antibiotics reduce septic complications of colon operations. *Ann. Surg.* **186**:251–259, 1977.
4. Committee on Pre- and Postoperative Care, American College of Surgeons: *Manual of Preoperative and Postoperative Care*. Philadelphia, Saunders, 1971, ch. 19.

5. Cooper, P.: Abdominal trauma, penetrating and nonpenetrating. In: *The Craft of Surgery.* Boston, Little, Brown, 1971.

6. Goldring, J., McNaught, W., Scott, A., et al.: Prophylactic oral antimicrobial agents in elective colonic surgery. *Lancet* **2**:997–1000, 1975.

7. Graham, J.B., and Villalba, R.J.: Damage to the small intestine by radiotherapy. *Surg. Obstet. Gynecol.* **116**:665–668, 1963.

8. Irvin, T.T., Hayter, C.J., Warren, K.E., et al.: The effect of intestinal preparation on fluid and electrolyte balance. *Br. J. Surg.,* **60**:484–488, 1973.

9. Peacock, E.E., and Van Winkle, W.: Healing and Repair of Viscera. In: *Wound Repair.* Philadelphia, Saunders, 1976, ch. 12.

10. Photopulos, G.: Personal communication.

11. Swan, R.W.: Stagnant loop syndrome resulting from small-bowel irradiation injury and intestinal by-pass. *Gynecol. Oncol.* **2**:441–445, 1974.

12. Trimpi, H., Khubchandani, I.T., Sheets, J.A., et al.: Advances in intestinal anastomosis. *Dis. Colon Rectum* **20**:107–117, 1977.

13. Wheeless, C.R.: Small bowel bypass for complications related to pelvic malignancy. *Obstet. Gynecol.* **42**:661–666, 1973.

20 Incidental Appendectomy

Removal of the normal appendix during abdominal pelvic surgery has been carefully studied for a number of years. Waters, in 1977, reviewed his personal experience with 830 patients in whom elective appendectomy was performed.[3] He found no increase in morbidity or mortality with an appendectomy rate of 47% in abdominal hysterectomies performed over a 47-year period. Others have noted no increase in morbidity or mortality in incidental appendectomy with vaginal hysterectomy, ectopic pregnancy, and cesarean section.[1,3] Removal of the appendix when the patient is explored and is found to have acute pelvic inflammatory disease likewise does not increase mortality or morbidity rates over those for acute pelvic inflammatory disease managed without appendectomy.[2]

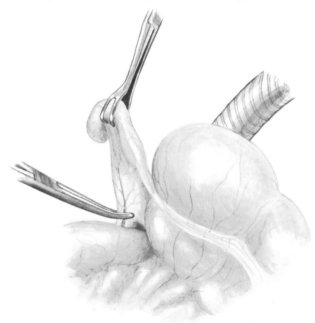

FIGURE 20.1.   Pull the appendix well into the wound, isolate the appendiceal mesentery, and place a Gemini clamp through the mesentery; ligate the appendiceal mesentery with 3-0 Nurolon suture and then cut the mesentery. Should an additional vessel be present, it may be clamped and carefully ligated.

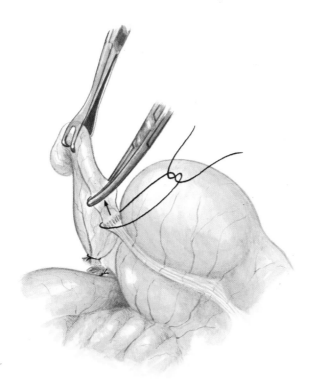

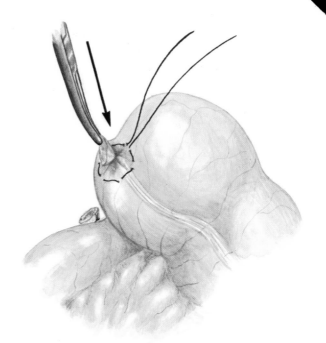

FIGURE 20.2. Place a straight clamp across the base of the appendix; crush the base and move the clamp 5 mm distal on the appendix. Tie the crushed area of the appendix with 2-0 absorbable suture and cut sharply along the margin of the straight clamp.

FIGURE 20.3. Place a purse-string suture of 4-0 Nurolon about the stump. Grasp the stump with a small straight clamp and invert into the cecum. Do not grasp the tie around the appendix as it may loosen, producing an open appendiceal stump. Tie the purse-string to approximate serosa over the defect. After the cecum is replaced in its normal position, check the appendiceal mesentery again for bleeding. Occasionally tension will prevent blood flow in the mesentery, which will become apparent when tension is removed from the right colon and ileocecal arteries.

Incidental appendectomy is contraindicated in cases with poor exposure and in the patient in whom the additional 10 min of operating time would pose some risk.

While some have suggested inversion of the appendix when the patient has free blood in the peritoneal cavity, such as with cesarean section, others have found simple crushing and ligation of the stump to be equal to inversion and treatment of the stump with phenol and alcohol.[3] The author has inverted the stump with a single Z-stitch or purse-string for a number of years and no complications have been noted in a large series of varied pelvic and abdominal surgical procedures (Figures 20.1 through 20.3).

References

1. Massoudnia, N.: Incidental appendectomy in vaginal surgery. *Int. Surg.* **60:** 89–96, 1975.
2. Thal, E.R., Guzzetta, P.C., Krupski, W.C., et al.: Morbidity of appendectomy in patients with acute salpingitis. *Am. Surg.* **43:**403–406, 1977.
3. Waters, E.G.: Elective appendectomy with abdominal and pelvic surgery. *Obstet. Gynecol.* **50:**511–517, 1977.

Marshall-Marchetti-Krantz Procedure

Kermit E. Krantz

True anatomic stress incontinence accounts for roughly three-fourths of all female urinary incontinence and should be relieved by a properly selected and executed surgical procedure in 90% of patients. However, approximately one-fourth of women who complain of uncontrollable loss of urine do not have anatomic stress incontinence, but one of several other conditions that adversely affect the continence mechanism, including urgency incontinence, bladder neuropathies, congenital or acquired urinary tract anomalies, psychogenic incontinence, and "detrussor" dyssynergia. Therefore, a careful differential diagnosis of all the various abnormalities leading to urinary incontinence is mandatory before concluding that surgical correction is indicated.

Urinary stress incontinence is the involuntary loss of an embarrassing amount of urine through an intact urethra as a result of sudden increases in intra-abdominal pressure. In pure anatomic incontinence, urine is not lost as a result of bladder muscle contraction, and the imminency of urinary loss is not preceded by the sensation of urinary urgency. Patients with anatomic incontinence experience loss of urine in spurts, synchronous with and ending abruptly after the peak of increased intra-abdominal pressure. Patients suffering from bladder neuropathies present quite different symptoms. These patients tend to dribble or leak urine during and after stress, often with a lag time of 10 to 20 sec. Furthermore, the instability may be accentuated by exposing such patients to the sound of running water, immersing their hands in water, or having them assume the erect position with bladder full. Accordingly, a careful, well-organized history is extremely important as a part of the diagnostic workup. By adherence to a rigid definition of true stress incontinence as immediate loss of urine without warning upon coughing, sneezing, laughing, or other activities that may result in an increase in intra-abdominal pressure, performance of various and complicated preoperative procedures such as cystoscopy or chain cystography may be avoided.

Physiology

Urinary continence is a function of suppression of the innate tendency of the smooth muscle of the bladder to contract as the bladder fills and the

232

ability of the urethra and vesical neck to remain closed except during voluntary voiding, thereby preventing accidental leakage of urine during times of increased abdominal pressure. In relation to one another, the urethra and the bladder function much like a torque system. The mechanical advantage is such a system is defined as the ratio of load to force (L/F) and is equal to the inverse ratio of the torque arms. Balance is achieved by multiplying the load times the length of one segment, which in turn equals the load times the length of the other segment. As applied to the urethra and bladder, the fulcrum of the torque is at the external urethral meatus, force is at the vesical neck near the puboprostatic (pubourethral) ligaments and the levator ani muscles, and load equals the capacity of the bladder or the volume of urine it contains. The distance of the first segment is measured from the fulcrum to the point of force as distance $A-F$. The second segment is measured from the fulcrum to the base of the bladder or load as distance $A-L$.

Normally, segments $A-F$ and $A-L$ are the same length, and utilizing the anterior vaginal wall as a horizontal plane of reference, the angle of function is approximately 35 degrees. If the urethra is of normal length (3.5 to 5.25 cm), function of the system will depend upon the balance between or the ratio of the puboprostatic ligaments and the puborectalis muscle (F) to urine volume in the bladder (L) and the tonus advantage of the smooth outer circumferential muscle of the urethra over the inner longitudinal muscle fibers. However, increased intra-abdominal pressure as a result of closure of the glottis and contraction of the abdominal musculature, with concomitant contracture of all the smooth muscle of the bladder and the urethra, results in a markedly increased load factor. This condition in turn results in the puboprostatic ligaments being forced downward toward the horizontal, and if the ratio of load to force becomes greater than 1, balance of the system is lost. Moreover, as the smooth longitudinal muscle of the urethra contracts, an additional reduction in the capacity of the puboprostatic ligaments occurs, decreasing the length of the urethra, making the hypotenuse of the triangle equal to the base, and reducing the angle of function to zero. With contraction of the bladder musculature adding to the load, urine is expressed via the only direction available, through the urethra to the outside. Any factor—the length of the urethra, a weakness in the puboprostatic ligaments or adjacent levator ani muscles, overdistention of the bladder as measured by the load factor, or a decrease in the angle of the urethra—may singularly or collectively contribute to stress incontinence.

Preoperative Evaluation

Physical examination is an important facet of preoperative evaluation. Urethral detachment should be demonstrated during physical examination, and the physician should be alert to the presence of a cystocele, urethral diverticula, vaginal scarring, or other abnormalities. However, because there is a considerable overlap among the symptoms associated with common causes of urinary incontinence, objective testing is necessary as a confirmatory measure.

The standard procedure for patients with true stress incontinence who have not had previous surgery should include a cystometrogram, a check of residual urine, observation of the presence or absence of incontinence with a full bladder, and demonstrated correction of stress incontinence through elevation of the vesical neck. The latter may be achieved by placing the patient in a dorsolithotomy position and filling the bladder with 250 to 350 ml water. If incontinence with coughing and straining is observed either in the prone position or when the patient is asked to stand, the physician may insert two fingers into the vagina from the posterior and, with one finger on either side, elevate the vesical neck. If incontinence upon further coughing and straining ceases, indications are favorable for surgery. If no incontinence is observed when the patient stands, the test is repeated at 100-ml increments until a level of 500 ml is reached. The bladder is then examined for perception of pain and cold.

Cystometric testing utilizing the carbon dioxide urethroscope yields characteristic findings in patients with anatomical incontinence. The urethral opening pressure is ordinarily low and the bladder filling pressure and bladder volume are normal. Observation of the vesical neck reveals a funneling and opening of the physiological sphincter mechanism under the challenge of coughing and straining. In addition, the vesical neck will drop depending upon the degree to which support has been lost.

Chain cystography may be used to measure the angle of urethral inclination and posterior urethrovesical angles. However, because chain cystograms are radiographic, they are not practical as a routine office procedure and should be reserved for complicated cases in which more information is needed.

If the patient does not meet the criteria for true stress incontinence, then other preoperative assessment tests should be considered, including cystoscopy for determining urethral length, evidence of trigonitis, urethral abnormalities, or the presence of urethral and bladder diverticula. For those patients who demonstrate recurring incontinence following previous corrective surgery for symptoms of the upper tract, an intravenous pyelogram may be performed.

Operative Strategy

A variety of vaginal and abdominal operations have been devised over the years for the correction of urinary stress incontinence. Nearly all, however, are designed to restore the normal urethrovesical anatomical relationship.

In 1949, Marshall, Marchetti, and Krantz described a urethrovesical suspension in a 54-year-old male who had developed urinary stress incontinence following an abdominal perineal resection; they also reported a subsequent 82% success rate performing the same procedure on 44 women who had urinary stress incontinence.[1]

The author has gradually modified the original operation over his 26 years of clinical practice. The use of multiple absorbable sutures has been discarded and now only one nonabsorbable suture is used on each side of the urethrovesical junction. The cystopexy has also been discarded as it contributes little to success.

Precise suture placement and permanent fixation are the critical factors and the cornerstones of long-term success in surgery for stress incontinence. Many of the author's patients have been referrals whose suprapubic uretheral suspension operations of one type or another had failed. Some patients have persistent urinary leakage because of nonanatomic types of incontinence and were selection errors. Another group did have anatomic incontinence, but at reoperation were found to have little or no scarring in the area of the urethrovesical junction. Often the anterior bladder was densely adherent to the symphysis in these patients.

234

The patient is placed in a low dorsolithotomy position, allowing the surgeon to operate with one hand in the vagina and the other suprapubically in the space of Retzuis. After standard preparation solutions have been applied to both the vagina and the hypogastric and ilioinguinal regions, the patient is draped in a fashion permitting easy access to the lower abdomen and the introitus. A size 20 Foley catheter with a 5-ml bag is inserted into the bladder through a plastic drape placed over the abdominoperineal area. The procedure is illustrated in Figures 21.1 through 21.4.

Postoperative Management

Following surgery, the vagina is packed with gauze to help reduce hematomas and disruption of the operation due to postanesthetic coughing. The packing is removed when the patient is fully awake. If the bladder was entered and repaired, the catheter is left in place until the urine is microscopically clear of blood. It may otherwise be removed on the day following surgery.

The patient is advised about straining, coughing, and lifting. When indicated, antibiotics and chemotherapeutics are employed to control infec-

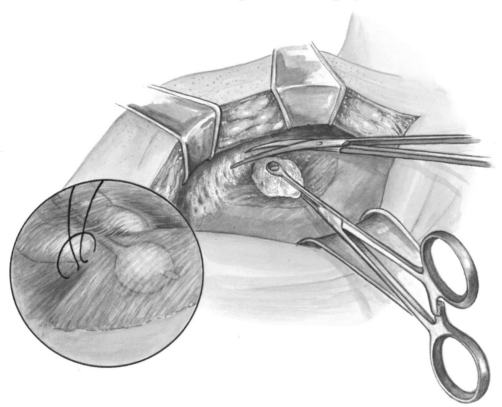

FIGURE 21.1. Make a Pfannenstiel incision in the abdomen and carry the incision through the subcutaneous tissue and fascia with sharp dissection. Separate the rectus muscles in the midline and tent and divide the posterior fascia. Place approximately 100 ml diluted methylene blue in the bladder through the Foley catheter and clamp the Foley until the end of the procedure. Dissect the space of Retzius and identify the vesical neck and urethra. Keep the balloon of the Foley catheter at the vesical neck by mild traction of the catheter. Inset: With the tips of the index and middle fingers of the assistant elevating the anterior vaginal wall on each side of the proximal urethra, make a double bite of the vaginal wall with 2-0 Mersilene on each side of the urethra at the region of the vesical neck (urethrovesical angle).

235

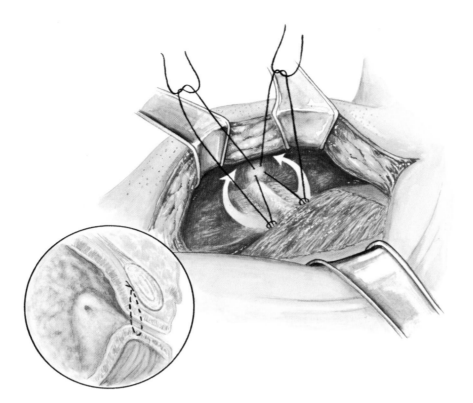

FIGURE 21.2.   Anchor the sutures to the periosteum on the posterior surface of the symphysis pubis, elevating the urethrovesical junction with the index and third fingers, and tie the suture to immobilize it. If there is venous bleeding it is controlled by pressure with a sponge stick. After satisfactory hemostasis, approximate the rectus abdominis muscles with a horizontal mattress suture of 2-0 chromic catgut. Close the rectus sheath with an interlocking suture of 2-0 absorbable suture. Close the subcutaneous tissue with a 3-0 chromic catgut placed in Scarpa's fascia, and close the skin with a subcuticular stitch of 4-0 absorbable suture or 5-0 nylon. These sutures are removed in 6 days.

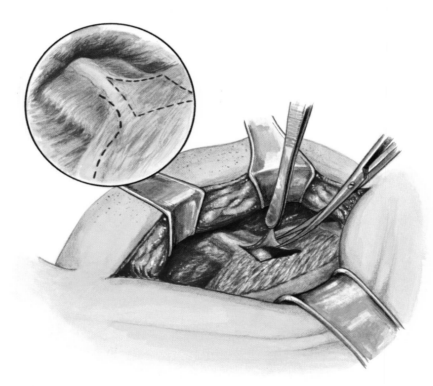

FIGURE 21.3.   Urethral lengthening is indicated in those patients who are operative failures and have a good urethrovesical angle, have a urethral length of 1.4 cm or less, and are incontinent with a volume greater than 100 to 125 ml. Such patients have usually had multiple vaginal and abdominal operations. Dotted line: new urethral position. Inset: Resect the area shown to lengthen the urethra anatomically. Make the incision by cutting or resecting a diamond-shaped piece of urethrovesical wall. The muscularis and mucosal apex in the urethrovesical junction extend laterally, terminating approximately 1 to 2.5 cm from the origin.

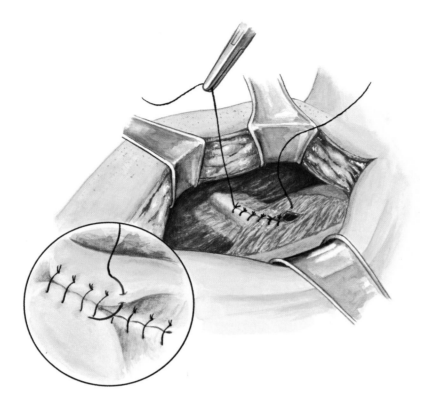

FIGURE 21.4. After the diamond-shaped tissue has been removed, close the mucosa with continuous or interrupted 4-0 chromic sutures. Note that the sutures are retro-mucosal and do not enter into the bladder. Place the second layer of interrupted sutures in the muscularis with 3-0 or 4-0 sutures. The urethra measured should increase 1 cm in length with the Foley bulb in place. Proceed with the urethral suspension, preferably using 2-0 chromic catgut suture.

tion, primarily if positive bacteriuria was present prior to surgery. In 3 to 4 weeks the patient may resume normal activity but is cautioned to refrain from lifting heavy objects. Eighty-nine percent of patients will have permanent relief of stress incontinence with this operative technique. Pregnancy may be anticipated without difficulty and vaginal delivery is not contraindicated.

References

1. Marshall, V.T., Marchetti, A.A., and Krantz, K.E.: The correction of stress incontinence by simple vesico-urethral suspension. *Surg. Gynecol. Obstet.* **88:**509–518, 1949.

Selected Bibliography

Green, T.H.: Urinary stress incontinence: Differential diagnosis, pathophysiology, and management. *Am. J. Obstet. Gynecol.* **22:**368–398, 1975.

Hodgkinson, C.P.: Stress urinary incontinence—1970. *Am. J. Obstet. Gynecol.* **108:**1141–1168, 1970.

Krantz, K.E.: Anatomy of the urethra and anterior vaginal wall. *Am. Assoc. Obstet. Gynecol. Abdom. Surg.* **61:**31–59, 1950.

Krantz, K.E.: Anatomy of the urethra and anterior vaginal wall. *Am. Assoc. Obstet. Gynecol.* **62:**382–396, 1951.

Krantz, K.E.: The anatomy and physiology of the vulva and vagina and the anatomy of the urethra and bladder. In Philipp, E., Barnes, J., and Newton, M. (eds.): *Scientific Foundations of Obstetrics and Gynecology.* London, Heinemann, 1970.

Marshall, V.T., Marchetti, A.A., and Krantz, K.E.: The correction of stress incontinence by simple vesico-urethral suspension. *Surg. Gynecol. Obstet.* **88:**509–518, 1949.

Shingleton, H.M., and Davis, R.O.: Stress incontinence in perspective. *Obstet. Gynecol. Dig.* **19:**15–25, 1977.

Ureteral Injury

22

The intimate relationship between the ureter and the female genital tract must be considered in the planning of any gynecologic surgical procedure. Preoperative intravenous pyelograms must be obtained in any patient with an abdominal mass, pelvic malignancy, or lower genital tract anomaly and are indicated in all patients undergoing hysterectomy or other major pelvic surgery. Cystoscopy, retrograde pyelography, renal scans, sonography, and other urinary studies may be needed in some instances to complete preoperative evaluation. Patients with cervical leiomyomas and endometriosis are particularly prone to ureteral injury and the common anomaly of ureteral reduplication must always be considered. St. Martin et al. found that 10.8% of patients having routine gynecologic surgical procedures had hydronephrosis and hydroureter prior to surgery and 33 of 36 resolved after pelvic operation.[11]

Conger et al. noted that 12% of patients had hydronephrosis and all resolved spontaneously after operation to remove the pelvic mass or other lesion compressing the ureter.[2]

Postoperative cystoscopy with indigo carmine administration following vaginal procedures in which ureteral injury might easily occur is recommended. The absence of a large mass, obesity, or endometriosis does not, however, provide protection against ureteral injury. Symmonds noted that most of the cases of ureteral injury resulted from "easy" abdominal hysterectomies.[12] The author consistently performs cystoscopy following vaginectomy, total vaginal prolapse repair, vesicovaginal fistula repair, and excision of vaginal cyst or urethral diverticulum. It is reassuring to see indigo carmine ejected from each ureter following such procedures. Immediate retrograde pyelography is performed if the dye fails to appear. The use of indigo carmine administration intravenously is indicated during ovarian cancer debulking, where ascitic fluid and the presence of large amounts of tumor may obscure ureteral injury.

Anuria is seen, of course, with bilateral ureteral obstructions. When the more common causes of postoperative anuria such as a clamped Foley catheter and hypovolemia have been ruled out, prompt investigation with cystoscopy and retrograde pyelograms is mandatory.

More significant than immediate detection, of course, is the prevention of the injury, and several measures are worthwhile. The use of the sur-

239

gical procedures outlined in this volume will minimize ureteral injuries. They are all designed to provide early exposure of the ureters and direct visualization during operations performed near them.

Technical Considerations

Isolate the ovarian vessels with the ureter under direct visualization and use free ties instead of large clamps. Leave the ureter on the peritoneum to maintain the integrity of its blood supply and make any ligation of the hypogastric or uterine vessels distal to the origin of the small vessels providing blood supply to the ureter if possible. Dissect the bladder down before placing any clamps on the uterine artery or paracervical tissue. Carefully locate and visualize the ureter when closing the pelvic peritoneum (Figure 22.1).

The basic surgical technique of fine suture, small portions of tissue in clamps, delicate artery forceps, nontraumatic parametrial clamps, and maximum exposure through an adequate incision is the most significant measure in reducing ureteral injury to an absolute minimum.

One of the more common mistakes in ureter identification is confusion between it and the obliterated hypogastric artery. The ureter and this structure run a similar course, appear at superficial inspection to be similar, and feel alike. They are differentiated by position, by the presence of periureteral vascular sheath, by the relationship between the uterine artery coursing over the ureter and arising in conjunction with the distal portion of the obliterated hypogastric artery, and by peristalsis. One elicits such peristalsis by a very gentle stroking of the ureter, taking care not to crush the ureter. The use of palpation alone for ureteral detection has misled many an experienced surgeon in situations where intense endometriosis, ovarian cancer, severe radiation reaction, or cervical leiomyomas have grossly disturbed the normal anatomic relationships.

Many ureteral injuries in radical hysterectomy result when the delicate periureteral sheath and its anastomosis between renal, aortic, hypogastric, ovarian, uterine, vaginal, and superior vesical arteries are needlessly sacrificed. Placing rubber drains on tension about the ureter and constantly elevating and manipulating them, thereby avulsing the vascular sheath, is a poor substitute for adequate exposure and leaving the ureter attached in its bed when possible. While the use of ureteral catheters is suggested by some to prevent ureteral injury, the author advises careful identification, wide retroperitoneal exposure with direct ureteral visualization, fine instruments, and suture as a much more effective technique.

The occurrence of ureteral injury reported in the literature varies from 0.05%[9] to 30%[11] depending on the material and types of procedures studied. Very high figures are noted with radical hysterectomy performed in the face of heavy radiation therapy. Those series with almost no ureteral injuries eliminated surgical procedures of any complexity. A more realistic figure for ureteral injury is that of Solomons et al., who performed preoperative and postoperative intravenous pyelograms following routine gynecologic surgical procedures in 200 consecutive patients.[10] They found a postoperative ureteral injury rate of 2.5% and no fistulas were observed. Three injuries were associated with abdominal hysterectomy and two with vaginal hysterectomy. One patient had ureterolysis with relief of hydronephrosis, two patients' hydronephrosis resolved under observation, one was lost to follow-up, and hydronephrosis persisted untreated in the upper pole of one kidney drained by a duplicate ureter. Ureteral injuries are usually silent; if infection does not occur, the patient will notice little and silent renal unit loss will occur. None of Solomons' five patients had particularly alarming symptoms or physical findings.

If the ureteral injury is one of transection or of significant injury near the vault, ureterovaginal fistula may occur. If unrecognized, ureteral injury produces extravasation of urine into the peritoneal cavity and signs of peri-

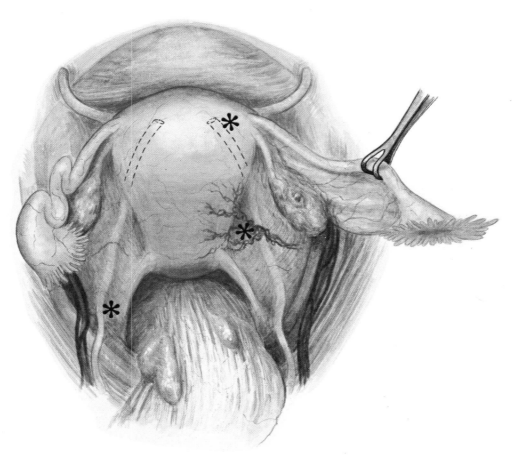

FIGURE 22.1. The pelvic surgeon must always be aware of the position of the ureter to avoid injuring it. Always visualize and palpate the ureter before dividing the ovarian vessels. Placement of large clamps blindly across these structures is a common cause of ureteral injury. Note the asterisk where the uterine arteries cross the ureter. Injury most commonly occurs at this site during abdominal hysterectomy. Avoid this injury by carefully visualizing and identifying the ureter as it lays laterally in the parametria prior to ligating the uterine artery. Equally important in avoiding injury is thorough dissection of the bladder downward and the use of Deaver retractors to keep the bladder out of the field during uterine artery ligation. Another site of injury is the terminal portion of the ureter as it courses over the upper third of the vagina. This area is commonly injured during vaginectomy and radical hysterectomy. Careful and repeated visual ureteral identification before division of the vagina minimizes ureteral trauma. Another type of injury is inclusion of the ureter in reperitonealization of the pelvic peritoneum. It is not worthwhile surgically to attempt to pull together torn and injured isolated segments of peritoneum at the risk of ureteral injury when the ureter cannot be identified. If pelvic peritoneum remains, close it with constant reference to the ureter.

toneal irritation rapidly develop, i.e., a rigid abdomen, rapid pulse, and ileus. If extravasation is retroperitoneal and undrained, abscess formation usually occurs.

Repair of Injury

The ideal time for repair of ureteral injury is at the time it occurs, and the gynecologist will be the only surgeon in attendance in most instances. It is therefore necessary that he have available the basic data on wound healing, operative techniques, and the outcome of such repairs. The detection of suspected ureteral injury is illustrated in Figure 22.2.

Uroepithelium of the ureter has great regenerative powers and will seal its leaks in 48 hr in the absence of obstruction. While the ureteral muscle seems to have little ability to regenerate, the submucosa has considerable inductive power over the surrounding mesenchymal cells. Intense fibrosis progressing to stricture formation and even osteogenesis with bone formation may occur and are promoted by urine. Fibrosis is diminished by diversion of the urinary stream during healing and does not occur if immediate nephrectomy follows ureteral injury.

The importance of the delicate periureteral vascular sheath and the ureteral bed of retroperitoneal fat in resumption of normal function cannot be overemphasized. Gentle and delicate handling of the ureter and these tissues is vital to the success of any reconstructive procedure. The reader is referred to the text by Peacock and Van Winkle for a more detailed discussion of this subject.[8]

Distal Ureter

If the ureter is crushed with a hemostat, the hemostat may simply be removed with no expected disability. Mannes et al. crushed dog ureters with Kelly clamps approximately 5 cm from the entrance into the bladder for a period of 5 sec to 60 min.[6] Intravenous pyelograms were done at 1 week and at monthly intervals thereafter. No fistulas or urinary extravasation resulted and serial intravenous pyelograms demonstrated progressive dilatation only after a 60-min crush. Although some abnormality in peristalsis was noted, in general all renal units were preserved. Note that Mannes et al. did not dissect the ureter out of its bed but rather crushed it in situ. John Masterson traumatized canine ureters by rubbing them with gauze, handling them with forceps, or ligating both hypogastric arteries; no fistulas were noted.[7] Some researchers feel that canine ureters have different healing qualities and we should be somewhat reserved in our acceptance of such data. Higgins observed seven patients with ureteral clamping without urologic abnormalities and observed that temporary clamp application did not seem to be a factor in fistula formation in his series.[3] Should the ureter be included in a tie, the ligature may usually be removed without injury.

The importance of using nontraumatic instruments in pelvic surgery is again emphasized. If one crushes and devitalizes ureteral tissue, such as may occur with a Heaney-Ballentine clamp or other grossly injurious instrument, as opposed to a less traumatic clamp, then considerable clinical judgment must be employed as to the viability of such tissue. It may be necessary to pass a ureteral catheter through this area and leave it in place for 7 to 14 days.

If the ureter has been transected, then implantation is indicated (Figures 22.3 and 22.4). The ureter is followed back to unquestionably normal and well-vascularized ureter. The bladder can be mobilized and fixed to the psoas muscle to avoid any tension. A simple mucosa-to-mucosa implantation into the bladder has produced far superior results as compared to ureteroureteral anastomosis. A Boari flap is rarely needed as an initial procedure and antireflux anastomosis, while crucial in children and theoretically superior, seems not to be necessary for satisfactory long-term results in

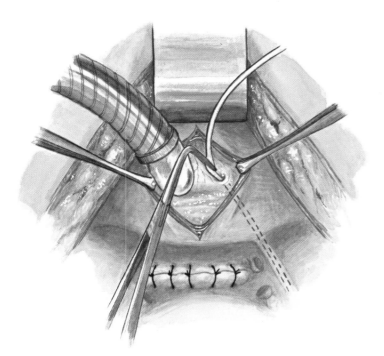

FIGURE 22.2. If ureteral injury is suspected, dissect the pelvic ureter in its entirety, beginning at the pelvic brim where positive identification is possible. An additional method of establishing its injury is to pass a polyethylene tube or No. 5 ureteral catheter in a retrograde fashion up the ureteral orifice in the trigone of the bladder. Grasp the dome of the bladder between Allis clamps and sharply enter the bladder. Enlarge the defect to produce adequate exposure of the trigone. Replace the Allis clamps to include full thickness of the bladder muscle and mucosa. Aspirate any urine present with a neurosuction tip and place a fiberoptic light source into the bladder. The ureteral orifices are usually located just lateral to the Foley catheter and are easily observed as small slits intermittently expelling urine. If the patient has had irradiation injury with bullous edema, visualization may be difficult. If the ureters cannot be easily located, inject 5 ml indigo carmine intravenously and observe its appearance in the bladder. Place 5 to 10 ml saline in the bladder with intermittent aspiration to make identification of the spurts or urine containing indigo carmine easier. Use care not to traumatize the mucosa as this will make placement of the ureteral catheter more difficult. After the ureters have been identified, grasp the polyethylene tubing or ureteral catheter with fine long right-angle forceps, enclosing the end of the catheter in the jaws of the instrument; place it through the ureteral orifice in the direction of the ureter. The tube is easily identified as it passes into the ureter and upward into the retroperitoneum. Any obstruction or division is easily identified. If the ureter has been divided, the passage of indigo carmine from any site will be observed as well. Retrograde passage of a catheter is useful if the surgeon is called in for consultation when the operator may have crushed large portions of tissue with mass ligatures during pelvic surgery.

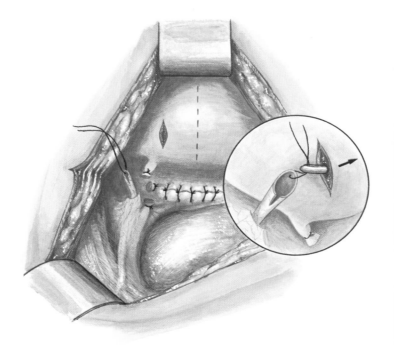

FIGURE 22.3. Significant injuries in the pelvic ureter are best managed by reimplanting the ureter into the bladder. This is done by mobilizing the bladder, dissecting the space of Retzius, and continuing the dissection laterally, freeing that margin of the bladder to be pulled upward. The obliterated hypogastric artery may be divided if it retards bladder mobilization. Suture the bladder well up on the iliopsoas muscle with several sutures of 2-0 absorbable suture. Make certain the ureter reaches and extends 1 to 2 cm beyond the bladder without tension. Use the incision made into the dome of the bladder to facilitate retrograde catheter passage for ureteral reimplantation site formation. Identify the proper site, which is generally in the most superior portion where the ureter reaches the bladder without tension. Place a right-angle clamp through the opening in the bladder to this site, open it, and produce a defect of 5 to 6 mm through all layers. Trim any ureter that does not appear entirely viable after the initial trimming and spatulate it with Potts right-angle scissors. Make every effort to preserve the periureteral vascular sheath and minimally handle the ureter by its peritoneal covering if any remains. Place a suture through the side opposite the spatulation incision and use it for a traction suture. Grasp this traction suture with right-angle forceps and pull the ureter into the bladder. Use four sutures of absorbable 4-0 Vicryl or chromic catgut. Place these through all layers of the ureter, bladder mucosa, and inner muscularis. Place one stay suture of 4-0 chromic catgut between the periureteral sheath and outer bladder muscularis and suture any remaining peritoneal covering against the bladder surface. There must be no tension on this anastomosis and the ureter should lie loosely against the bladder. Observe the blood supply of this anastomosis. If the blood supply is questionable redo the anastomosis. Close the bladder with two layers of 2-0 absorbable suture. Make certain the initial layer imbricates the mucosa. No bladder mucosa should be visible when the second layer is completed. No stint is required in the ureter for the anastomosis. Place a retroperitoneal suction drain and leave the Foley catheter in place for 1 week. The suction catheter should not be in contact with the anastomosis site. It may be removed in 5 days or, if the anastomosis leaks, leave it in place until urine drainage ceases. The presence of urine or serum in the suction catheter can be established with the injection of indigo carmine. Do not use wall suction; instead use Hemovac-type suction that uses low pressures.

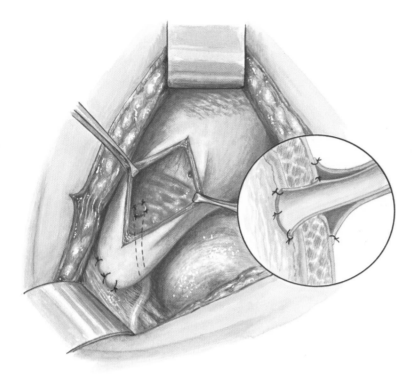

FIGURE 22.4. The anastomosis through the bladder wall is a straight, simple anastomosis without any tunnel formation. No antireflux procedure is necessary. If the surgeon provides an adequate blood supply, creates a tension-free anastomosis, and employs minimal suture material in a nontraumatic fashion, the results will be excellent. Expect some calyceal blunting and mild hydronephrosis in the initial intravenous pyelogram following ureteral reimplantation. This resolves in 2 to 3 months on follow-up study.

adult females.[5,12] Owing to the incidence of stricture and peristalic dysfunction of the distal ureteral segment, it is better to err on the side of implantation rather than do an end-to-end anastomosis. Most of the pelvic surgical injuries can be handled by implantation as the bladder can be mobilized to the pelvic brim and good results may be anticipated.

Middle Third

Injuries in the middle third of the ureter such as passage of suture through the ureter or incision require no therapy. Excision of a margin of the ureteral tube can be handled by simple suture repair. Experimentally, the ureter will heal defects of one-half its circumference if not obstructed. If, however, the ureter is transected in its upper middle third, then the area should be freshened and a spatula-type end-to-end anastomosis performed (Figure 22.5). Weinberg has carefully studied this ureteral anastomosis and its reported poor results. His recommendations are incorporated in this technique and his writings merit review.[13]

In all reconstructive procedures the presence of an adequate blood supply and the absence of tension are absolutely essential. If the ureter has been shortened, mobilizing the kidney downward is of benefit to relieve any tension at the site as well as mobilizing the bladder and suturing it to the psoas muscle. An extraperitoneal drain may be placed to drain the urine at this site. The drain should be in place for 10 days to allow a well-formed tract for drainage. Suction catheters, while preferable, must not be in contact with the anastomosis and may be sutured into position with fine chromic catgut or other absorbable suture. From an experimental standpoint, it is better that the anastomosis not be splinted.[8]

A 2.5-cm ureterotomy 5 cm above the anastomosis to divert the urine will decrease the incidence of stricture. The drain leading to the ureterotomy site can be removed in 10 to 14 days. The incidence of problems following ureterotomy is minimal and stricture at the ureterotomy site is rare.

245

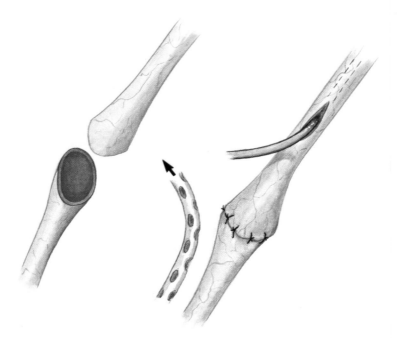

FIGURE 22.5. Freshen the transected upper middle third of the ureter by cutting the severed ends diagonally with Potts scissors. Spatulate when necessary. Touch the ureter as little as possible. Do not dissect the periureteral sheath. Close the ureter with 5-0 absorbable suture on a swaged needle through and through using a wedge-type suture incorporating more muscularis than mucosa. Four to five sutures will usually suffice. Inject indigo carmine at the onset of repair to make certain it is watertight. Make an incision in the ureter 4 cm above the anastomosis and pass a soft No. 5 catheter or infant feeding tube up the ureter to divert the urine flow. Pass this out a stab wound and suture it to the adjacent fascia with 4-0 chromic catgut. Place a suction catheter in the area and suture it in position such that it is not in contact with the ureter. Do not use wall suction. Remove the ureterotomy and drains in 10 to 14 days.

Upper Third

Injuries of the upper third of the ureter are usually not associated with gynecologic procedures but are often a result of gunshot wounds or other major trauma. Ureteroureterostomy is the procedure of choice. While these cases are not usually seen on a gynecologic service, should a long stricture occur as a result of radical hysterectomy or irradiation injury, a ureteroureterostomy may be performed as indicated or ileal diversion may be considered.

Postoperative Management

Careful follow-up of patients with ureteral injuries is very important. Ihse reported 39 reconstructive procedures for surgical injuries of the ureter.[4] The majority were located in the distal ureter and were repaired in 16 instances by ureteroneocystostomy. Three of these progressed to stricture formation: 2 were reimplanted, and 1 Boari flap was constructed. Ten end-to-end anastomoses were fashioned and 5 required reoperation: 2 were implanted into the bladder, and 2 were managed by nephrectomy and 1 by Boari flap. A wide variety of other reconstructive procedures were employed and it is noted that while 4 patients died of associated malignant disease, there was no operative mortality. Of the 33 patients followed, 25 were symptom free at follow-up examination for 0.5 to 10 years after surgery. Four patients had had urinary tract infections.

Even better results were noted by Beland.[1] He reported on the management of 34 ureteral injuries in 25 patients after gynecologic surgical procedures. Except for temporary urinary fistulas, the immediate postoperative course was benign. No kidneys were lost and no urologic reoperation was required.

The injury should be repaired when it occurs, before the process of fibrosis and stricture formation begins. Simple ligation of the proximal ureter with loss of the kidney is rarely indicated in modern gynecologic surgery.

References

1. Beland, G.: Early treatment of ureteral injuries found after gynecological surgery. *J. Urol.* **118:**25–27, 1977.
2. Conger, K., Beecham, C.T., and Horrax, T.M.: Ureteral injury in pelvic surgery. *Obstet. Gynecol.* **3:**343–357, 1954.
3. Higgins, C.C.: Ureteral injuries during surgery. *J.A.M.A.* **199:**118–124, 1967.
4. Ihse, I.: Surgical injuries of the ureter. *Scand. J. Urol. Nephrol.* **9:**39–44, 1975.
5. Lee, R.A., and Symmonds, R.E.: Ureterovaginal fistual. *Am. J. Obstet. Gynecol.* **109:**1032–1035, 1971.
6. Mannes, H., Zimskind, P.D., Subbarao, Y., et al.: Crush injury of the lower ureter: An experimental study. *J. Urol.* **108:**548–552, 1972.
7. Masterson, J.G.: An experimental study of ureteral injuries in radical pelvic surgery. *Am. J. Obstet. Gynecol.* **73:**359–370, 1957.
8. Peacock, E.E., Jr., and Van Winkle, W., Jr.: Healing and repair of viscera. In: *Wound Repair.* Philadelphia, Saunders, 1976, ch. 12.
9. Rusche, C.F., and Bacon, S.K.: Injury of the ureter. *J.A.M.A.* **114:**201–207, 1940.
10. Solomons, E., Levin, E.J., Bauman, J., et al.: A pyelographic study of ureteric injuries sustained during hysterectomy for benign conditions. *Surg. Gynecol. Obstet.* **111:**41–48, 1960.
11. St. Martin, E.C., Trichel, B.E., Campbell, J.H., et al.: Ureteral injuries in gynecologic surgery. *J. Urol.* **70:**51–57, 1953.
12. Symmonds, R.E.: Ureteral injuries associated with gynecologic surgery: Prevention and management. *Clin. Obstet. Gynecol.* **19:**623–644, 1976.
13. Weinberg, S.R.: Injuries of the ureter. In Bergman, H. (ed.): *The Ureter.* Harper & Row, New York, 1967.

Selected Bibliography

Peacock, E.E., and Van Winkle, W.: *Wound Repair.* Philadelphia, Saunders, 1976.

Selected Bibliography

Blaustein, A. (ed.): *Pathology of the Female Genital Tract*. New York, Springer-Verlag, 1977.

Boileau, J.C.: *Grant—An Atlas of Anatomy*, 7th ed. Baltimore, Williams & Wilkins, 1978.

Krantz, K.E.: Anatomy of the female reproductive system. In Benson, R.C. (ed.): *Current Obstetrics and Gynecologic Diagnosis and Treatment*. Los Altos, Lang, 1976.

Plentl, A.A., and Friendman, E.A.: *Lymphatic Systemic of the Female Genitalia*. Philadelphia, Saunders, 1971.

Sobotta, J.: *Atlas of Human Anatomy*, 8th ed., vols. 1–3 (revised by Figge, F.H.J.). New York, Hafner, 1963.

Thorek, P.: *Anatomy in Surgery*, 2nd ed. Philadelphia, Lippincott, 1962.

Uhlenhuth, E.: *Problems in the Anatomy of the Pelvis, An Atlas*. Philadelphia, Lippincott, 1953.

Index